T0358863

Pediatric Neuroimaging: State-of-the-Art

Editor

MAI-LAN HO

MAGNETIC RESONANCE IMAGING CLINICS OF NORTH AMERICA

www.mri.theclinics.com

Consulting Editors
SURESH K. MUKHERJI
LYNNE S. STEINBACH

November 2021 • Volume 29 • Number 4

ELSEVIER

1600 John F. Kennedy Boulevard • Suite 1800 • Philadelphia, Pennsylvania, 19103-2899

http://www.mri.theclinics.com

MRI CLINICS OF NORTH AMERICA Volume 29, Number 4
November 2021 ISSN 1064-9689, ISBN 13: 978-0-323-79320-9

Editor: John Vassallo (j.vassallo@elsevier.com)
Developmental Editor: Arlene Campos

© **2021 Elsevier Inc. All rights reserved.**

This periodical and the individual contributions contained in it are protected under copyright by Elsevier, and the following terms and conditions apply to their use:

Photocopying

Single photocopies of single articles may be made for personal use as allowed by national copyright laws. Permission of the Publisher and payment of a fee is required for all other photocopying, including multiple or systematic copying, copying for advertising or promotional purposes, resale, and all forms of document delivery. Special rates are available for educational institutions that wish to make photocopies for non-profit educational classroom use. For information on how to seek permission visit www.elsevier.com/permissions or call: (+44) 1865 843830 (UK)/ (+1) 215 239 3804 (USA).

Derivative Works

Subscribers may reproduce tables of contents or prepare lists of articles including abstracts for internal circulation within their institutions. Permission of the Publisher is required for resale or distribution outside the institution. Permission of the Publisher is required for all other derivative works, including compilations and translations (please consult www.elsevier.com/permissions).

Electronic Storage or Usage

Permission of the Publisher is required to store or use electronically any material contained in this periodical, including any article or part of an article (please consult www.elsevier.com/permissions). Except as outlined above, no part of this publication may be reproduced, stored in a retrieval system or transmitted in any form or by any means, electronic, mechanical, photocopying, recording or otherwise, without prior written permission of the Publisher.

Notice

No responsibility is assumed by the Publisher for any injury and/or damage to persons or property as a matter of products liability, negligence or otherwise, or from any use or operation of any methods, products, instructions or ideas contained in the material herein. Because of rapid advances in the medical sciences, in particular, independent verification of diagnoses and drug dosages should be made.

Although all advertising material is expected to conform to ethical (medical) standards, inclusion in this publication does not constitute a guarantee or endorsement of the quality or value of such product or of the claims made of it by its manufacturer.

Magnetic Resonance Imaging Clinics of North America (ISSN 1064-9689) is published quarterly by Elsevier Inc., 360 Park Avenue South, New York, NY 10010-1710. Months of issue are February, May, August, and November. Business and Editorial Offices: 1600 John F. Kennedy Blvd., Ste. 1800, Philadelphia, PA 19103-2899. Customer Service Office: 3251 Riverport Lane, Maryland Heights, MO 63043. Periodicals postage paid at New York, NY and additional mailing offices. Subscription prices are $404.00 per year (domestic individuals), $1037.00 per year (domestic institutions), $100.00 per year (domestic students/residents), $450.00 per year (Canadian individuals), $1063.00 per year (Canadian institutions), $567.00 per year (international individuals), $1063.00 per year (international institutions), $100.00 per year (Canadian students/residents), and $275.00 per year (international students/residents). International air speed delivery is included in all *Clinics* subscription prices. All prices are subject to change without notice. **POSTMASTER:** Send address changes to *Magnetic Resonance Imaging Clinics*, Elsevier Health Sciences Division, Subscription Customer Service, 3251 Riverport Lane, Maryland Heights, MO 63043. Customer Service (orders, claims, online, change of address): Elsevier Health Sciences Division, Subscription **Customer Service, 3251 Riverport Lane, Maryland Heights, MO 63043. Tel:1-800-654-2452 (U.S. and Canada); 314-447-8871 (outside U.S. and Canada). Fax: 314-447-8029. E-mail: journalscustomerservice-usa@elsevier.com (for print support); journalsonlinesupport-usa@elsevier.com (for online support).**

Reprints. For copies of 100 or more of articles in this publication, please contact the Commercial Reprints Department, Elsevier Inc., 360 Park Avenue South, New York, NY 10010-1710. Tel.: 212-633-3874; Fax: 212-633-3820; E-mail: reprints@elsevier.com.

Magnetic Resonance Imaging Clinics of North America is covered in the *RSNA Index of Imaging Literature, MEDLINE/PubMed (Index Medicus),* and *EMBASE/Excerpta Medica.*

Contributors

CONSULTING EDITORS

SURESH K. MUKHERJI, MD, MBA, FACR
Clinical Professor, Marian University, Director of Head and Neck Radiology, ProScan Imaging, Regional Medical Director, Envision Physician Services, Carmel, Indiana, USA

LYNNE S. STEINBACH, MD, FACR
Emeritus Professor of Radiology on Full Recall, Department of Radiology and Biomedical Imaging, University of California, San Francisco, San Francisco, California, USA

EDITOR

MAI-LAN HO, MD
Associate Professor of Radiology, Director of Research, Department of Radiology, Director, Advanced Neuroimaging Core, Faculty Lead, Imaging Genomics Research Affinity Group, Chair, Asian Pacific American Network, Secretary, Association for Staff and Faculty Women, Nationwide Children's Hospital, The Ohio State University, Columbus, Ohio, USA

AUTHORS

JAYAPALLI RAJIV BAPURAJ, MD
Radiology Department, Neuroradiology Division, University of Michigan, Ann Arbor, Michigan, USA

SVEN BAMBACH, PhD
Data Scientist II, Abigail Wexner Research Institute at Nationwide Children's Hospital, Columbus, Ohio, USA

M. ALEJANDRA BEDOYA, MD
Department of Radiology, Boston Children's Hospital, Boston, Massachusetts, USA

STEFAN BLUML, PhD
Associate Professor of Research, Department of Radiology, Children's Hospital Los Angeles, Keck School of Medicine of USC, University of Southern California, Los Angeles, California, USA; Rudi Schulte Research Institute, Santa Barbara, California, USA

YONG CHEN, PhD
Department of Radiology, Case Western Reserve University, Cleveland, Ohio, USA

DINESH KUMAR DEELCHAND, PhD
Department of Radiology, Assistant Professor, Center for Magnetic Resonance Research, University of Minnesota, Minneapolis, Minnesota, USA

TEJASWINI DESHMUKH, MBBS, MD
Department of Radiology, Medical College of Wisconsin, Children's Wisconsin, Milwaukee, Wisconsin, USA

JUDY A. ESTROFF, MD
Section Chief, Department of Radiology, Maternal Fetal Care Center, Boston Children's Hospital, Boston, Massachusetts, USA

TALHA UL GHAZI, BS
Michigan State University, College of Human Medicine, Lansing, Michigan, USA

P. ELLEN GRANT, MD, MSc
Departments of Radiology and Pediatrics,
Fetal and Neonatal Neuroimaging and
Developmental Science Center, Boston
Children's Hospital, Boston, Massachusetts,
USA

MAI-LAN HO, MD
Associate Professor of Radiology, Director of
Research, Department of Radiology, Director,
Advanced Neuroimaging Core, Faculty Lead,
Imaging Genomics Research Affinity Group,
Chair, Asian Pacific American Network,
Secretary, Association for Staff and Faculty
Women, Nationwide Children's Hospital, The
Ohio State University, Columbus, Ohio, USA

SHENG-CHE HUNG, MD, PhD
Clinical Assistant Professor, Department of
Radiology, Biomedical Research Imaging
Center, School of Medicine, The University of
North Carolina at Chapel Hill, Chapel Hill, North
Carolina, USA

MOHANNAD IBRAHIM, MD
Radiology Department, Neuroradiology
Division, University of Michigan, Ann Arbor,
Michigan, USA

NAOHARU KOBAYASHI, PhD
Assistant Professor of Radiology, Center for
Magnetic Resonance Research, University of
Minnesota, Minneapolis, Minnesota, USA

ARUNARK KOLIPAKA, PhD, FAHA, FSCMR
Associate Professor, Department of Radiology,
The Ohio State Wexner Medical Center,
Columbus, Ohio, USA

RAM KRISHNAMURTHY, PhD
MRI Physicist, Department of Radiology,
Nationwide Children's Hospital, Columbus,
Ohio, USA

DENIS LE BIHAN, MD, PhD
Director, NeuroSpin, Centre d'études de
Saclay, Gif-sur-Yvette, France

ERIC C. LEUTHARDT, MD
Department of Neurosurgery, Washington
University, St Louis, Missouri, USA

WEILI LIN, PhD
Professor, Department of Radiology,
Biomedical Research Imaging Center, School

of Medicine, The University of North Carolina at
Chapel Hill, Chapel Hill, North Carolina, USA

MOHIT MAHESHWARI, MBBS, MD
Department of Radiology, Medical College of
Wisconsin, Children's Wisconsin, Milwaukee,
Wisconsin, USA

TOSHIO MORITANI, MD, PhD
Professor and Director of Clinical Neuroradiology
Research, Division of Neuroradiology,
Department of Radiology, University of Michigan,
Ann Arbor, Michigan, USA

MAHMUD MOSSA-BASHA, MD
Professor, Vice Chair of Clinical Operations,
Chief of Service, Medical Director of MRI,
Department of Radiology, University of
Washington, Seattle, Washington, USA

MANJUNATHAN NANJAPPA, PhD
Research Associate, Department of Radiology,
The Ohio State University Wexner Medical
Center, Columbus, Ohio, USA

IGOR NESTRASIL, MD, PhD
Assistant Professor, Masonic Institute for the
Developing Brain, Division of Clinical
Behavioral Neuroscience, Department of
Pediatrics, University of Minnesota,
Minneapolis, Minnesota, USA

YUN PENG, MD, PhD
Department of Radiology, Beijing Children's
Hospital, Capital Medical University,
National Center for Children's Health,
Beijing, China

SANJAY P. PRABHU, MBBS, DCH, FRCR, DABR
Staff Pediatric Neuroradiologist, Department of
Radiology, Clinical Director, SIMPeds3D Print,
Director, Advanced Image Analysis Lab,
Boston Children's Hospital, Assistant
Professor of Radiology, Harvard Medical
School, Boston, Massachusetts, USA

JOSHUA S. SHIMONY, MD, PhD
Mallinckrodt Institute of Radiology,
Washington University, St Louis, Missouri, USA

MARK SMITH, MS, RT(R) (MR)
MRI Physicist, Department of Radiology,
Nationwide Children's Hospital, Columbus,
Ohio, USA

ASHOK SRINIVASAN, MD
Radiology Department, Neuroradiology Division, University of Michigan, Ann Arbor, Michigan, USA

JEFFREY N. STOUT, PhD
Fetal and Neonatal Neuroimaging and Developmental Science Center, Boston Children's Hospital, Boston, Massachusetts, USA

DANNY J.J. WANG, PhD
Professor of Neurology and Radiology, USC Institute for Neuroimaging and Informatics, SHN, Los Angeles, California, USA

MATTHEW T. WHITEHEAD, MD
Associate Professor of Pediatrics and Radiology, Vice Chief of Academic Affairs, Department of Radiology, Children's National Hospital, Prenatal Pediatrics Institute, Children's National Hospital, The George Washington University School of Medicine and Health Sciences, Washington, DC, USA

LEI WU, MD
Assistant Professor, Department of Radiology, University of Washington, Seattle, Washington, USA

PEW-THIAN YAP, PhD
Associate Professor, Department of Radiology, Biomedical Research Imaging Center, School of Medicine, The University of North Carolina at Chapel Hill, Chapel Hill, North Carolina, USA

HONG ZHANG, MD, PhD
Department of Radiology, Beijing Children's Hospital, Capital Medical University, National Center for Children's Health, Beijing, China

JINYUAN ZHOU, PhD
Department of Radiology, Johns Hopkins University, Baltimore, Maryland, USA

CHENGCHENG ZHU, PhD
Assistant Professor, Department of Radiology, University of Washington, Seattle, Washington, USA

Contents

Functional MR imaging (fMRI) is a valuable tool for presurgical planning and is well established in adult patients. The use of task-based fMRI is increasing in pediatric populations because it provides similar benefits for pre-surgical planning in children. This article reviews special adaptations that are required for successful applications of task-based fMRI in children, especially in the motor and language systems. The more recently introduced method of resting state fMRI is reviewed and its relative advantages and disadvantages discussed. Common pitfalls and other systems and networks that may be of interest are reviewed.

Magnetic resonance spectroscopy (MRS) is a valuable adjunct to structural brain imaging and has benefited greatly from recent technical advancements. Neurometabolic alterations in pediatric brain diseases have implications for diagnosis, prognosis, and therapy. Herein, the authors discuss MRS technical considerations and applications in the setting of various pediatric disease processes including tumors, metabolic diseases, hypoxic-ischemic encephalopathy, stroke, epilepsy, demyelinating disease, and infection.

MR imaging is used in conjunction with ultrasound screening for fetal brain abnormalities because it offers better contrast, higher resolution, and multiplanar capabilities that increase the accuracy and confidence of diagnosis. Fetal motion can severely limit the quality of MR imaging examinations. We outline the current acquisition strategies for fetal brain MR imaging and discuss near term advances that will improve study reliability. Prospective and retrospective motion correction will make the complement of MR neuroimaging modalities available for fetal diagnosis, improve the performance of existing technologies, and open new horizons to understanding in utero brain development.

Bone MR imaging techniques use extremely rapid echo times to maximize detection of short-T2 tissues with low water concentrations. The major approaches used in clinical practice are ultrashort echo-time and zero echo-time. Synthetic CT generation is feasible using atlas-based, voxel-based, and deep learning approaches. Major clinical applications in the pediatric head and neck include evaluation for craniosynostosis, sinonasal and jaw imaging, trauma, interventional planning, and postoperative follow-up. In this article, we review the technical background and practical utility of bone MR imaging with key clinical case examples.

Vessel wall MR imaging (VWI) has gained traction in clinical diagnostic applications for evaluation of intracranial and extracranial vasculopathies, with increasing use in pediatric populations. The technique has shown promise in detection, differentiation, and characterization of both inflammatory and noninflammatory vasculopathies. In this article, optimal techniques for intracranial and extracranial VWI as well as applications and value for pediatric neurovascular disease evaluation are discussed.

Magnetic resonance fingerprinting (MRF) is a new quantitative MR imaging technique for rapid and simultaneous quantification of multiple tissue properties. MRF can be used to reliably and accurately characterize intrinsic tissue properties, such as T1 and T2 relaxation times. This is a powerful tool with promising potential applications in children, such as the evaluation of brain development and differentiation of normal from pathologic tissues.

Magnetic resonance elastography (MRE) enables noninvasive quantitative assessment of biomechanical tissue properties. In MRE, tissue stiffness information is obtained by a 3-step process: propagating mechanical waves in tissues, measuring wave propagation using modified magnetic resonance (MR) pulse sequences, and generating quantitative stiffness maps from MR images. MRE is clinically used in patients with liver diseases, whereas applications in brain and other organs are still being investigated. At present, pediatric studies are in early stages and preliminary results promise to provide added value for clinical neuroimaging applications.

Amide proton transfer-weighted (APTw) imaging is a molecular MR imaging technique that can detect concentrations of the amide protons in mobile cellular proteins and peptides or pH changes in vivo. Previous studies have indicated that APTw MR imaging can be used to detect malignant brain tumors, stroke, and other neurologic diseases, although clinical applications are still emerging in pediatric patients. The authors briefly introduce the basic principles of APTw imaging. Then, they review early clinical applications of this approach to pediatric central nervous system diseases, including pediatric brain development, hypoxic-ischemic encephalopathy, intracranial infection, and brain tumors.

Neuroimaging with ultra-high-field magnets ($\geq$7T) provides superior signal-to-noise, spatial resolution and tissue contrast; but also greater safety concerns, longer scanning times, and increased distortion and field inhomogeneity. Brain and spinal cord anatomic microstructure and function imaged in greater detail offers improved lesion detection, delineation, and characterization. Ongoing development of novel imaging contrasts and translation of cutting-edge sequences will aid more accurate,

MAGNETIC RESONANCE IMAGING CLINICS OF NORTH AMERICA

SERIES OF RELATED INTEREST

Advances in Clinical Radiology
Available at: www.advancesinclinicalradiology.com

Neuroimaging Clinics of North America
Available at: www.neuroimaging.theclinics.com

Radiologic Clinics of North America
Available at: www.radiologic.theclinics.com

VISIT THE CLINICS ONLINE!
Access your subscription at:
www.theclinics.com

PROGRAM OBJECTIVE

The goal of Magnetic Resonance Imaging Clinics of North America is to keep practicing physicians up to date with current clinical practice by providing timely articles reviewing the state of the art in patient care.

TARGET AUDIENCE

All practicing physicians and healthcare professionals who provide patient care utilizing findings from Magnetic Resonance Imaging.

LEARNING OBJECTIVES

Upon completion of this activity, participants will be able to:

1. Review the application and significance of advances such as diffusion-weighted imaging (DWI) sequences, diffusion-tensor imaging (DTI), and fiber tractography (FT) in pediatric brain and spine.
2. Discuss applications of MR perfusion, with and without contrast, in investigating cerebrovascular diseases and cerebral neoplastic processes in pediatric patients.
3. Recognize current and potential use cases for virtual reality (VR) and augmented reality (AR) applications in a pediatric neuroimaging setting.

ACCREDITATION

The Elsevier Office of Continuing Medical Education (EOCME) is accredited by the Accreditation Council for Continuing Medical Education (ACCME) to provide continuing medical education for physicians.

The EOCME designates this journal-based CME activity enduring material for a maximum of 13 *AMA PRA Category 1 Credit*(s)™. Physicians should claim only the credit commensurate with the extent of their participation in the activity.

All other healthcare professionals requesting continuing education credit for this enduring material will be issued a certificate of participation.

DISCLOSURE OF CONFLICTS OF INTEREST

The EOCME assesses conflict of interest with its instructors, faculty, planners, and other individuals who are in a position to control the content of CME activities. All relevant conflicts of interest that are identified are thoroughly vetted by EOCME for fair balance, scientific objectivity, and patient care recommendations. EOCME is committed to providing its learners with CME activities that promote improvements or quality in healthcare and not a specific proprietary business or a commercial interest.

The planning committee, staff, authors and editors listed below have identified no financial relationships or relationships to products or devices they or their spouse/life partner have with commercial interest related to the content of this CME activity:

Jayapalli Rajiv Bapuraj, MD; Sven Bambach, PhD; M. Alejandra Bedoya, MD; Stefan Bluml, PhD; Regina Chavous-Gibson, MSN, RN; Dinesh Kumar Deelchand, PhD; Tejaswini Deshmukh, MBBS, MD; Judy A. Estroff, MD; Talha Ul Ghazi, BS; P. Ellen Grant, MD, MSc; Mai-Lan Ho, MD; Sheng-Che Hung, MD, PhD; Mohannad Ibrahim, MD; Naoharu Kobayashi, PhD; Arunark Kolipaka, PhD, FAHA, FSCMR; Ram Krishnamurthy, PhD; Pradeep Kuttysankaran; Denis Le Bihan, MD, PhD; Eric C. Leuthardt, MD; Weili Lin, PhD; Mohit Maheshwari, MBBS, MD; Toshio Moritani, MD, PhD; Mahmud Mossa-Basha, MD; Manjunathan Nanjappa, PhD; Yun Peng, MD, PhD; Sanjay P. Prabhu, MBBS, DCH, FRCR, DABR; Joshua S. Shimony, MD, PhD; Mark Smith, MS, RT(R) (MR); Ashok Srinivasan, MD; Jeffrey N. Stout, PhD; Matthew T. Whitehead, MD; Lei Wu, MD; Pew-Thian Yap, PhD; Hong Zhang, MD, PhD; Chengcheng Zhu, PhD

The planning committee, staff, authors and editors listed below have identified financial relationships or relationships to products or devices they or their spouse/life partner have with commercial interest related to the content of this CME activity:

Yong Chen, PhD: Research support: Siemens Healthineers

Igor Nestrasil, MD, PhD: Consultant/advisor: ICON plc, Quantim; Research support: BioMarin, Sanofi, Takeda Pharmaceutical Company Limited

Danny J.J. Wang, PhD: Ownership Interest: Translational MRI, LLC

Jinyuan Zhou, PhD: Speakers Bureau, Patents and/or Royalties: Philips Healthcare

UNAPPROVED/OFF-LABEL USE DISCLOSURE

The EOCME requires CME faculty to disclose to the participants:

1. When products or procedures being discussed are off-label, unlabelled, experimental, and/or investigational (not US Food and Drug Administration [FDA] approved); and
2. Any limitations on the information presented, such as data that are preliminary or that represent ongoing research, interim analyses, and/or unsupported opinions. Faculty may discuss information about pharmaceutical agents that is outside of FDA-approved labelling. This information is intended solely for CME and is not intended to promote off-label use of these

medications. If you have any questions, contact the medical affairs department of the manufacturer for the most recent prescribing information.

TO ENROLL
To enroll in the *Magnetic Resonance Imaging Clinics of North America* Continuing Medical Education program, call customer service at 1-800-654-2452 or sign up online at http://www.theclinics.com/home/cme. The CME program is available to subscribers for an additional annual fee of USD 281.00.

METHOD OF PARTICIPATION
In order to claim credit, participants must complete the following:
1. Complete enrolment as indicated above.
2. Read the activity.
3. Complete the CME Test and Evaluation. Participants must achieve a score of 70% on the test. All CME Tests and Evaluations must be completed online.

CME INQUIRIES/SPECIAL NEEDS
For all CME inquiries or special needs, please contact elsevierCME@elsevier.com.

Foreword

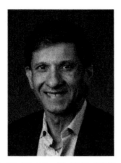

Suresh K. Mukherji, MD, MBA, FACR
Consulting Editor

I have always found pediatric neuroimaging one of the most daunting yet rewarding specialties of neuroradiology. Although my passion is head and neck imaging, I have always had a certain affinity toward anything involving children since I have been married to a pediatrician for almost 30 years!

This important issue of *Magnetic Resonance Imaging Clinics of North America* is dedicated to pediatric neuroradiology with a specific emphasis on advanced imaging techniques. There are specific articles devoted to diffusion, noncontrast perfusion, contrast perfusion, functional imaging, spectroscopy, fetal and placental imaging, ultrashort echo time, vessel wall imaging, fingerprinting, elastography, chemical exchange saturation transfer, ultra-high field imaging, and 3D modeling and advanced visualization. Although this issue is focused on advanced imaging, the articles are very practical and emphasize the clinical applications of these important techniques.

I would like to thank all the article authors for their wonderful contributions. The content is superb, and the images are exquisite. I would also like to especially thank Dr Mai-Lan Ho for guest editing this wonderful issue. I have known Mai-Lan for many years and have enjoyed watching her evolve into one of the most respected pediatric neuroradiologists in our field. Thank you, Mai-Lan, for your numerous contributions and the positive impact you are having on your patients.

Suresh K. Mukherji, MD, MBA, FACR
Marian University, Head and Neck Radiology,
ProScan Imaging, Carmel, IN, USA

E-mail address:
sureshmukherji@hotmail.com

Magn Reson Imaging Clin N Am 29 (2021) xv
https://doi.org/10.1016/j.mric.2021.08.003
1064-9689/21/© 2021 Published by Elsevier Inc.

Preface
Advanced Pediatric Neuroimaging: *"Better, Stronger, Faster"*

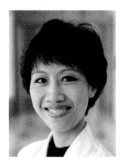

Mai-Lan Ho, MD
Editor

Pediatric neuroimaging is a fascinating discipline that combines human neuroanatomy and neurodevelopment with ongoing advances in imaging hardware and software. Our understanding of embryology, genomics, and disease pathogenesis continues to evolve amid an ever-expanding array of available imaging technologies. Advanced MR imaging techniques can serve as noninvasive biomarkers of microstructural, functional, and metabolic changes in normal development as well as in disease processes. Many MR imaging sequences are well established for adult clinical and translational neuroimaging applications. However, scanning of children is practically limited by smaller anatomy, rapidly changing structure and function, lower scan tolerance, and safety considerations.

The added value of pediatric MR imaging arises at the intersection of effectiveness (diagnostic information) and efficiency (diagnostic throughput). When discussing the evolution of pediatric neuro MR imaging, I like to invoke the catchphrase of *The Six Million Dollar Man*: *"Better, Stronger,*

Faster." Better refers to new and improved MR imaging techniques, especially those that provide information beyond standard neuroanatomic macrostructure. *Stronger* refers to improved MR imaging hardware, particularly magnetic field strengths and coil configurations that augment image quality. *Faster* refers to abbreviated or accelerated software approaches that enable rapid image acquisition, workflow, and reconstruction.

This special issue of *Magnetic Resonance Imaging Clinics of North America*, "Pediatric Neuroimaging: State-of-the-Art," is dedicated to the latest and greatest MR imaging advances poised to impact pediatric neuroimaging practice. We present cutting-edge content from leaders in the field covering a variety of current and novel imaging technologies. Each article is coauthored by imaging scientists and radiologists, reflecting the translational process from MR imaging technical development to clinical application. Our 13 articles cover advanced diffusion, noncontrast perfusion, contrast perfusion, functional, spectroscopy, fetal and placental imaging, ultrashort echo-time,

Magn Reson Imaging Clin N Am 29 (2021) xvii–xviii
https://doi.org/10.1016/j.mric.2021.07.001
1064-9689/21/© 2021 Published by Elsevier Inc.

vessel wall imaging, fingerprinting, elastography, chemical exchange saturation transfer, ultra-high-field imaging, and 3D modeling and advanced visualization.

It is my greatest hope that this issue will elevate the global interest and implementation of advanced MR imaging in the pediatric head, neck, and spine. Pediatric and adult radiologists, imaging scientists, and clinical practitioners can all benefit from the cutting-edge team science exemplified in these articles, which will undoubtedly influence the future of radiology and precision medicine as a whole.

Thank you so much to Drs Suresh Mukherji and Lynne Steinbach for their mentorship and interest in this topic; as well as John Vassallo, Arlene Campos, and Pradeep Kuttysankaran for administrative and editorial support. This issue of *Magnetic Resonance Imaging Clinics of North America* is dedicated to our global medical community, particularly those who worked ceaselessly during the pandemic to improve children's care; my friends and colleagues who contributed such wonderful content; and my parents, Huong and Sa Ho.

Mai-Lan Ho, MD
Department of Radiology
Nationwide Children's Hospital
The Ohio State University
Columbus, OH, USA

E-mail address:
mailanho@gmail.com

Advanced Diffusion of the Pediatric Brain and Spine

Toshio Moritani, MD, PhD

KEYWORDS

- Diffusion • Tensor • Kurtosis • DSI • Q-space • IVIM • NODDI • OGSE

KEY POINTS

- Diffusion-weighted imaging (DWI), diffusion tensor imaging (DTI), and fiber tractography (FT) have established clinical significance in the pediatric brain and spine.
- Multi-shot echo planar imaging (EPI) and non-EPI DWI provide higher spatial resolution with less susceptibility artifact, and are thus replacing conventional single-shot EPI.
- Advanced diffusion imaging includes diffusion kurtosis imaging (DKI), neurite orientation dispersion and density imaging (NODDI), diffusion spectrum imaging (DSI), intravoxel incoherent motion (IVIM), and oscillating-gradient spin-echo (OGSE) DWI.

INTRODUCTION

In vivo diffusion phenomena using magnetic resonance (MR) techniques were first described by Stejskal and Tanner[1] in 1965. In 1986, Le Bihan and colleagues[2] applied diffusion techniques for the first time in MR imaging. Progress in diffusion imaging is occurring at a very fast pace, with numerous articles in the last 20 years. Diffusion-weighted imaging (DWI) has been one of the routine MR sequences for more than 20 years because of its tremendous clinical usefulness with unique information and short acquisition time.[3] MR imaging is attractive in pediatric imaging, with a lack of ionizing radiation making it a suitable modality for multiple scans in longitudinal follow-ups. DWI is crucial in the evaluation of the pediatric brain and spine, especially for ischemic disease, trauma, infectious disease, toxic metabolic disease, and tumors.

Recently developed new techniques of DWI, such as multishot (MS) echo planar imaging (EPI) and non-EPI sequences, provide higher spatial resolution with less susceptibility artifact and distortion compared with single-shot (SS) EPI sequence with shorter acquisition time. Likewise, diffusion tensor imaging (DTI) and fiber tractography (FT) are available on clinical scanners with diffusion sequences and are useful tools in evaluation of white matter structures and visualization of nerve fibers.[4–8]

Advanced diffusion imaging, including diffusion kurtosis imaging (DKI),[9] neurite orientation dispersion and density imaging (NODDI),[10] q-space imaging (QSI),[11] intravoxel incoherent motion (IVIM),[2,12] and oscillating-gradient spin-echo (OGSE),[13] has been reported in the application of pediatric brain and spine. Advanced diffusion imaging potentially provides quantitative parameter measurement with more specific information of underlying disorder and pathophysiology, such as microstructures and microcirculations.

This article covers the application and significance of new and advanced diffusion imaging in pediatric brain and spine with brief explanation of the physics and with the discussion of underlying disorders and pathophysiology, using case examples of infarction/ischemia and secondary degeneration, encephalopathy, encephalomyelitis, demyelinating and toxic metabolic diseases, tumors, and congenital anomalies.

Underlying Disorders and Pathophysiology of Diffusion Imaging

Diffusion imaging has been investigated not only for its clinical usefulness, such as disease

Division of Neuroradiology, Department of Radiology, University of Michigan, 1500 East Medical Center Drive, UH B2 A209K, Ann Arbor, MI 48109, USA
E-mail address: tmoritan@med.umich.edu

Magn Reson Imaging Clin N Am 29 (2021) 465–492
https://doi.org/10.1016/j.mric.2021.06.001
1064-9689/21/© 2021 Elsevier Inc. All rights reserved.

diagnosis or evaluation of the treatment effect, but also for the understanding of underlying disorders and pathophysiology based on seeking information on tissue microstructures and microcirculations. Water diffusion can provide unique information on the functional architecture of tissues, because, during their random displacements, water molecules probe tissue structure at a microscopic scale.[2,14] There are 2 main barriers that obstruct water molecule movement in biological tissues: (1) membranous structures, and (2) macromolecules (**Fig. 1**).[15]

There are many different types of membranous structures in the cells, including the outer cell membrane, axonal membrane, membranes of the myelin sheath, and intracellular organelle membranes. In the central nervous system (CNS), the gray matter is mainly composed of neurons and glial cells (astrocytes), whereas the white matter is mainly composed of glial cells, axons, and myelin sheaths. In the gray matter, cytotoxic edema occurs mainly in neurons and glial cells

(astrocytes, oligodendrocytes). However, in the white matter, the edema occurs in glial cells, axons (axonal swelling), and myelin sheaths (intramyelinic edema).[15,16]

Myelin is a lipid-rich substance that surrounds nerve cell axons to insulate and increase the rate of electrical impulses (called action potentials) along the axon. Myelin comprises approximately 40% water; the dry mass comprises between 60% and 75% lipid and between 15% and 25% protein. Axons are mainly composed of neurofilaments and microtubules in the axoplasm with higher water content (approximately 90%). Myelin sheaths are composed of inner and outer membranes and loops, the cell processes of oligodendrocytes in the CNS (**Fig. 2**).[17] Axons are located in the center and surrounded by multiple layers of myelin sheaths. There is a periaxonal space between the axonal membrane (axolemma) and myelin sheath.

Based on Cs[133] nuclear MR (NMR) studies with global CNS ischemia in rat brain, decrease in water apparent diffusion coefficient (ADC) arises

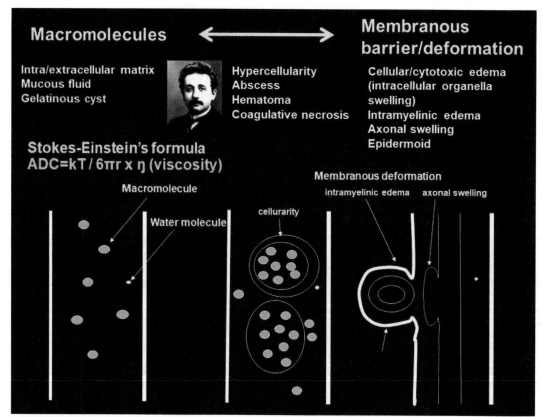

Fig. 1. Water molecule diffusion is restricted by macromolecules and/or membranous barrier/deformation in tissues. Water molecule diffusion restriction by macromolecules is also known as viscosity. Diffusion coefficient and viscosity have negative correlation based on the Stokes-Einstein formula, which originated from Albert Einstein's PhD thesis. Many of the biological and pathologic tissues, such as mucous fluid, tumor, hematoma, abscess, necrosis, and edema, consist of the combination of macromolecules and membranous structures. (*From* Moritani T. Brain Edema. In: Moritani T, Capizzano AA, editors. Diffusion Weighted MR Imaging of the Brain, Head and Neck, and Spine, 3rd eds. Springer; 2021.)

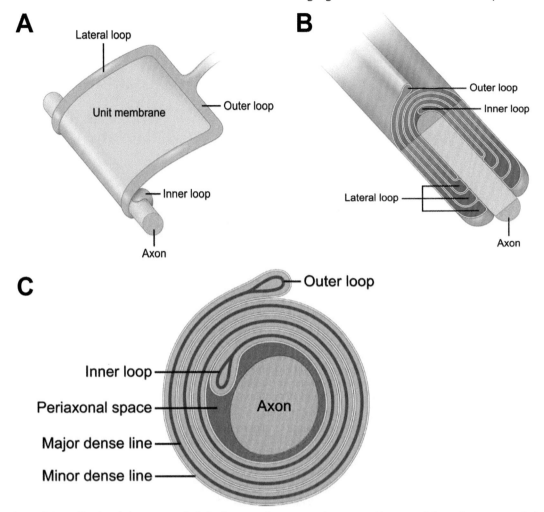

Fig. 2. (*A*) Myelin sheath is composed of the inner and outer membranes and loops and the cell processes of oligodendrocytes. (*B*) Fusion of the inner membranes forms the major dense line made by part of the cytoplasm (intracellular space). Fusion of the outer membranes forms the minor dense line (intraperiod line), which is potentially the extracellular space. (*C*) Intramyelinic edema usually occurs in the closed extracellular space in the myelin sheath, which can cause restricted diffusion likely related to the geometric distortion of membranous structures. There is a periaxonal space between axonal membrane and myelin sheath. (*From* Moritani T. Brain Edema. In: Moritani T, Capizzano AA, editors. Diffusion Weighted MR Imaging of the Brain, Head and Neck, and Spine, 3rd eds. Springer; 2021.)

largely from the changes in the intracellular space.[18] However, the observed 40% reduction of ADC cannot be explained by an increase in intracellular water alone, even if all extracellular fluid is intracellular.[19] Decrease in the energy-dependent intracellular circulation, cytoplasmic streaming, or axoplasmic flow is too slow (less than 1 μm/s) to affect the ADC values.[20]

Membranous geometric deformation of axons and myelin sheaths is one of the important causes of water molecule diffusion restriction. Neurite beading has recently been proposed as a mechanism for the diffusion changes after ischemic stroke and traumatic brain injury (**Fig. 3**).[21–25] The neurite refers to any projection from the cell body of a neuron. This projection can be either an

axon or a dendrite, and it has been studied using complex geometric models of nonuniformed swollen neurites (ie, beading) and OGSE diffusion.[21–24] Beading-induced changes in cell-membrane morphology were sufficient to significantly hinder water mobility and decrease ADC after ischemic stroke. Electron microscopy of axonal swelling in traumatic axonal injury shows microtubule breakage and varicose axonal swellings after dynamic stretch injury of axons (see **Fig. 3**).[25]

In intramyelinic edema, trapped water mainly accumulates between the intraperiod lines of the myelin sheath, the widened potential space of the extracellular space, rather than the cytoplasm. The edema, even in the closed extracellular space in the myelin sheath, can cause restricted

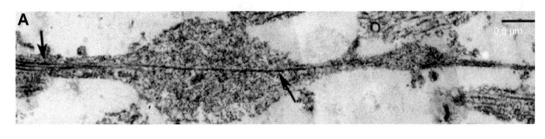

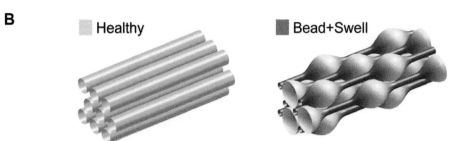

Fig. 3. (*A*) Electron microscopy of axonal swelling (neurite beading) in traumatic axonal injury. Microtubule breakage and varicose axonal swellings after dynamic stretch injury of axons. Transmission electron microscopy shows a solitary intact microtubule traversing a large swelling (*right arrow*), whereas multiple microtubules can be observed in the adjacent nonswollen region from which it emerged (*left arrow*). (*B*) Neurite beading has recently been proposed as a mechanism for the diffusion restriction in ischemia and traumatic brain injury. Healthy and beaded and swelled cylinders are shown for Monte-Carlo simulations. ([A] *Courtesy of* Min D. Tang-Schomer, PhD [From[25]]; [B] *Courtesy of* Corey Allan Baron, PhD [From[21]].)

diffusion, probably related to the geometric distortion of the membranous structures. It may be inappropriate to continue to label this phenomenon cytotoxic.[26] Intramyelinic edema is thought to be related to the complete reversibility of diffusion-restricted lesions.[15,16] Pure intramyelinic edema can occur in an acute cytotoxic plaque of multiple sclerosis, acute disseminated encephalomyelitis, vigabatrin-associated vacuolar myelinopathy (**Fig. 4**), spectrum of reversible splenial lesion of corpus callosum (**Fig. 5**), and metabolic and toxic leukoencephalopathies.[16,27–29]

The macromolecule is another cause of water molecule diffusion restriction, which is called viscosity (see **Fig. 1**). A decrease in intracellular ADC can be related to an increase in cytoplasmic viscosity from a swelling of intracellular organelles.[30] Diffusion coefficient and viscosity have the negative correlation based on the Stokes-Einstein formula, which originated from Albert Einstein's PhD thesis[31]:

$$D = kT / 6\pi r \times \eta$$

where *D* is diffusion coefficient, *K* is constant, *T* is temperature, *r* is radius of macromolecule, and η is viscosity.

Many of the biological and pathologic tissues are consistent in the combination of macromolecules and membranous structures, including hyperviscous fluid (mucous fluid, abscess, hematoma), neoplasm (increased cell density), inclusion cysts (composed of membranous structures), and edema of various cellular components (see **Fig. 1**).

DWI is crucial in the evaluation of the pediatric brain and spinal cord. The water content of the brain and spinal cord is considerably higher in neonates and early infants than in adults.

During brain development (perinatal, early infant), the pediatric brain is more vulnerable to excitotoxic injury than the adult brain.[32] The pediatric brain during the first 2 years of life has abundant excitotoxic amino acid receptors. *N*-Methyl-D-aspartate (NMDA) receptors dominate in the immature brain. However, non-NMDA receptors (α-amino-3-hydroxy-5-methyl-4-isoxazolepropionic acid [AMPA] receptors and kainic receptors) predominate during maturation. Secondary degeneration in the pediatric brain tends to be more widely distributed via prewallerian and transsynaptic degeneration and therefore presents earlier compared with adults.[33,34] Prewallerian and transsynaptic degeneration show diffusion restriction along the areas that comprise excitotoxic circuits (**Fig. 6**). Electron microscopy shows axonal swelling and intramyelinic edema in prewallerian degeneration (**Fig. 7**).[35] Gamma-aminobutyric acid (GABA) receptors are excitatory in early infants, whereas they are inhibitory in adults. The distribution of the lesions of vigabatrin-induced vacuolar myelinopathy corresponds to distribution of abundant areas of GABA

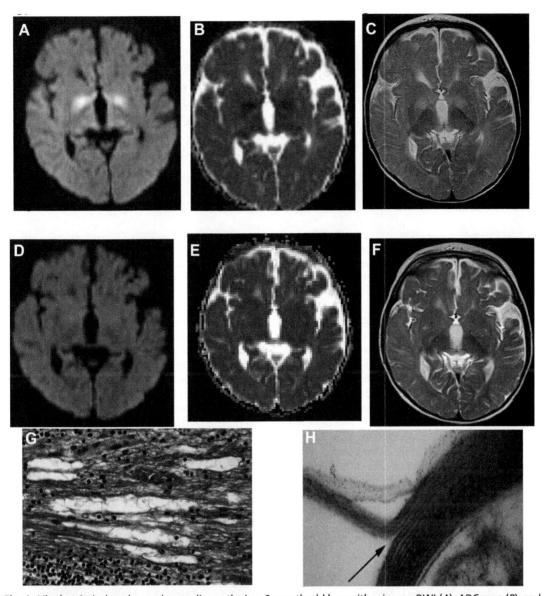

Fig. 4. Vigabatrin-induced vacuolar myelinopathy in a 9-month-old boy with seizures. DWI (*A*), ADC map (*B*), and T2-weighted image (*C*) show symmetric high signal and diffusion restriction in the globi pallidi and thalami bilaterally. Three-month follow-up MR imaging (*D–F*) shows complete reversibility of the lesions. The lesion distribution corresponds to the distribution of abundant areas of gamma-aminobutyric acid (GABA) receptors. (*G*) In a different patient, light micrograph shows vacuoles 25 to 50 mm in diameter in white matter. (*H*) Electron microscopy shows splitting myelin (*arrow*) at minor dense (intraperiod) line, which is a potential extracellular space. (*Courtesy of* Myles Horton, MD, and Marc R Del Bigio, MD, PhD [from[27]]; and *From* Moritani T. Brain Edema. In: Moritani T, Capizzano AA, editors. Diffusion Weighted MR Imaging of the Brain, Head and Neck, and Spine, 3rd eds. Springer; 2021.)

receptors. These lesions pathologically represent intramyelinic edema (see **Fig. 4**).[27]

Various Techniques of Diffusion-Weighted Imaging Sequences

In DWI, the SS EPI technique is often used clinically because of its short acquisition time, with only 1 repetition time to fill the k space. However, SS EPI suffers from greater susceptibility effects, geometric distortion, and reduced spatial resolution. The artifacts are especially prominent in spine and head and neck areas, and are prominent using a higher-tesla magnet.

There are various approaches to improve these artifacts, related to strong magnetic field gradients,

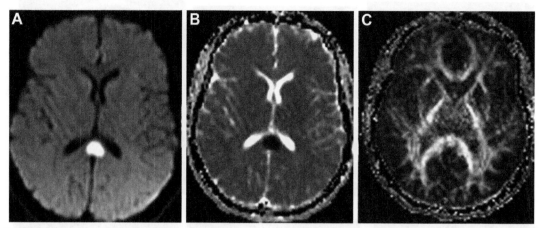

Fig. 5. A focal lesion of the splenium of the corpus callosum related to seizure medication. (*Left*) Trace DWI shows an ovoid hyperintense lesion in the splenium of the corpus callosum with decreased ADC (*middle*). (*Right*) Fractional anisotropy (FA) is slightly increased in the lesion. The lesion is completely resolved on follow-up MR imaging (not shown).

maintenance of a reliable magnetic field environment during rapid gradient switching, and postacquisition correction techniques. Thin-sliced sagittal, coronal, or axial SS DWI provide high-resolution images with better detection of the lesion (**Fig. 8**).[36,37] The zonally magnified oblique multislice EPI (ZOOM-EPI) DWI with reduced field of view (FOV) (**Fig. 9**) provides superior MR diffusion image quality compared with the full-FOV SS EPI sequence.[38–40] MS EPI sequences such as two-dimensional navigated interleaved MS EPI DWI with image reconstruction using image-space sampling (IRIS) DWI, or readout segmentation of long variable echo-trains (RESOLVE) DWI (**Fig. 10**), are not only largely free of distortions but can also deliver sharp imaging at higher spatial resolution.[38] Non-EPI DWI techniques include SS fast spin-echo DWI, half-Fourier-acquired SS turbo spin-echo DWI, and MS turbo spin-echo sequences such as turbo spin-echo XD DWI (split acquisition of first spin-echo signals) with or without multivane (non-cartesian k-space filling using radial rectangular blades), PROPELLER (periodically rotated overlapping parallel lines with enhanced reconstruction) and BLADE DWI (see **Fig. 10**).[40] Non-EPI DWI techniques have less susceptibility artifact and higher spatial resolution, but at the cost of longer acquisition time and lower signal to noise ratio.

Diffusion Tensor Imaging

DTI is available on clinical scanners with diffusion sequences. DTI can detect not only the magnitude but the directionality of water diffusion and allows

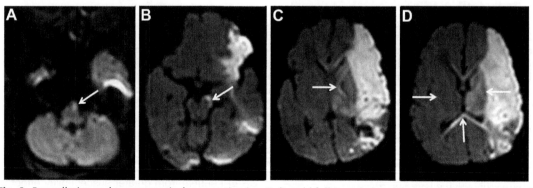

Fig. 6. Prewallerian and transsynaptic degeneration in a 6-day-old full-term baby with acute infarction in the left middle cerebral artery territory. (*A, B*) DWI shows acute infarcts involving the left middle cerebral artery territory with prewallerian degeneration along the left corticospinal tract (*arrows*), and anterior and posterior corpus callosum, and internal capsule (*arrows*). (*C, D*) Mild diffusion hyperintensities in the left basal ganglia and thalamus (*arrows*) are likely caused by transsynaptic degeneration via striatocortical and thalamocortical connections, which comprise secondary changes via excitotoxic circuits. (*From* Moritani T. Brain Edema. In: Moritani T, Capizzano AA, editors. Diffusion Weighted MR Imaging of the Brain, Head and Neck, and Spine, 3rd eds. Springer; 2021.)

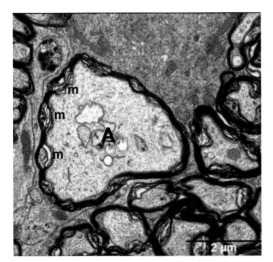

Fig. 7. Electron microscopy of axonal swelling and in-tramyelinic edema in prewallerian degeneration after NMDA injection. Electron microscopy shows swollen axons (A) with abnormal collection of altered tubulo-vesicular structures and surrounding multilayered myelin sheath (m). (*Courtesy of* Sarabjit K Saggu, MD and Robert J Casson, MD [from[35]].)

the investigation of CNS microstructure. The water molecules in white matter are mainly restricted by membranous structures of the myelin sheaths and axons in the white matter bundles. The movement of water molecules is less impeded along the direction of white matter bundles than perpendicular to the bundles. The net effect is high directionality (high anisotropy) of movement. In areas of high concentration of fluid (ie, ventricles filled with cerebrospinal fluid [CSF]), there is little preferential

directionality of movement (low anisotropy) and minimal hindrance to diffusion (high diffusivity). DTI is a method using gaussian distribution of water molecules in the white matter and is based on a mathematical ellipsoid model (**Fig. 11**).[41]

Fractional anisotropy (FA) and mean diffusivity (MD) are used to measure microscopic motion of tissue water. In a DTI measurement, 6 or more DWI measurements are required, tensor eigenvalues (λ_1, λ_2, λ_3) and eigenvectors are derived from these measurements.[4] Maps of MD and FA can then be generated from the eigenvalues with the following relations:

$$MD = \frac{\lambda_1 + \lambda_2 + \lambda_3}{3}$$

$$FA = \sqrt{\frac{2}{3}} \sqrt{\frac{(\lambda_1 - MD)^2 + (\lambda_2 - MD)^2 + (\lambda_3 - MD)^2}{\lambda_1^2 + \lambda_2^2 + \lambda_3^2}}$$

A useful representation of DTI measurement results is given by a color FA map, which represents the orientation of the largest eigenvalue from left to right as red, anterior to posterior (AP) as green, and superior to inferior (SI) directions as blue, respectively, whereas image intensity represents FA values (**Figs. 12–14**).

In tissue with dense fibers, the diffusivity in the direction perpendicular to the fiber is suppressed and the FA is increased. When the fiber structure is damaged by degenerative disease, the diffusivity in the direction perpendicular to the fiber is increased and the FA value is decreased. However, decreased FA is nonspecific and also seen in extracellular edema (vasogenic and interstitial edema) (see **Fig. 12**), cystic change, gliosis,

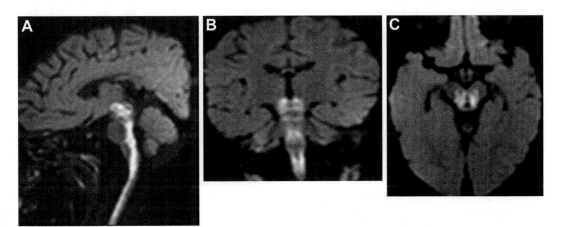

Fig. 8. Acute flaccid myelitis caused by Enterovirus 71 in a 6-month-old boy who presented with increased secretions, vomiting, and concern for aspiration. (*A*) Sagittal and (*B*) coronal thin slice (2 mm, gapless) and (*C*) axial SS EPI DWI clearly shows diffusion restriction affecting the dorsal brainstem and the gray matter of the spinal cord with less distortion on 3 T.

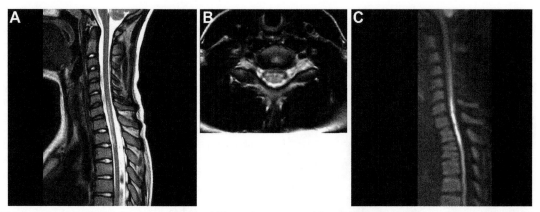

Fig. 9. Spinal cord infarction in an 11-year-old boy who presented for weakness of his extremities and chest pain after playing outside on the trampoline. (*A*) Sagittal and (*B*) axial T2-weighted images show high-signal-intensity lesions in the spinal cord at the level of C6/7 through T2/3. (*C*) ZOOM-EPI DWI clearly shows restricted diffusion in the lesions consistent with spinal cord infarction, most likely caused by fibrocartilaginous emboli.

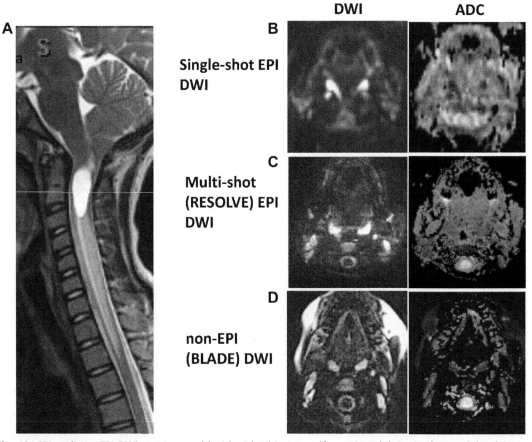

Fig. 10. EPI and non-EPI DWI. A 13-year-old girl with Chiari 1 malformation. (*A*) Sagittal T2-weighted image shows low-lying tonsils, syrinx at C2-C3 levels, and diffuse high signal intensity in the cord from C4 to T2 level, representing presyrinx state. (*B–D*) SS EPI DWI (*B*), MS EPI DWI (*C*), and non-EPI (BLADE) DWI (*D*) with the ADC maps are shown. SS EPI DWI has the lowest spatial resolution with image distortion but shorter acquisition time (40 seconds), whereas MS (RESOLVE) EPI DWI has better spatial resolution with less distortion but longer acquisition time (3 minutes), and with no distortion but the longest acquisition time (7 minutes) in non-EPI (BLADE) DWI.

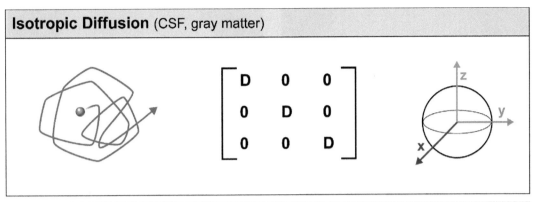

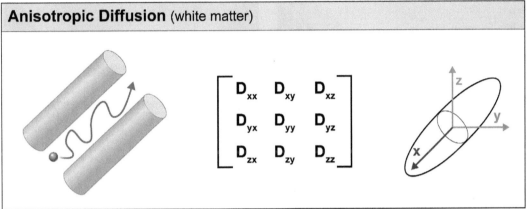

Fig. 11. Diffusion and corresponding diffusion tensor and ellipsoid. Upper row illustrates the case with unrestricted diffusion, forming a spherical probability distribution. Lower row shows restricted diffusion, as is the case in white matter. The diffusion ellipsoid is elongated along the direction of maximum diffusion. Note that the more elliptical the ellipsoid is, the higher the measured FA.

demyelination, and so forth in the white matter. In contrast, in cytotoxic edema, FA is preserved or increased likely because of increased tortuosity of the extracellular space and movement of water into the more restricted environment of the intracellular space (see **Fig. 5**).

DTI is useful for evaluating the myelination and premyelination states of the infant brain by showing anisotropy earlier than conventional MR imaging.[42] Normal reference data of brain and spinal cord of FA and ADC values have been reported in utero and in newborns (preterm, term), infants, and early childhood.[43–47] FA and ADC values dramatically change during the in utero period (32 weeks) in the pyramidal tract and the corpus callosum.[45] In the first 3 months, the early rate of ADC decrease is twice as great for peripheral white matter as for deep white matter, whereas the rate of FA increase is half as great for peripheral white matter as for deep white matter (**Fig. 15**). The anisotropy of the corpus callosum is already visible by DTI as early as the 28th gestational week. This process occurs even though the corpus callosum is composed of nonmyelinated

fibers at this stage. The phenomenon has been called premyelination anisotropy.[42] The anisotropic effect in the immature brain is more likely to be related to structural changes of the axonal membrane. In Pelizaeus-Merzbacher disease, the FA has high values throughout the white matter, which is likely caused by the axonal structure of the white matter (**Fig. 16**).

The anisotropic pattern depends on the irregularity of axonal orientation as well as the degree of myelination. In Sturge-Weber syndrome in neonates, abnormal hypermyelination is shown as increased FA and is decreased on DTI (**Fig. 17**), which is useful for the early diagnosis of the extent of brain abnormality.[48] Axons control the formation and thickness of myelin. If ischemia occurs in the cortex, it could interfere with normal neuronal function and lead to premature axonal release of a myelinogenic trophic factor.[49] Structural and functional alterations of the axons and oligodendrocytes that may affect diffusion anisotropy include an increase of the axonal diameter, increase in the concentration of the microtubule-associated proteins and microperoxisome,

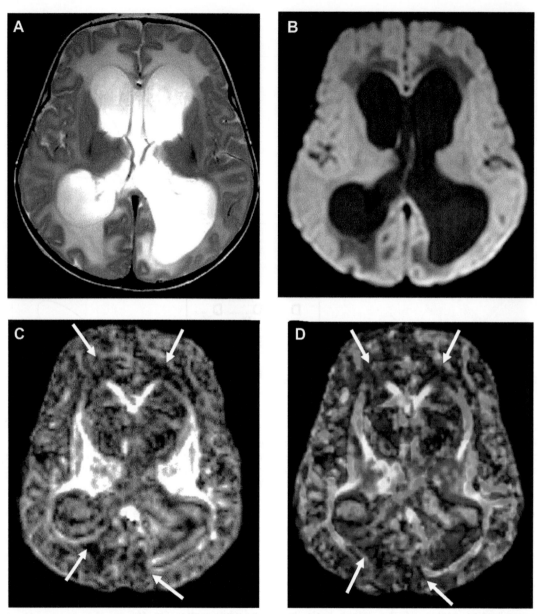

Fig. 12. Acute hydrocephalus. A 3-month-old girl with posterior fossa mass (atypical teratoid/rhabdoid tumor). (*A*) T2-weighted image shows hydrocephalus and diffuse periventricular hyperintensity consistent with interstitial edema. (*B*) Trace DWI shows hypointensity in the periventricular interstitial edema with decreased FA on the FA map (*arrows*) (*C*), and with decreased directional anisotropy on the color map (*arrows*) (*D*). (*From* Moritani T. Brain Edema. In: Moritani T, Capizzano AA, editors. Diffusion Weighted MR Imaging of the Brain, Head and Neck, and Spine, 3rd eds. Springer; 2021.)

activity of Na^+/K^+-ATPase, and ion fluxes secondary to action potentials.[50] DTI allows earlier detection of specific anatomic microstructural abnormalities in infants at risk for neurologic abnormalities and disability.[45]

Diffusion tensor (DT) FT is a method to estimate white matter structural anatomy from DTI. DT-FT can provide detailed imaging of white matter tracts and connectivity between different regions of the brain not easily appreciated with other imaging

methods. DT-FT has been widely used to assess the neuroanatomical basis of congenital brain malformations by the evaluation of the integrity of the adjacent white matter and its aberrant fiber networks. DT-FT findings have been reported in cortical dysplasia, heterotopia of gray matter, hemimegalencephaly, holoprosencephaly, schizencephaly, polymicrogyria, lissencephaly, callosal agenesis/dysgenesis, rhombencephalosynapsis, Moebius syndrome, Joubert syndrome, and other

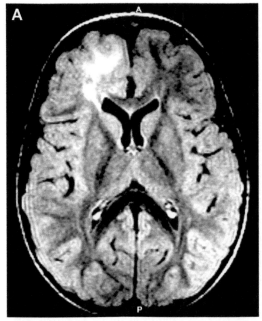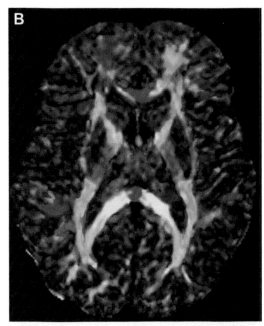

Fig. 13. Cortical dysplasia in a 5-year-old boy with right frontal spikes. (*A*) Fluid-attenuated inversion recovery (FLAIR) image shows cortical thickening and white matter hyperintensity in the right frontal lobe. (*B*) DTI color map shows decreased anisotropy in the right frontal abnormal area, which may represent decreased fiber connection between deep white matter and dysplastic cortex. (*Courtesy of* Noriko Salamon, MD, PhD [From[3]].)

brainstem malformations.[51–55] DTI is useful to detect focal cortical dysplasia (FCD) by the evaluation of the integrity of the adjacent white matter. Reduced values of FA are seen in the subcortical white matter of FCD (see **Fig. 13**). In hemimegalencephaly, DTI shows increased FA and slightly decreased ADC in the hemispheric area with accentuated myelination. DT-FT also shows an aberrant midsagittal fiber tract that passes anteroposteriorly through between the 2 anterior horns of the lateral ventricles (see **Fig. 14**) and disruption of corticopontocerebellar pathway.[56,57] In callosal agenesis, DT-FT shows the Probst bundle and related fiber connections to the gyri (**Fig. 18**).[58]

DT-FT represents a noninvasive technique for assessing tumor tissue characteristics in the preoperative surgical planning for tumor biopsy or debulking procedures for pediatric brain tumors and gives information about white matter integrity of structures contiguous to the lesions before and after surgery (**Fig. 19**).[59–61] Preoperative tractography of the corticospinal tract involvement has been correlated with motor deficits. Normalization of postoperative tractography is predictive of improvement of function.

Diffusion Kurtosis Imaging

DTI is a method using gaussian distribution of water molecules in the white matter. Gaussian distribution is only applicable to free diffusion in sufficiently large and uniform regions of fluid (**Fig. 20**).[62] However, neuronal tissues are highly heterogeneous microstructures. Diffusion kurtosis is a method to analyze the nongaussian distribution of water molecules within tissues.[9,63] DKI can provide useful information on tissue microstructure in ischemia, brain tumor, epilepsy, traumatic brain injury, demyelinating disease, white matter development, and cortical microstructural maturation.[64–78] DKI has been applied to the pediatric spinal cord in 1 study.[79]

Increased diffusion kurtosis means the distribution has a larger deviation from gaussian and is more sharply peaked, which is closely associated with diffusional heterogeneity (see **Fig. 20**).[9,62,80,81] DKI is less susceptible to free fluid contamination compared with the MD or FA by DTI.[82] The parameters in DKI include radial kurtosis (Krad), axial kurtosis (Kax), and mean kurtosis (MK). DKI parameters correlated well with age, and kurtosis parameters showed a potential advantage in detecting the normal brain development of children.[64–67] Largely increased Kax and mildly increased Krad in acute infarction could be caused by a large change in the intra-axonal diffusivity, which can be related to axonal varicosities or alterations in the endoplasmic reticulum.[68] DKI parameters show significant differences in high-grade and low-grade gliomas with better separation than conventional diffusion

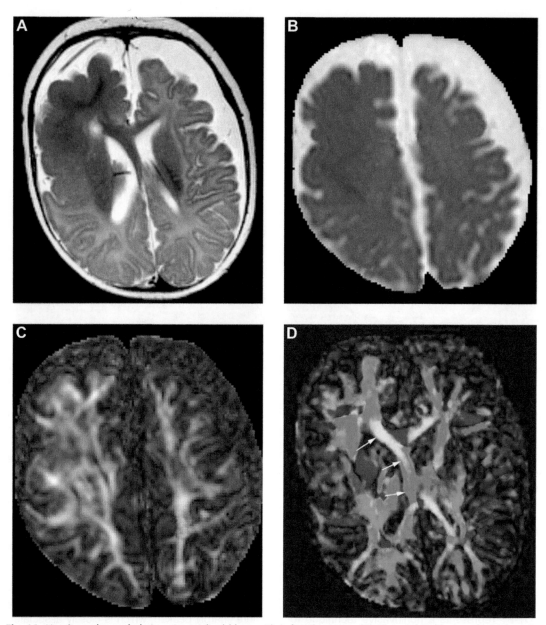

Fig. 14. Hemimegalencephaly in a 4-month-old boy with infantile spasm. (*A*) T2-weighted image shows hypointense areas in the right frontal cortex and white matter, which probably represents abnormally advanced myelination associated with hemimegalencephaly. (*B, C*) DTI shows increased FA and slightly decreased ADC suggesting accentuated myelination in the right hemisphere. (*D*) DTI color map shows an aberrant midsagittal fiber tract passing anteroposteriorly between the 2 anterior horns of the lateral ventricles (*arrows*). (*Courtesy of* Noriko Salamon, MD, PhD [From³].)

parameters.⁷²,⁷³ DKI provides more detailed information of tissue microstructures such as changes in myelination than DTI. Krad and MK have stronger correlations with myelin content compared with diffusion tensor metrics.⁸³ Decreased Krad without change of Kax may indicate that the pathologic change in the demyelinating lesion is mainly caused

by the breakdown of myelin structure (see **Fig. 16**). In Pelizaeus-Merzbacher disease, higher Krad is observed in the bilateral pyramidal tracts and corpus callosum compared with Kax and MK, which may indicate that the myelinic structure is present in the pyramidal tract and the corpus callosum (**Fig. 21**). The metrics of DKI are not specific to axon density

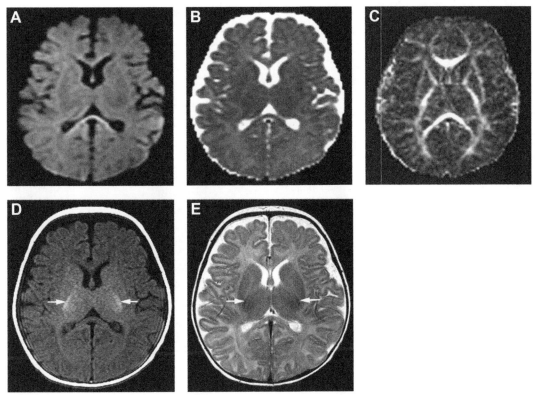

Fig. 15. Normal MR image in a 2-month-old girl. (*A, B*) DWI shows grossly homogeneous signal intensity in the brain. The ADC values in the gray matter and corpus callosum appear slightly lower than in the other white matter. (*C*) FA map shows anisotropy noted not only in the corpus callosum and internal capsules but also the entire white matter, including U fibers (premyelination state). (*D, E*) T1-weighted and T2-weighted images show myelination mainly in the posterior limb of the internal capsules (*arrows*).

and diameters; therefore, the change in the metrics in diseases is sometimes difficult to explain.

Neurite Orientation Dispersion and Density Imaging

NODDI is used as a microstructural DWI model, composed of 3 compartments: (1) restricted intracellular compartment (neurite density index [NDI]), (2) hindered extracellular compartment, and (3) CSF with free diffusion.[84] NDI is attributed to the density of neurites, which are composed of axon and dendrites. NDI has a stronger relationship with age and is more sensitive to microstructural changes in late childhood and adolescence than DTI.[10,85,86] NODDI provides directional information on neurites as an orientation dispersion index (ODI). NODDI is more robust for estimating the volume of axons than DTI. Neurite density images (intracellular volume fraction [Ficv]) can visualize hypomyelination better than FA images (see **Fig. 21**). In tuberous sclerosis, neurite density image (Ficv) from NODDI reflects microstructural

abnormality such as hypomyelination, gliosis, or heterotopic cells in white matter in tuberous sclerosis complex more sensitively compared with FA map by conventional DTI method (**Fig. 22**).

By combining DWI on modeling and myelin imaging, g ratio and axon volume fraction can be estimated.[87] G ratio is the ratio of the inner to the outer diameter of myelinated axon, which is associated with speed of conduction. Larger axons and thicker myelin sheaths give rise to faster conduction of electrochemical information.[88] Changes in the g ratio with age and development in infants have been shown in the literature.[89,90] G ratio can differentiate between demyelination and axonal degeneration. Normal-appearing white matter in patients with multiple sclerosis (MS) had diffusely lower NDI than healthy controls.[91] In patients with idiopathic normal-pressure hydrocephalus, ODI can capture the reversible straightening of nerve fibers in the corticospinal tract, whereas decreased NDI suggests irreversible microstructural damage.[92,93] NODDI has also

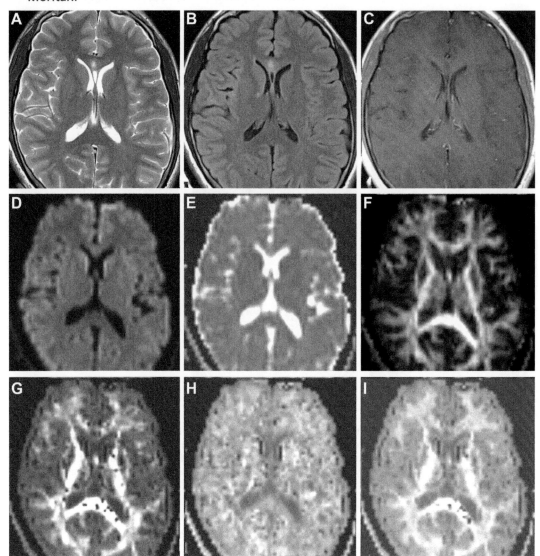

Fig. 16. Multiple sclerosis in a 15-year-old boy. T2-weighted (*A*) and T1-weighted image (*B*) shows a lesion in the genu of the corpus callosum. Postcontrast T1-weighted image (*C*) does not show any enhancement of the lesion. DWI (*D*) shows slightly high signal intensity; however, the ADC image (*E*) shows equal value to the surrounding tissue, indicating T2 shine-through. The FA image (*F*) shows reduced FA in the lesion. The radial kurtosis image (*G*) shows obvious low values in the lesion; however, the axial kurtosis image (*H*) shows little difference, and the mean kurtosis image (*I*) seems to indicate intermediate values. These findings may indicate that the pathologic change in the lesion is mainly caused by the breakdown of myelin structure. (*From* Panesar SS, Abhinav K, Yeh FC, et al. Tractography for surgical neuro-oncology planning: towards a gold standard. Neurotherapeutics 2019;16(1):36-51.)

been applied to the spinal cord.[94–98] NODDI is superior to DTI in terms of fitting and reproducibility.

Diffusion Spectrum Imaging

To acquire probability distributions for complicated wall structures in the neuronal tissue, dedicated model-free methods such as diffusion spectrum imaging (DSI) have been introduced.

DSI has high demand on scanner hardware and a long acquisition time.[99,100] One method of DSI is q-space (multishell) imaging (see **Fig. 19**).[11,62] QSI is performed by acquiring a large number of diffusion encodings, and can provide a probability density function of water molecules. The q value represents the strength of the multiaxis motion probing gradients (MPGs), such as a b value, and the definition is as follows: $q = \gamma/2\pi \; G\delta$, where γ is gyromagnetic ratio, G is strength of

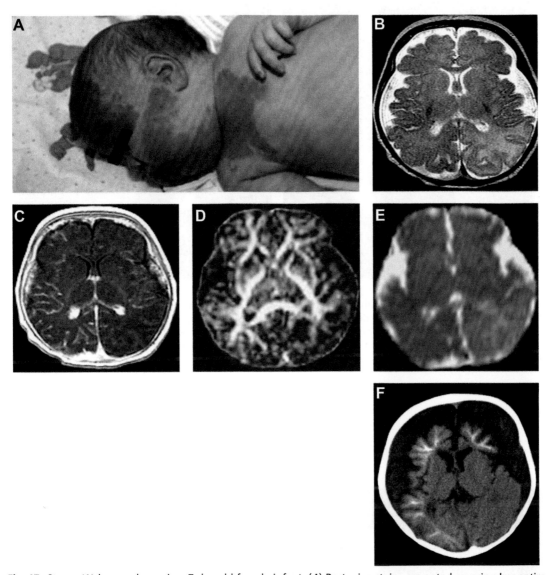

Fig. 17. Sturge-Weber syndrome in a 7-day-old female infant. (*A*) Port wine stains are noted covering her entire head and extending onto her back and shoulders. (*B*) T2-weighted image shows hypointensity in the white matter of the entire right hemisphere and left frontotemporoparietal areas, compared with the left parieto-occipital white matter. (*C*) Postcontrast T1-weighted image shows extensive leptomeningeal enhancement in the right hemisphere and left frontotemporoparietal areas consistent with leptomeningeal angiomatosis. (*D*) FA shows homogeneously increased anisotropy in the right cerebral hemisphere and left frontotemporoparietal areas, compared with the left parieto-occipital white matter, likely representing abnormal hypermyelination. (*E*) The ADC map shows decreased ADC in the white matter in the entire right hemisphere and left frontotemporoparietal areas, compared with the left parieto-occipital white matter. (*F*) A 6-month follow-up noncontrast computed tomography scan shows diffuse cortical and subcortical calcifications and atrophy in the right hemisphere and left frontal lobe with sparing of the left temporo-occipital and parietal regions. (*From*[3]).

the MPG, and δ is duration of the MPG. QSI enables investigation of tissue microstructure in more detail. For example, QSI with low q-value shows increased mean axon diameter and decreased intra-axonal space volume fraction in splenium and genu of the corpus callosum compared with those in the body of the corpus callosum.[101] This finding may explain why a reversible diffusion restriction tends to occur in the splenium of the corpus callosum. Although QSI is theoretically superior to conventional gaussian distribution analysis, the main limitation is a long acquisition time caused by the large number of sampling processes.

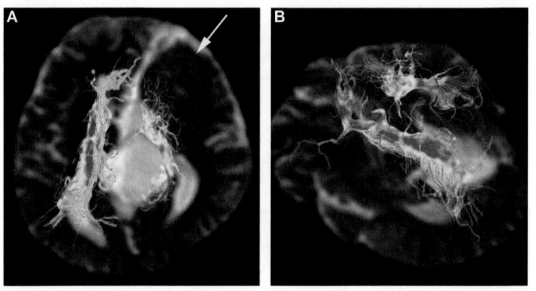

Fig. 18. Complete callosal agenesis and cortical dysplasia in the left frontal lobe in a 34-year-old man. (*A*) DTI FT (2-region-of-interest method) shows that although the Probst bundle in the right hemisphere is well developed, that in the left hemisphere is poorly developed. Cortical dysplasia is shown in the left frontal lobe (*arrow*). The fibers from the right prefrontal area run along the innermost side of the Probst bundle (*blue lines*). (*B*) The fibers from the right orbital gyrus run along the outermost side in Probst bundle (*green lines*). (*Courtesy of* Hidetsuna Utsunomiya, MD, PhD [From[3,58]].)

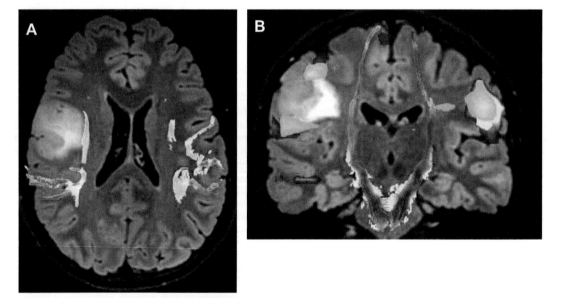

Fig. 19. Glioblastoma with H3 G34 R isocitrate dehydrogenase wild-type in a 16-year-old girl who presented with episodes of left facial twitching. (*A*) Fiber tracking overlying axial FLAIR image and (*B*) fiber tracking overlying coronal FLAIR image with motor tasks including left finger tapping and lip smacking show bilateral corticospinal tracts are unremarkable reaching up to activated primary motor cortex. The right corticospinal tract and associated projection fibers are separated from the FLAIR hyperintense mass lesion.

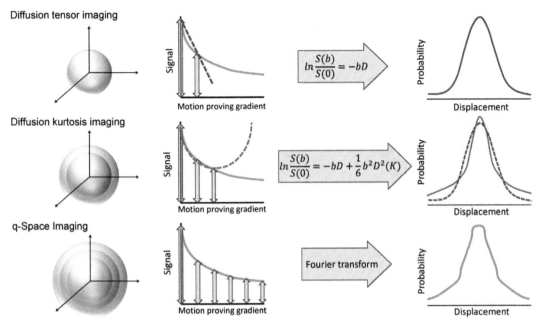

Fig. 20. DTI, DKI, and q-space (multishell) diffusion imaging. DTI can be obtained by a set of multiaxis motion probing gradients (MPGs). Because DTI is based on the assumption that water diffusion obeys a gaussian distribution, only a single set of b values is required: $ln\frac{S(b)}{S(0)} = -bD$, where S is signal intensity, b is b value, and D is diffusivity. To acquire DKI, the following approximation can estimate both the diffusivity and kurtosis when the b values of the MPGs are sufficiently small. Kurtosis is a dimensionless statistical metric for quantifying the non-gaussianity of an arbitrary probability distribution. $ln\frac{S(b)}{S(0)} = -bD + \frac{1}{6}b^2D^2(K)$, where K is kurtosis. Large kurtosis means a high peak and a fat tail in the probability distribution. QSI is a method to measure the probability distribution of a detailed water molecule. The main principle in q-space analysis is that a Fourier transformation of the signal intensity with respect to the MPGs provides a probability density function. QSI is performed by the measurement of a large amount of diffusion encoding. (*Courtesy of* Toshiaki Taoka, MD, PhD [From[62]].)

Intravoxel Incoherent Motion

Intravoxel incoherent motion (IVIM) was first proposed by Le Bihan and colleagues[2,12] in 1986. IVIM refers to the microscopic incoherent motion of water molecules within the voxel, which includes true diffusion and pseudodiffusion (capillary perfusion) (**Fig. 23**).[102] IVIM can evaluate diffusion and capillary perfusion simultaneously without contrast administration, by applying a biexponential model to DWI with multiple b values. In the IVIM model, signal intensity is described using a biexponential equation (**Fig. 24**)[102]:

$$Sb/S0 = f \cdot exp\ (-bD^*) + (1-f) \cdot exp(-bD)$$

where $S0$ and Sb are signal intensities with b values of 0 and b; f is volume fraction of perfusion component, proportional to cerebral blood volume; D^* is pseudodiffusion coefficient, inversely proportional to mean transit time; D is true diffusion coefficient; and $f \times D^*$ is proportional to cerebral blood flow.

The true diffusion coefficient, D, can provide a more accurate measure of tissue microstructure than conventional ADC by eliminating contaminating effects of perfusion. The use of multiple b values needs more imaging acquisition time. This additional time is a particular concern when scanning pediatric patients. Diffusion and perfusion MR imaging have been used for pediatric brain tumors in order to characterize the cellularity and vascularity. In IVIM, the true diffusion coefficient (D) represents tumor cell density and the volume fraction of perfusion component (f) represents tumor vascularity. Increased perfusion fraction (f) and decreased true diffusion coefficient (D) have been reported in high-grade gliomas compared with low-grade gliomas[103-105] (**Figs. 25 and 26**). D* is generally a less reproducible index than D or f.[106] IVIM can be useful in differentiating tumor progression and treatment effect, reflecting the tumor microenvironment.[107] True diffusion coefficient (D) and perfusion fraction (f) have been significantly decreased in the acute infarction.[108,109] Decreased perfusion fraction (f) and f·D* were predictive for the development of delayed cerebral ischemia caused by vasospasm in patients with ruptured cerebral aneurysm.[110]

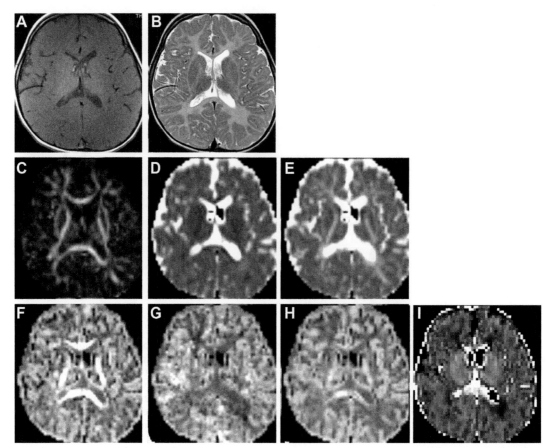

Fig. 21. Pelizaeus-Merzbacher disease in a 2-year-old boy with spastic paralysis and vertical nystagmus. T1-weighted (A) and T2-weighted (B) images show hypomyelination in the white matter, including the pyramidal tracts. FA image (C) has high values throughout the white matter, which may be caused by the axonal structure of the white matter. The radial diffusivity (D) and axial diffusivity (E) images indicate that the diffusivity in the white matter is greater in the direction of the fiber bundles. On the radial kurtosis image (F), higher kurtosis can be observed in the bilateral pyramidal tracts and in the corpus callosum, which are not obvious on the axial (G) and mean (H) kurtosis images. This combination of results on the kurtosis images may indicate that the myelinic structure is present in the pyramidal tract and the corpus callosum. Neurite density image (intracellular volume fraction [Ficv]) (I) can visualize hypomyelination better than FA image. (*Courtesy of* Toshiaki Taoka, MD, PhD.)

Estimated f and D* is influenced by the settings of echo time and the presence of CSF.[111,112] Controlling the effects by gating can improve the reproducibility of IVIM measurement.[113]

Oscillating-Gradient Spin-Echo Diffusion-Weighted Imaging

OGSE DWI enables acquisitions with shorter diffusion times (<10 milliseconds), whereas conventional pulsed-gradient spin-echo (PGSE) DWI with longer diffusion times (35–67 milliseconds).[84] Interference with water molecule movement is caused by in 2 main barriers: membranous structures and macromolecules (see **Fig. 1**). Although the membranous structures obstruct water

molecule movement, the water molecules move faster between the membranous structures. In contrast, the water molecule movement in viscous fluid is continuously slower because of the presence of macromolecules. Spatial barriers of membranous structures (fibers or cell membranes) in the tissue lead to nongaussian diffusion in which, if diffusion time of DWI decreases, the ADC increases.[114] The number of studies using OGSE DWI has been increasing recently.[13,19,20,115–123] Most of the reported OGSE applications focus on brain imaging. It is essential for radiologists to know how the diffusion time affects DWI.

DWI reveals acute cerebral infarction as less signal using OSGE.[13,19,20,115] The reduction of ADC in white matter in stroke is likely caused by

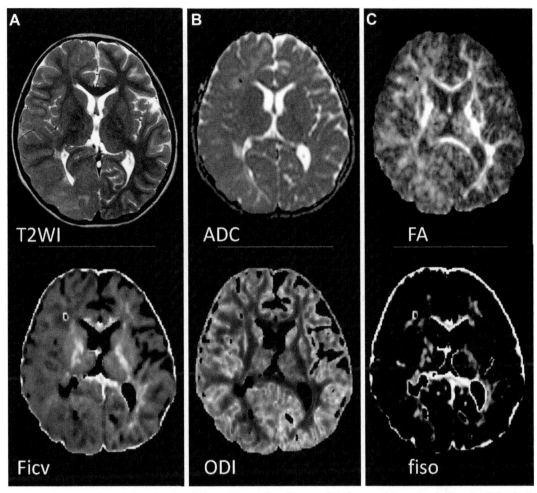

Fig. 22. Tuberous sclerosis in a 6-year-old boy. T2-weighted image (*A*) shows white matter abnormalities in the right frontal and temporo-occipital regions as mildly hyperintense. ADC map (*B*) shows mildly increased ADC. FA map (*C*) shows low values in the white matter abnormalities. Neurite density image (Ficv) from NODDI reflects microstructural abnormality such as hypomyelination, gliosis, or heterotopic cells in white matter in tuberous sclerosis complex more sensitively compared with FA map by conventional DTI method. Fiso, isotropic fraction; T2WI, T2-weighted image. (*Courtesy of* Toshiaki Taoka, MD, PhD and Noriko Aida, MD, PhD.)

neurite beading and axonal swelling (**Fig. 27**).[19] Similar findings have been reported in neonates with hypoxic-ischemic encephalopathy[118] and reversible corpus callosum lesions[119] (**Fig. 28**).

Epidermoid cyst (**Fig. 29**) and choroid plexus cyst show higher ADC values with shorter diffusion times on OGSE DWI than those with longer diffusion times on PGSE DWI, which is likely related to histologically dense membranous structures in the lesions.[120] High DWI signal of epidermoid is not only caused by T2 shine-through effect but is also related to diffusion time on DWI.

OGSE DWI has been reported in the differential diagnosis between malignant and benign tumors in the brain and head and neck.[121,122] High-grade tumors show significant difference in ADC values between OGSE (short diffusion time) and PGSE (long diffusion time) compared to low-grade tumors (**Fig. 30**), which is probably related to the cellular density, cell size, membranous integrity, and tumor microstructure. OGSE DWI potentially can provide quantitative evaluation of treatment response and differential diagnosis of tumors.[123] Technical advances of MR scanners with higher maximum gradients enable more reduction of diffusion time, which will help in understanding the microstructures of tissues in the future.

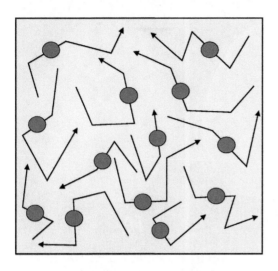 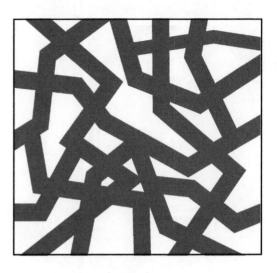

True molecular diffusion   **Capillary perfusion**

Fig. 23. IVIM refers to microscopic incoherent motion of water molecules within each imaging voxel that affects signal intensity on diffusion-weighted images. IVIM includes both true molecular diffusion caused by random brownian motion and pseudodiffusion caused by capillary perfusion. (*Courtesy of* Takashi Yoshiura, MD, PhD [From[102]].)

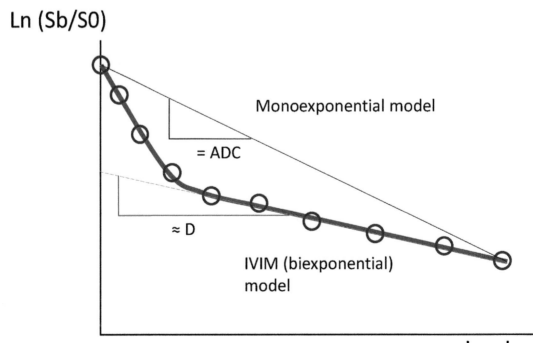

Fig. 24. Monoexponential and biexponential models of DWI. With the conventional monoexponential diffusion model, the ADC is calculated from signal intensities at 2 b values. In IVIM imaging, signal intensities at multiple b values are fitted to a biexponential function including both perfusion and true diffusion components. A steeper slope at low b values reflects the contribution of perfusion (D*) in addition to the true diffusion (D). At higher b values, the contribution of perfusion components becomes negligible. Slope over high b values thus closely approximates the true diffusion coefficient D. (*Courtesy of* Takashi Yoshiura, MD, PhD [From[102]].)

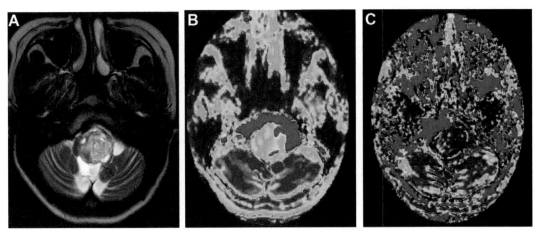

Fig. 25. Pilocytic astrocytoma in a 15-year-old girl. T2-weighted image (*A*) shows a heterogeneous hyperintensity mass in the medulla oblongata. True diffusion coefficient D map (*B*) shows increased value in the tumor. Perfusion fraction f map (*C*) shows decreased value in the tumor. (*Courtesy of* Kiyohisa Kamimura, MD, PhD and Takashi Yoshiura, MD, PhD.)

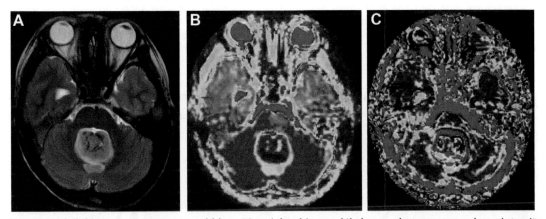

Fig. 26. Medulloblastoma in an 11-year-old boy. T2-weighted image (*A*) shows a heterogeneous hyperintensity mass in the fourth ventricle. True diffusion coefficient D map (*B*) shows decreased value in the tumor. Perfusion fraction f map (*C*) shows increased value in the tumor. (*Courtesy of* Kiyohisa Kamimura, MD, PhD and Takashi Yoshiura, MD, PhD.)

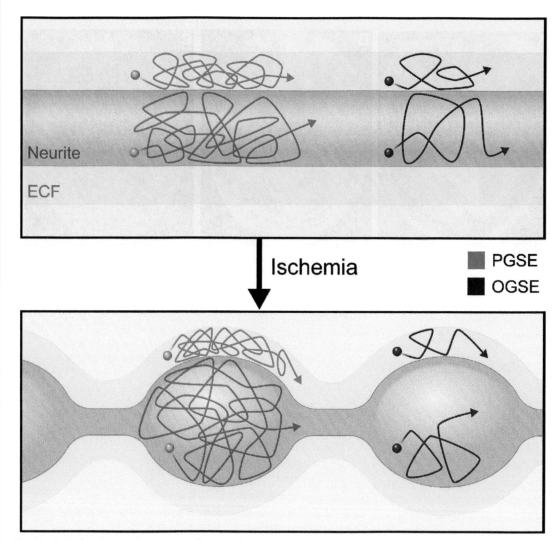

Fig. 27. On ischemia, neurites may swell nonuniformly (ie, beading). These constrictions of the neuron membrane inhibit the ability of water to diffuse along the axon (in both neurite and extracellular fluid). Therefore, beading is a plausible mechanism for the marked decrease of the mean ADC of water within a lesion after stroke observed using traditional PGSE DWI. The PGSE (*blue*) technique measures mean ADC after a long diffusion time, where the molecules have enough time to interact with all the barriers in the vicinity. The shorter diffusion time of OGSE (*orange*) lessens interactions with boundaries, thereby reducing the effect of beading on the diffusion measurement. ECF, extracellular fluid. (*Courtesy of* Corey Allan Baron, PhD [From[21]].)

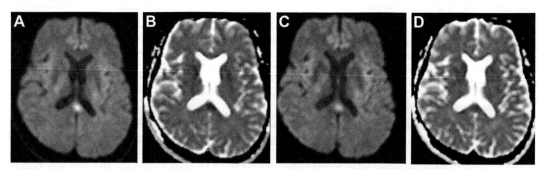

Fig. 28. Reversible splenial lesion. DWI (*A, C*) and ADC maps (*B, D*) for PGSE (*left*) and OGSE (*right*). The lesion showed reduced diffusivity on both PGSE (longer diffusion time) and OGSE (shorter diffusion time). The reduction was weaker in OGSE. (*Courtesy of* Tomoko Maekawa, MD, PhD [From[119]].)

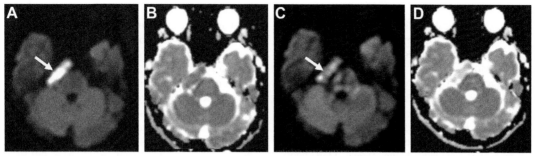

Fig. 29. Epidermoid cyst. DWIs (*A*, *C*) and ADC maps (*B*, *D*) for PGSE (*left*) and OGSE (*right*). PGSE DWI (longer diffusion time) (*A*) and the ADC maps (*B*) show higher signal intensity (*arrow*) with lower ADC values than those in OGSE DWI (shorter diffusion time) (*C*) (*arrow*) and the ADC map (*D*) in the epidermoid cyst located in the right cerebellopontine angle and prepontine cistern. (*Courtesy of* Christina Andica MD, PhD [From[120]].)

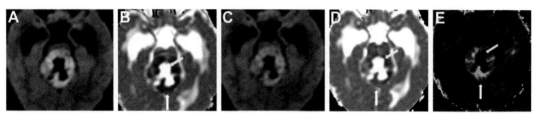

Fig. 30. Atypical teratoid/rhabdoid tumor in a 2-year-old boy. DWI (*A*, *B*) and the ADC map (*C*, *D*) with PGSE (long diffusion time, Δeff of 35.2 milliseconds) and OGSE (short diffusion time, Δeff of 6.5 milliseconds). The ADC values in the tumor appear higher at short diffusion time than at long diffusion time (*white arrows*). The fluid in the tumor has a similar high ADC value at both a Δeff of 6.5 milliseconds and a Δeff of 3.5 milliseconds (*yellow arrows*). (*E*) The ADC color subtraction map provides excellent delineation of the tumor (*white arrows*) and decreased visualization of fluid (*yellow arrows*). (*Courtesy of* Tomoko Maekawa, MD, PhD [From[121]].)

SUMMARY

The major highlights of this article are the application and significance of new and advanced diffusion imaging sequences. MS EPI, non-EPI DWI, and DTI/FT have already been established as clinically useful sequences in pediatric brain and spine. Advanced diffusion imaging, such as DKI, NODDI, DSI, IVIM, and, OGSE, provide quantitative parameter measurements with more specific information about underlying pathophysiology such as tissue microstructure and microcirculation. The main limitations of advanced diffusion imaging are clinical usefulness compared with other modalities, feasibility, longer acquisition time, repeatability, reliability (because of variations in vendors, sites, or software), and lack of normal brain reference data. Wider dissemination of guidelines and better availability of support systems will help promote advanced diffusion imaging sequences in the future.

CLINICS CARE POINTS

- MS EPI DWI, non-EPI DWI, and DTI/FT have already been established as clinically useful sequences in pediatric brain and spine.

- Pitfalls of advanced diffusion imaging are feasibility, repeatability, reliability, longer acquisition time, and lack of normal brain reference data.

REFERENCES

1. Stejskal EO, Tanner JE. Spin diffusion measurements: spin echoes in the presence of a time-dependent field gradient. J Chem Phys 1965;42:288–92.
2. Le Bihan D, Breton E, Lallemand D, et al. MR imaging of intravoxel incoherent motions: application to diffusion and perfusion in neurologic disorders. Radiology 1986;161(2):401–7.
3. Moritani T, Capizzano AA, editors. Diffusion weighted MR imaging of the brain, head and neck, and spine. 3rd edition. Switzerland: Springer Nature AG; 2021.
4. Basser PJ, Mattiello J, Le Bihan D. Estimation of the effective self-diffusion tensor from the NMR spin echo. J Magn Reson 1994;B103:247–54.
5. Mori S, Crain BJ, Chacko VP, et al. Three-dimensional tracking of axonal projections in the brain by magnetic resonance imaging. Ann Neurol 1999;45:265–9.
6. Basser PJ, Pajevic S, Pierpaoli C, et al. In vivo fiber tractography using DT-MRI data. Magn Reson Med 2000;44:625–32.

7. Kose K. Physical and technical aspects of human magnetic resonance imaging: present status and 50 years historical review. Adv Phys X 2021;6(1): 1885310.

8. Utsunomiya H. Diffusion MRI abnormalities in pediatric neurological disorders. Brain Dev 2011;33(3):235–42.

9. Jensen JH, Helpern JA, Ramani A, et al. Diffusional kurtosis imaging: the quantification of non-gaussian water diffusion by means of magnetic resonance imaging. Magn Reson Med 2005; 53(6):1432–40.

10. Zhang H, Schneider T, Wheeler-Kingshott CA, et al. NODDI: practical in vivo neurite orientation dispersion and density imaging of the human brain. Neuroimage 2012;61(4):1000–16.

11. King MD, Houseman J, Roussel SA, et al. q-Space imaging of the brain. Magn Reson Med 1994;32(6): 707–13.

12. Le Bihan D, Lima M, Federau C, et al. Intravoxel Incoherent Motion (IVIM) MRI. Principles and applications. Singapore: Pan Stanford Publishing Pte Ltd; 2019.

13. Schachter M, Does MD, Anderson AW, et al. Measurements of restricted diffusion using an oscillating gradient spin-echo sequence. J Magn Reson 2000;147(2):232–7.

14. Le Bihan D. Diffusion MRI: what water tells us about the brain. EMBO Mol Med 2014;6(5):569–73.

15. Moritani T, Smoker WR, Sato Y, et al. Diffusion-weighted imaging of acute excitotoxic brain injury. AJNR Am J Neuroradiol 2005;26(2):216–28.

16. Moritani T. Brain edema. In: Moritani T, Capizzano AA, editors. Diffusion weighted MR imaging of the brain, head and neck, and spine. 3rd edition. Switzerland: Springer Nature AG; 2021. p. 113–54.

17. Hirano A. The role of electron microscopy in neuropathology. Acta Neuropathol 2005;109(1):115–23.

18. Goodman JA, Ackerman JJ, Neil JJ. Cs + ADC in rat brain decreases markedly at death. Magn Reson Med 2008;59(1):65–72.

19. Duong TQ, Ackerman JJ, Ying HS, et al. Evaluation of extra- and intracellular apparent diffusion in normal and globally ischemic rat brain via 19F NMR. Magn Reson Med 1998;40(1):1–13.

20. Mussel M, Inzelberg L, Nevo U. Insignificance of active flow for neural diffusion weighted imaging: A negative result. Magn Reson Med 2017;78(2): 746–53.

21. Baron CA, Kate M, Gioia L, et al. Reduction of diffusion-weighted imaging contrast of acute ischemic stroke at short diffusion times. Stroke 2015;46(8):2136–41.

22. Budde MD, Frank JA. Neurite beading is sufficient to decrease the apparent diffusion coefficient after ischemic stroke. Proc Natl Acad Sci U S A 2010; 107(32):14472–7.

23. Landman BA, Farrell JA, Smith SA, et al. Complex geometric models of diffusion and relaxation in healthy and damaged white matter. NMR Biomed 2010;23(2):152–62.

24. Portnoy S, et al. Oscillating and pulsed gradient diffusion magnetic resonance microscopy over an extended b-value range: implications for the characterization of tissue microstructure. Magn Reson Med 2013;69(4):1131–45.

25. Tang-Schomer MD, Johnson VE, Baas PW, et al. Partial interruption of axonal transport due to microtubule breakage accounts for the formation of periodic varicosities after traumatic axonal injury. Exp Neurol 2012;233(1):364–72.

26. Rosenblum WI. Cytotoxic edema: monitoring its magnitude and contribution to brain swelling. J Neuropathol Exp Neurol 2007;66(9):771–8.

27. Horton M, Rafay M, Del Bigio MR. Pathological evidence of vacuolar myelinopathy in a child following vigabatrin administration. J Child Neurol 2009;24(12):1543–6.

28. de Oliveira AM, Paulino MV, Vieira APF, et al. Imaging patterns of toxic and metabolic brain disorders. Radiographics 2019;39(6):1672–95.

29. Starkey J, Kobayashi N, Numaguchi Y, et al. Cytotoxic lesions of the corpus callosum that show restricted diffusion: mechanisms, causes, and manifestations. Radiographics 2017;37(2):562–76.

30. van der Toorn A, Syková E, Dijkhuizen RM, et al. Dynamic changes in water ADC, energy metabolism, extracellular space volume, and tortuosity in neonatal rat brain during global ischemia. Magn Reson Med 1996;36(1):52–60.

31. Einstein A. A new determination of molecular dimensions. In: Furth R, editor. Investigations on the theory of the Brownian movement. New York: Dover Publications, INC; 1956. p. 37–62.

32. Johnston MV. Excitotoxicity in perinatal brain injury. Brain Pathol 2005;15(3):234–40.

33. Domi T, deVeber G, Shroff M, et al. Corticospinal tract pre-wallerian degeneration: a novel outcome predictor for pediatric stroke on acute MRI. Stroke 2009;40(3):780–7.

34. Bekiesinska-Figatowska M, Duczkowska A, Szkudlinska-Pawlak S, et al. Diffusion restriction in the corticospinal tracts and the corpus callosum in neonates after cerebral insult. Brain Dev 2017;39(3): 203–10.

35. Saggu SK, Chotaliya HP, Blumbergs PC, et al. Wallerian-like axonal degeneration in the optic nerve after excitotoxic retinal insult: an ultrastructural study. BMC Neurosci 2010;11:97.

36. Schönfeld MH, Ritzel RM, Kemmling A, et al. Improved detectability of acute and subacute brainstem infarctions by combining standard axial and thin-sliced sagittal DWI. PLoS One 2018; 13(7):e0200092.

37. Treit S, Steve T, Gross DW, et al. High resolution in-vivo diffusion imaging of the human hippocampus. Neuroimage 2018;182:479–87.

38. Alizadeh M, Poplawski MM, Fisher J, et al. Zonally magnified oblique multislice and non-zonally magnified oblique multislice DWI of the cervical spinal cord. AJNR Am J Neuroradiol 2018;39(8):1555–61.

39. Riffel P, Michaely HJ, Morelli JN, et al. Zoomed EPI-DWI of the head and neck with two-dimensional, spatially-selective radiofrequency excitation pulses. Eur Radiol 2014;24(10):2507–12.

40. Andre JB, Bammer R. Advanced diffusion-weighted magnetic resonance imaging techniques of the human spinal cord. Top Magn Reson Imaging 2010;21(6):367–78.

41. Venkataraman A, Zhong J. Basics of diffusion measurements by MRI. In Moritani T, Capizzano AA, editors. Diffusion weighted MR imaging of the brain, head and neck, and spine, 3rd edition. Switzerland: Springer Nature AG; 2021. p. 3-10.

42. Wimberger DM, Roberts TP, Barkobich AJ, et al. Identification of "premyelination" by diffusion-weighted MRI. JCAT 1995;19:28–33.

43. Neil JJ, Shiran SI, McKinstry RC, et al. Normal brain in human newborns: apparent diffusion coefficient and diffusion anisotropy measured by using diffusion tensor MR imaging. Radiology 1998;209:57–66.

44. Hermoye L, Saint-Martin C, Cosnard G, et al. Pediatric diffusion tensor imaging: normal database and observation of the white matter maturation in early childhood. Neuroimage 2006;29:493–504.

45. Arzoumanian Y, Mirmiran M, Barnes PD, et al. Diffusion tensor brain imaging findings at term-equivalent age may predict neurologic abnormalities in low birth weight preterm infants. AJNR Am J Neuroradiol 2003;24:1646–53.

46. Provenzale JM, Liang L, DeLong D, et al. Diffusion tensor imaging assessment of brain white matter maturation during the first postnatal year. AJR Am J Roentgenol 2007;189:476–86.

47. Singhi S, Tekes A, Thurnher M, et al. Diffusion tensor imaging of the maturing paediatric cervical spinal cord: from the neonate to the young adult. J Neuroradiol 2012;39(3):142–8.

48. Moritani T, Kim J, Sato Y, et al. Abnormal hyper-myelination in a neonate with Sturge-Weber syndrome demonstrated on diffusion-tensor imaging. J Magn Reson Imaging 2008;27:617–20.

49. Evans AC, Brain Development Cooperative Group. The NIH MRI study of normal brain development. Neuroimage 2006;30:184–202.

50. Prayer D, Barkovich AJ, Kirschner DA, et al. Visualization of nonstructural changes in early white matter development on diffusion-weighted MR images: evidence supporting premyelination anisotropy. AJNR Am J Neuroradiol 2001;22:1572–6.

51. Spalice A, Nicita F, Papetti L, et al. Usefulness of diffusion tensor imaging and fiber tractography in neurological and neurosurgical pediatric diseases. Childs Nerv Syst 2010;26(8):995–1002.

52. Rollins NK. Clinical applications of diffusion tensor imaging and tractography in children. Pediatr Radiol 2007;37(8):769–80.

53. Arrigoni F, Peruzzo D, Mandelstam S, et al. Characterizing white matter tract organization in polymicrogyria and lissencephaly: a multifiber diffusion MRI modeling and tractography study. AJNR Am J Neuroradiol 2020;41(8):1495–502.

54. Arrigoni F, Romaniello R, Peruzzo D, et al. The spectrum of brainstem malformations associated to mutations of the tubulin genes family: MRI and DTI analysis. Eur Radiol 2019;29(2):770–82.

55. Huisman TA, Bosemani T, Poretti A. Diffusion tensor imaging for brain malformations: does it help? Neuroimaging Clin N Am 2014;24(4):619–37.

56. Sato N, Ota M, Yagishita A, et al. Aberrant midsagittal fiber tracts in patients with hemimegalencephaly. AJNR Am J Neuroradiol 2008;29(4):823–7.

57. Enokizono M, Sato N, Ota M, et al. Disrupted cortico-ponto-cerebellar pathway in patients with hemimegalencephaly. Brain Dev 2019;41(6):507–15.

58. Utsunomiya H, Yamashita S, Takano K, et al. Arrangement of fiber tracts forming Probst bundle in complete callosal agenesis: report of two cases with an evaluation by diffusion tensor tractography. Acta Radiol 2006;47(10):1063–6.

59. Cinalli G, Aguirre DT, Mirone G, et al. Surgical treatment of thalamic tumors in children. J Neurosurg Pediatr 2018;21(3):247–57.

60. Lober RM, Guzman R, Cheshier SH, et al. Application of diffusion tensor tractography in pediatric optic pathway glioma. J Neurosurg Pediatr 2012;10(4):273–80.

61. Panesar SS, Abhinav K, Yeh FC, et al. Tractography for surgical neuro-oncology planning: towards a gold standard. Neurotherapeutics 2019;16(1):36–51.

62. Taoka T. Diffusion tensor and kurtosis. In: Moritani T, Capizzano AA, editors. Diffusion weighted MR imaging of the brain, head and neck, and spine. 3rd edition. Switzerland: Springer Nature AG; 2021. p. 43–66.

63. Hori M, Fukunaga I, Masutani Y, et al. Visualizing non-gaussian diffusion: clinical application of q-space imaging and diffusional kurtosis imaging of the brain and spine. Magn Reson Med Sci 2012;11(4):221–33.

64. Shi J, Yang S, Wang J, et al. Detecting normal pediatric brain development with diffusional kurtosis imaging. Eur J Radiol 2019;120:108690.

65. Ouyang M, Jeon T, Sotiras A, et al. Differential cortical microstructural maturation in the preterm human brain with diffusion kurtosis and tensor imaging. Proc Natl Acad Sci U S A 2019;116.

66. Paydar A, Fieremans E, Nwankwo JI, et al. Diffusional kurtosis imaging of the developing brain. AJNR Am J Neuroradiol 2014;35(4):808–14.

67. Grinberg F, Maximov II, Farrher E, et al. Diffusion kurtosis metrics as biomarkers of microstructural development: A comparative study of a group of children and a group of adults. Neuroimage 2017;144(Pt A):12–22.

68. Jensen JH, Falangola MF, Hu C, et al. Preliminary observations of increased diffusional kurtosis in human brain following recent cerebral infarction. NMR Biomed 2011;24(5):452–7.

69. Taoka T, Fujioka M, Sakamoto M, et al. Time course of axial and radial diffusion kurtosis of white matter infarctions: period of pseudonormalization. AJNR Am J Neuroradiol 2014;35(8):1509–14.

70. Taoka T, Fujioka M, Kashiwagi Y, et al. Time course of diffusion kurtosis in cerebral infarctions of transient middle cerebral artery occlusion rat model. J Stroke Cerebrovasc Dis 2016;25(3):610–7.

71. Yin J, Sun H, Wang Z, et al. Diffusion kurtosis imaging of acute infarction: comparison with routine diffusion and follow-up MR imaging. Radiology 2018;287(2):651–7.

72. Raab P, Hattingen E, Franz K, et al. Cerebral gliomas: diffusional kurtosis imaging analysis of microstructural differences. Radiology 2010;254(3):876–81.

73. Van Cauter S, Veraart J, Sijbers J, et al. Gliomas: diffusion kurtosis MR imaging in grading. Radiology 2012;263(2):492–501.

74. Zhang Y, Gao Y, Zhou M, et al. A diffusional kurtosis imaging study of idiopathic generalized epilepsy with unilateral interictal epileptiform discharges in children. J Neuroradiol 2016;43(5):339–45.

75. Sours C, Raghavan P, Medina AE, et al. Structural and functional integrity of the intraparietal sulcus in moderate and severe traumatic brain injury. J Neurotrauma 2017;34(7):1473–81.

76. Davenport EM, Apkarian K, Whitlow CT, et al. Abnormalities in diffusional kurtosis metrics related to head impact exposure in a season of high school varsity football. J Neurotrauma 2016;33(23):2133–46.

77. Spampinato MV, Kocher MR, Jensen JH, et al. Diffusional kurtosis imaging of the corticospinal tract in multiple sclerosis: association with neurologic disability. AJNR Am J Neuroradiol 2017;38(8):1494–500.

78. Yoshida M, Hori M, Yokoyama K, et al. Diffusional kurtosis imaging of normal-appearing white matter in multiple sclerosis: preliminary clinical experience. Jpn J Radiol 2013;31(1):50–5.

79. Conklin CJ, Middleton DM, Alizadeh M, et al. Spatially selective 2D RF inner field of view (iFOV) diffusion kurtosis imaging (DKI) of the pediatric spinal cord. Neuroimage Clin 2016;11:61–7.

80. Hui ES, Cheung MM, Qi L, et al. Towards better MR characterization of neural tissues using directional diffusion kurtosis analysis. Neuroimage 2008;42(1):122–34.

81. Jensen JH, Helpern JA. MRI quantification of non-Gaussian water diffusion by kurtosis analysis. NMR Biomed 2010;23(7):698–710.

82. Hui ES, Cheung MM, Qi L, et al. Advanced MR diffusion characterization of neural tissue using directional diffusion kurtosis analysis. Conf Proc IEEE Eng Med Biol Soc 2008;2008:3941–4.

83. Kelm ND, West KL, Carson RP, et al. Evaluation of diffusion kurtosis imaging in ex vivo hypomyelinated mouse brains. Neuroimage 2016;124(Pt A):612–26.

84. Obata T, Hagiwara A, Kershaw J, et al. Diffusion imaging in the future. In: Moritani T, Capizzano AA, editors. Diffusion weighted MR imaging of the brain, head and Neck, and spine. 3rd edition. Switzerland: Springer Nature AG; 2021. p. 877–89.

85. Genc S, Malpas CB, Holland SK, et al. Neurite density index is sensitive to age related differences in the developing brain. Neuroimage 2017;148:373–80.

86. Mah A, Geeraert B, Lebel C. Detailing neuroanatomical development in late childhood and early adolescence using NODDI. PLoS One 2017;12(8):e0182340.

87. Stikov N, Campbell JS, Stroh T, et al. In vivo histology of the myelin g-ratio with magnetic resonance imaging. Neuroimage 2015;118:397–405.

88. Rushton WA. A theory of the effects of fibre size in medullated nerve. J Physiol 1951;115(1):101–22.

89. Cercignani M, Giulietti G, Dowell NG, et al. Characterizing axonal myelination within the healthy population: a tract-by-tract mapping of effects of age and gender on the fiber g-ratio. Neurobiol Aging 2017;49:109–18.

90. Dean DC 3rd, O'Muircheartaigh J, Dirks H, et al. Mapping an index of the myelin g-ratio in infants using magnetic resonance imaging. Neuroimage 2016;132:225–37.

91. Granberg T, Fan Q, Treaba CA, et al. In vivo characterization of cortical and white matter neuroaxonal pathology in early multiple sclerosis. Brain 2017;140(11):2912–26.

92. Kamiya K, Hori M, Irie R, et al. Diffusion imaging of reversible and irreversible microstructural changes within the corticospinal tract in idiopathic normal pressure hydrocephalus. NeuroImage Clin 2017;14:663–71.

93. Irie R, Tsuruta K, Hori M, et al. Neurite orientation dispersion and density imaging for evaluation of corticospinal tract in idiopathic normal pressure hydrocephalus. Jpn J Radiol 2017;35(1):25–30.

94. Grussu F, Schneider T, Zhang H, et al. Neurite orientation dispersion and density imaging of the

healthy cervical spinal cord in vivo. Neuroimage 2015;111:590–601.

95. Grussu F, Schneider T, Tur C, et al. Neurite dispersion: a new marker of multiple sclerosis spinal cord pathology? Ann Clin Transl Neurol 2017;4(9): 663–79.

96. Schilling KG, By S, Feiler HR, et al. Diffusion MRI microstructural models in the cervical spinal cord - Application, normative values, and correlations with histological analysis. Neuroimage 2019;201:116026.

97. Iwama T, Ohba T, Okita G, et al. Utility and validity of neurite orientation dispersion and density imaging with diffusion tensor imaging to quantify the severity of cervical spondylotic myelopathy and assess postoperative neurological recovery. Spine J 2020;20(3):417–25.

98. Hori M, Hagiwara A, Fukunaga I, et al. Application of quantitative microstructural MR imaging with atlas-based analysis for the spinal cord in cervical spondylotic myelopathy. Sci Rep 2018;8(1):5213.

99. Wedeen VJ, Wang RP, Schmahmann JD, et al. Diffusion spectrum magnetic resonance imaging (DSI) tractography of crossing fibers. Neuroimage 2008;41(4):1267–77.

100. Reese TG, Benner T, Wang R, et al. Halving imaging time of whole brain diffusion spectrum imaging and diffusion tractography using simultaneous image refocusing in EPI. J Magn Reson Imaging 2009;29(3):517–22.

101. Suzuki Y, Hori M, Kamiya K, et al. Estimation of the mean axon diameter and intra-axonal space volume fraction of the human corpus callosum: diffusion q-space imaging with low q-values. Magn Reson Med Sci 2016;15(1):83–93.

102. Yoshiura T. Intravoxel incoherent motion and high b value. In: Moritani T, Capizzano AA, editors. Diffusion weighted MR imaging of the brain, head and Neck, and spine. 3rd edition. Switzerland: Springer Nature AG; 2021. p. 67–76.

103. Bisdas S, Koh TS, Order C, et al. Intravoxel incoherent motion diffusion-weighted MR imaging of gliomas: feasibility of the method and initial results. Neuroradiology 2013;55:1189–96.

104. Federau C, Meuli R, O'Brien K, et al. Perfusion measurement in brain gliomas with intravoxel incoherent motion MRI. AJNR Am J Neuroradiol 2014;35:256–62.

105. Togao O, Hiwatashi A, Yamashita K, et al. Differentiation of high-grade and low-grade diffuse gliomas by intravoxel incoherent motion MR imaging. Neuro-Oncol 2016;18:132–41.

106. Kim HS, Suh CH, Kim N, et al. Histogram analysis of intravoxel incoherent motion for differentiating recurrent tumor from treatment effect in patients with glioblastoma: Initial clinical experience. AJNR Am J Neuroradiol 2014;35:490–7.

107. Wu W-C, Chen Y-F, Tseng H-M, et al. Caveats of measuring perfusion indexes using intravoxel

incoherent motion magnetic resonance imaging in the human brain. Eur Radiol 2015;25:2485–92.

108. Federau C, Sumer S, Becce F, et al. Intravoxel incoherent motion perfusion imaging in acute stroke: initial clinical experience. Neuroradiology 2014; 56:629–35.

109. Suo S, Cao M, Zhu W, et al. Stroke assessment with intravoxel incoherent motion diffusion-weighted MRI. NMR Biomed 2016;29:320–8.

110. Heit J, Wintermark M, Martin BW, et al. Reduced intravoxel incoherent motion microvascular perfusion predicts delayed cerebral ischemia and vasospasm after aneurysm rupture. Stroke 2018;49: 741–5.

111. Federau C, O'Brien K. Increased brain perfusion contrast with T2-prepared intravoxel incoherent motion (T2prep IVIM) MRI. NMR Biomed 2015;28: 9–16.

112. Bisdas S, Klose U. IVIM analysis of brain tumors: an investigation of the relaxation effects of CSF, blood, and tumor tissue on the estimated perfusion fraction. Magn Reason Mater Phys 2015;28: 377–83.

113. Kang KM, Choi SH, Kim DE, et al. Application of cardiac gating to improve the reproducibility of intravoxel incoherent motion measurements in the head and neck. Magn Reson Med Sci 2017;16: 190–202.

114. Callaghan PT. 7.1.2 Diffusive diffraction in an enclosed pore. Translational dynamics and magnetic resonance, principles of pulsed gradient spin echo NMR. Oxford: Oxford University Press; 2011. p. 312–6.

115. Boonrod A, Hagiwara A, Hori M, et al. Reduced visualization of cerebral infarction on diffusion-weighted images with short diffusion times. Neuroradiology 2018;60(9):979–82.

116. Maekawa T, Hori M, Murata K, et al. Changes in the ADC of diffusion-weighted MRI with the oscillating gradient spin-echo (OGSE) sequence due to differences in substrate viscosities. Jpn J Radiol 2018; 36(7):415–20.

117. Maekawa T, Hori M, Murata K, et al. Choroid plexus cysts analyzed using diffusion-weighted imaging with short diffusion-time. Magn Reson Imaging 2019;57:323–7.

118. Gao F, Shen X, Zhang H, et al. Feasibility of oscillating and pulsed gradient diffusion MRI to assess neonatal hypoxia-ischemia on clinical systems. J Cereb Blood Flow Metab 2020. https://doi.org/ 10.1177/0271678X20944353. Epub ahead of print.

119. Maekawa T, Kamiya K, Murata K, et al. Time-dependent Diffusion in Transient Splenial Lesion: Comparison between Oscillating-Gradient Spin-echo Measurements and Monte-Carlo Simulation. Magn Reson Med Sci 2020. https://doi.org/10. 2463/mrms.bc.2020-0046. Epub ahead of print.

120. Andica C, Hori M, Kamiya K, et al. Spatial restriction within intracranial epidermoid cysts observed using short diffusion-time diffusion-weighted imaging. Magn Reson Med Sci 2018;17(3):269–72.

121. Maekawa T, Hori M, Murata K, et al. Differentiation of high-grade and low-grade intra-axial brain tumors by time-dependent diffusion MRI. Magn Reson Imaging 2020;72:34–41.

122. Iima M, Yamamoto A, Kataoka M, et al. Time-dependent diffusion MRI to distinguish malignant from benign head and neck tumors. J Magn Reson Imaging 2019;50(1):88–95.

123. Gore JC, Xu J, Colvin DC, et al. Characterization of tissue structure at varying length scales using temporal diffusion spectroscopy. NMR Biomed 2010; 23(7):745–56.

Noncontrast Pediatric Brain Perfusion
Arterial Spin Labeling and Intravoxel Incoherent Motion

Danny J.J. Wang, PhD[a], Denis Le Bihan, MD, PhD[b], Ram Krishnamurthy, PhD[c], Mark Smith, MS, RT(R) (MR)[c], Mai-Lan Ho, MD[c],*

KEYWORDS

- Arterial spin labeling • ASL • Cerebral blood flow • Cerebral blood volume • Diffusion
- Intravoxel incoherent motion • IVIM • Perfusion

KEY POINTS

- Noncontrast magnetic resonance imaging techniques for measuring brain perfusion include arterial spin labeling and intravoxel incoherent motion.
- Technical understanding is necessary for correctly identifying normal physiologic variants and pitfalls.
- Major clinical applications include tumors, stroke, vasculopathies, vascular malformations, epilepsy, and migraine.

INTRODUCTION

Arterial spin labeling (ASL) and intravoxel incoherent motion (IVIM) are techniques that provide noninvasive and repeatable assessment of cerebral blood flow (CBF) and cerebral blood volume (CBV), which serve as biomarkers of brain tissue physiologic status, metabolism, and neuronal activity. Noncontrast magnetic resonance (MR) imaging perfusion approaches are highly desirable for use in children to minimize unnecessary gadolinium administration and potential deposition. Furthermore, some individuals have relative or absolute contraindications to gadolinium, such as allergy or liver/renal failure predisposing to nephrogenic systemic fibrosis. Effective use and application of these techniques requires a solid understanding of the underlying physical principles, technical parameters, normal physiologic variants, and potential imaging artifacts.[1] This article reviews the physical principles of ASL and IVIM with important pediatric neuroimaging applications, including stroke, tumors, vascular malformations, epilepsy, and migraine.

ARTERIAL SPIN LABELING PRINCIPLES

ASL uses magnetically labeled arterial blood water as an endogenous and freely diffusible tracer. Radiofrequency inversion pulses are used to label mobile protons within arteries just below the skull base. Following a short postlabel delay (PLD), tagged protons flow into the head and undergo capillary exchange within brain parenchyma. The difference in signal before tagging (control image) and after tagging (label image) is proportional to

 a USC Institute for Neuroimaging and Informatics, SHN, 2025 Zonal Avenue, Health Sciences Campus, Los Angeles, CA 90033, USA; b NeuroSpin, Centre d'études de Saclay, Bâtiment 145, Gif-sur-Yvette 91191, France; c Department of Radiology, Nationwide Children's Hospital, 700 Children's Drive – ED4, Columbus, OH 43205, USA
* Corresponding author.
E-mail address: mai-lan.ho@nationwidechildrens.org

Magn Reson Imaging Clin N Am 29 (2021) 493–513
https://doi.org/10.1016/j.mric.2021.06.002
1064-9689/21/© 2021 Elsevier Inc. All rights reserved.

absolute CBF. Signal-to-noise ratio (SNR) is inherently limited by the small arterial blood volume fraction (~1%), which can be addressed by a combination of improved labeling, image acquisition, and scanning at higher magnetic fields for longer blood T1 decay time.[2] ASL techniques are classified into 4 general categories based on the labeling scheme: pulsed, continuous, pseudocontinuous, and velocity-selective ASL. Pseudocontinuous ASL (PCASL) has emerged as the preferred method for clinical imaging, combining the hardware compatibility of pulsed ASL with a longer tagging bolus and higher SNR approaching continuous ASL.[3–5] Three-dimensional acquisitions are preferred rather than two-dimensional acquisitions, because of higher imaging efficiency, SNR, resolution, and repeatability.[6,7] PCASL CBF measurements have been validated against several perfusion techniques with high test-retest reliability across a variety of imaging techniques, scanner environments, and patient ages.[8–12]

The 2015 white paper on ASL, a consensus of the International Society for Magnetic Resonance in Medicine (ISMRM) perfusion study group and the European consortium for ASL in dementia, provides general recommendations for ASL parameters and modeling across the lifespan.[13] In children, brain water content is higher and CBF increases with development, resulting in up to 70% increase in SNR compared with adults.[14–18] Labeling efficiency depends on blood flow velocities, which are also higher in children than in adults.[19] To achieve sufficient labeling efficiency, the flow-driven adiabatic condition needs to be met with higher radiofrequency amplitudes, albeit within the limitations of specific absorption rate, which increases quadratically with B1.[20] For a given patient, optimal PLD selection depends on arterial transit time (ATT), which correlates with patient age, brain region, and disease process. Overly short PLD does not provide adequate time for labeled blood to reach tissues, whereas too long PLD results in excessive signal decay.[21–23] In pathologic conditions that produce slow flow, the use of short PLDs yields a mixed pattern of low and artifactually high signal on ASL. The latter is known as arterial transit artifact, a characteristic feature of ischemia in which labeled signal remains trapped within arteries proximal to or surrounding the ischemic territory.[24–26] In these scenarios, long-delay or multidelay ASL can be used to acquire multiple PLDs for calculation of ATT and ATT-corrected CBF maps.[27–30]

For accurate perfusion quantification, it is important to account for age-dependent variations in blood T1 and hematocrit.[31–34] The single-compartment (blood pool) model[13] is preferred rather than the original 2-compartment perfusion model,[35] which incorrectly assumes that labeled water can freely and instantaneously exchange across the blood-brain barrier (BBB) from the vascular compartment into the tissue compartment once it arrives at capillaries. Recent evidence indicates that the BBB has limited permeability to water molecules, with trans-BBB water exchange occurring through both passive diffusion and active pathways, requiring measurement of the water exchange rate. Diffusion-weighted techniques have been used to differentiate the fraction of labeled water in capillary and brain tissue based on their distinctive pseudodiffusion. The curves can be well fitted by a biexponential diffusion model, in which the fraction of fast-decaying vascular water decreases with longer PLD as labeled water gradually exchanges into brain tissue with restricted diffusion[36–41] (**Fig. 1A**).

INTRAVOXEL INCOHERENT MOTION PRINCIPLES

IVIM MR imaging is an alternative approach to noncontrast perfusion that uses diffusion-weighted imaging (DWI) to model both molecular diffusion and blood microcirculation, physical phenomena with different spatial and temporal scales. Blood flow within the capillary microvascular network can be modeled as a pseudodiffusion process that yields deviations in signal decay at low b values, in addition to the overall tissue diffusion-driven signal decay. Based on known values for mean capillary segment length and blood velocity, the pseudodiffusion coefficient is about 10 times the true diffusion coefficient of water in brain tissue, around 10^{-2} mm^2/s. Because the fraction of flowing blood is small (1%–4% in the normal brain) compared with overall tissue water content, this deviation remains difficult to detect and requires high-SNR techniques. The most comprehensive and accurate approach is to acquire multiple DWI images with a range of b values: low (0–200 s/mm^2) to provide perfusion sensitivity, and high (200 to ideally >2000 s/mm^2) to account for tissue diffusion, including nongaussian diffusion effects. The number of b-value acquisitions determines total scan time, which should be balanced against motion sensitivity and artifacts in children.[42–45] Brain anisotropy adds additional complexity, which can be mitigated by taking the geometric mean of the diffusion-weighted signals acquired over different directions, or by the use of diffusion tensor imaging requiring longer scan times.[46] Physiologic variations in CBF can also affect serial measurements and repeatability.[47,48]

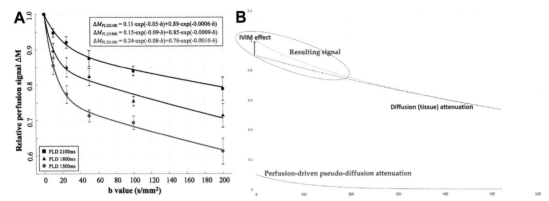

Fig. 1. Perfusion and diffusion interactions. (*A*) ASL perfusion signal at different b values and PLD. Using a biexponential model, the fraction of fast-decaying microvascular component decreases with greater PLD as labeled water gradually exchanges into brain tissue with restricted diffusion. (*B*) IVIM pseudodiffusion effects caused by capillary microcirculation produce measurable attenuation of diffusion-weighted signal at low b values. At high b values, tissue diffusion effects predominate.

IVIM model fitting can be performed in single or multiple stages, and should include correction for noise bias, especially at high b values.[49,50] In the classic biexponential model, water diffusion is assumed to follow a so-called free gaussian pattern, which is a fair approximation at moderately low b values (<600 s/mm^2).[51] However, many studies have revealed that diffusion in tissues is largely nongaussian because of anomalous interactions of water molecules with the local microenvironment.[52–56] Hence, more sophisticated models have been proposed, including polynomial or kurtosis, statistical, triexponential, stretched exponential, multicompartmental, and bayesian algorithms. Parameters that can be calculated after model fitting include vascular volume fraction (f); pseudodiffusion coefficient ascribed to blood random microcirculation (D*); water diffusion coefficient in tissue (D); the apparent diffusion coefficient corrected for perfusion effects (ADCo); and kurtosis parameter describing signal deviation from gaussian diffusion (K). A summative flow-related parameter fD* can be calculated from the product of f and D*, although accurate estimation of D* is often elusive. By identifying the low and high b-value thresholds that maximize sensitivity for tissue distinction based on IVIM, gaussian, and nongaussian diffusion effects, an absolute, normalized signature index (S index) can be computed to classify tissues (eg, benign and malignant lesions, cysts)[57–67] (**Fig. 1**B).

Compared with ASL, which monitors the transit of blood labeled outside of and arriving at the region of interest, IVIM attempts to measure the randomly flowing blood within each voxel. IVIM parameters can be mathematically related to classic perfusion measurements such as CBV; CBF, and mean transit time, via modeling of capillary network geometry with knowledge of water content fraction (f$_w$), total capillary length (from artery to vein), and mean capillary segment length. These quantities are constant for a given tissue, without the need to estimate an arterial input function or transit time in large feeding vessels, although sensitivity to vessel sizes depends on the range of b values used.[68–70] In addition, the IVIM principle can be used for virtual elastography to compute the mechanical driven effects of propagating shear waves in tissues or lesions without the use of mechanical vibrations. From a shifted ADC, tissue elasticity (diffusion-based shear modulus μ$_{diff}$) can be computed and used to simulate effects of various vibration frequencies and amplitudes beyond that of conventional MR elastography hardware, generating a new type of contrast.[70–72]

CLINICAL APPLICATIONS
Brain Tumors

Brain tumor perfusion is an important biomarker for neoangiogenesis, microvascular density, and arteriovenous shunting. MR imaging perfusion metrics can be correlated with various clinical, pathologic, and genomic features (for example histology, grade, molecular signature, and treatment response). Although dynamic susceptibility contrast (DSC) is the clinical reference standard for MR imaging perfusion of brain tumors, repeated administrations of contrast should be avoided in patients with absolute or relative contraindications to gadolinium, as well as children with greater lifetime risks of gadolinium deposition.[73,74] Furthermore, DSC is highly dependent on large vessel flow and requires computation of an arterial input function to compute ATT and relative CBV. Noncontrast perfusion techniques have been correlated with DSC in various neuro-oncologic studies for evaluation of tumor origin, histology, and grade, as well as differentiation of tumor recurrence from treatment effects. ASL enables the evaluation of absolute CBF, as well as ATT and CBV if multiple PLDs are used.[75–86] IVIM extracts both microstructure and microcirculation information to compute ADCo, f_{IVIM}, K, and μ_{diff}.[87–103] Combined or hybrid perfusion and diffusion techniques show great promise for neuro-oncologic imaging[104–115] (**Fig. 2**).

Head and Neck Tumors

Head and neck tumors can also be evaluated using MR imaging perfusion, although techniques are more limited because of the complex anatomy and physiologic motion. Both ASL and IVIM have been used to characterize multiple tumor histologies in various locations, including pharynx,[116–120] sinonasal cavity,[121–124] calvarium and skull base,[125–129] parotid,[130–133] and orbit[134–139]; to differentiate benign, low-grade, and high-grade malignant lesions; to distinguish tumor recurrence from treatment effects; and to evaluate nodal metastases.[140–145] Lesions with characteristic growth patterns, such as hemangiomas, can also be assessed in various stages of proliferation and involution[146] (**Fig. 3**).

Stroke

In patients with ischemic stroke, MR imaging can be used to evaluate both the infarct core (diffusion) and ischemic penumbra (perfusion). The perfusion pattern depends on the acuity of presentation (acute, subacute, chronic), and the type and distribution of vessels involved (large arteries, small arteries, veins). Collateral flow can be estimated based on core-penumbra mismatch[147–153] and the presence of arterial transit artifact on ASL.[24–26] Perfusion imaging can be performed repeatedly and noninvasively to collect longitudinal information in untreated stroke, or to assess reperfusion of treated stroke. Ischemic areas show decreased CBF, ADCo, f, D*, D, and fD*, particularly in the acute setting. For untreated subacute infarcts, ADCo, f, and fD* tend to increase and CBF decreases as the brain tissue becomes edematous and encephalomalacic.[154–165] Treated stroke can normalize in flow parameters or even evolve into cerebral hyperperfusion syndrome, caused by preexisting collaterals with risk for hemorrhagic transformation.[166,167] Other characteristic imaging signs include crossed cerebellar diaschisis associated with cerebral infarcts,[168–170] the border-zone sign of small vessel disease,[171] and the bright sinus appearance of venous thrombosis on ASL[172,173] (**Fig. 4**).

Global Anoxic Injury

Global anoxic injury patterns depend on the severity, duration, and mechanism of injury, as well as patient age, which determines developmental stage and brain regional vulnerability.[174] In neonates and infants, overall brain perfusion is low and blood relaxation parameters highly variable,[31,32] such that long-delay or multidelay ASL can be useful for evaluation.[30,175,176] Preterm neonates tend to develop periventricular white matter injury and intraventricular hemorrhage. In term neonates, hypoxic-ischemic injury can affect the vascular border zones when mild, or the basal ganglia and corticospinal tracts when severe. ASL helps to assess rebound hyperperfusion after the primary perinatal ischemic insult. This physiologic response leads to secondary energy failure with additional brain damage, and is therapeutically minimized by hypothermic treatment.[177–181] In older children and adolescents, diffuse anoxic injury can occur because of systemic emboli, drowning, or strangulation. Energetically active areas, including the cerebral cortex and basal ganglia, can be preferentially affected by ischemia with rebound hyperperfusion in the acute stage and diffuse hypoperfusion in the chronic stage.[174,182–185] Perfusion techniques can also be used to evaluate minimally conscious states and brain death, although care must be taken to correlate with the clinical presentation and exclude MR imaging artifacts that could lead to underestimation of intracranial perfusion.[186–188] Recently, ASL and IVIM have been explored for evaluation of optic neuropathies and chorioretinal ischemia[189–191] (**Fig. 5**).

Vasculopathies

Multiple vascular conditions can predispose to segmental or diffuse ischemia. In children, the differential includes connective tissue, inflammatory, infectious, coagulopathic, metabolic, toxic, and functional vascular disorders. Again, perfusion patterns depend on the time course, distribution, types, and sizes of vessels involved. One of the most common pediatric vasculopathies is moyamoya, a chronic progressive vaso-occlusive disorder that usually affects the distal internal carotid arteries and proximal branches, with varying degrees of moyamoya or so-called puff-of-smoke collaterals in the lenticulostriate, basal, and

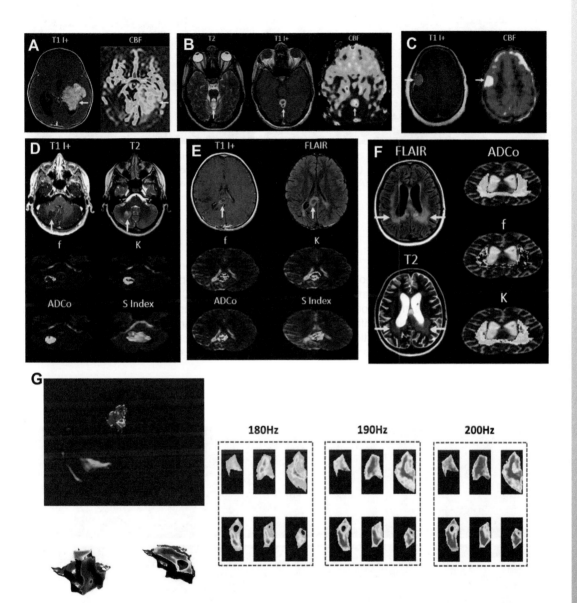

Fig. 2. Brain tumors. (*A*) ASL of choroid plexus papilloma. Hyperenhancing and hyperperfused frondlike mass in the left atrium (*arrows*) with associated ventricular enlargement and ependymal enhancement. (*B*) ASL of recurrent ganglioglioma. Lobulated mass with heterogeneous T2 hyperintensity, rim enhancement, and hyperperfusion in the superior vermis (*arrows*). (*C*) ASL of meningioma. Enhancing and hyperperfused extra-axial mass along the right frontal convexity (*arrows*). (*D*) IVIM of right cerebellar ganglioglioma (*arrows*) with heterogeneous T2 hyperintensity, mild peripheral enhancement, and low S index. (*E*) IVIM of recurrent right splenial glioblastoma (*arrows*) with heterogeneous signal and enhancement, central necrosis, and high S index. (*F*) IVIM of treated pineoblastoma with toxic leukoencephalopathy (*arrows*). (*G*) IVIM of right frontopolar tumor with virtual elastography performed at frequencies of 180, 190, and 200 Hz. FLAIR, fluid-attenuated inversion recovery; T1 I+, postcontrast T1 weighted MR imaging; T2, T2-weighted MR imaging.

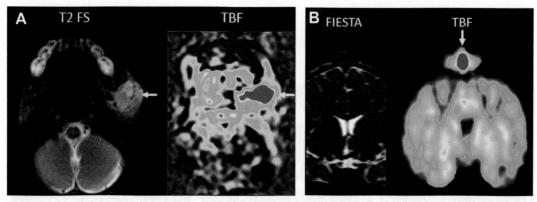

Fig. 3. Head and neck tumors. (*A*) ASL of left parotid infantile hemangioma in proliferative phase with T2-hyperintense signal and hyperperfusion (*arrows*). (*B*) ASL of scalp infantile hemangioma in proliferative phase with avid hyperperfusion (*arrow*). FIESTA, fast imaging employing steady-state acquisition; TBF, tumor blood flow; FS, fat suppression.

leptomeningeal distributions. Moyamoya disease refers to the isolated or primary form, whereas moyamoya disease reflects the secondary form associated with multiple genetic, inflammatory, prothrombotic, and iatrogenic conditions. Long-delay or multidelay ASL is helpful for assessing slow and time-dependent flow through collateral pathways.[192,193] Cerebrovascular reactivity (CVR) can also be assessed by ASL before and after acetazolamide administration to induce maximal vasodilation, which helps predict the need for and response to revascularization surgery.[194–197]

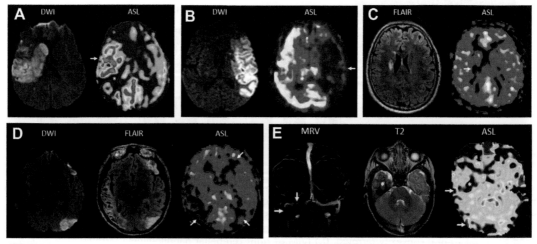

Fig. 4. Stroke. (*A*) Acute right middle cerebral artery (MCA) territory infarct with restricted diffusion on DWI. ASL shows surrounding hypoperfusion (*asterisk*) indicating ischemic penumbra, and overlying high signal representative of arterial transit artifact (*arrow*). (*B*) Subacute left MCA territory infarct with matched diffusion restriction and hypoperfusion on ASL (*arrow*). (*C*) Chronic lacunar infarct of the right centrum semiovale with wallerian degeneration and hypoperfusion of the right corticospinal tract (*arrow*). (*D*) Advanced vascular disease with acute-on-chronic infarcts showing restricted diffusion, encephalomalacia, and hypoperfusion of the external vascular border zones (*arrows*). (*E*) Right temporal lobe hemorrhagic venous infarct with hypoperfusion (*asterisks*) on ASL. MR venography (MRV) shows a partially thrombosed right vein of Labbe, sigmoid and transverse sinus with corresponding bright venous signal on ASL (*arrows*).

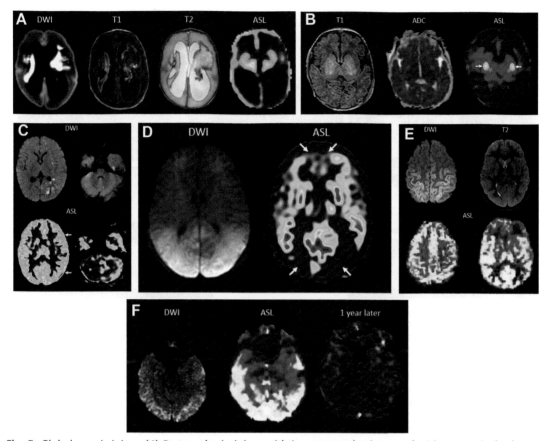

Fig. 5. Global anoxic injury. (*A*) Preterm brain injury with immature sulcation, grade 4 intraventricular hemorrhage with hydrocephalus, periventricular white matter T2 hyperintense signal, and hypoperfusion on ASL. (*B*) Term hypoxic-ischemic injury with abnormal T1 signal and restricted diffusion in the ventrolateral thalami, and rebound hyperperfusion of the basal ganglia on ASL (*arrows*). (*C*) Left cerebral and cerebellar shower emboli with multifocal restricted diffusion (*arrows*). ASL shows asymmetric hypoperfusion of left cerebral deep gray and white matter with overlying arterial transit artifact and crossed right cerebellar diaschisis (*asterisk*). (*D*) Near-drowning with diffuse cortical and basal ganglia infarction on DWI, as well as global and watershed hypoperfusion on ASL (*arrows*). (*E*) Cardiac arrest with diffuse cerebral edema, cortical restricted diffusion and rebound cerebral hyperperfusion on ASL. (*F*) Fat emboli with innumerable foci of restricted diffusion. ASL in the acute stage shows diffuse cerebral hyperperfusion, evolving to hypoperfusion in the chronic stage.

IVIM parameters can also be correlated with moyamoya vascular disease burden and severity of ischemia.[198]

Focal cerebral arteriopathy (FCA) of childhood is a typically monophasic and self-resolving condition that can result following varicella zoster and other herpesvirus infections. FCA usually presents with acute unilateral basal ganglia infarction and transient narrowing of the distal carotid, proximal anterior, and middle cerebral arteries.[199]

Posterior reversible encephalopathy syndrome is a functional vascular disorder thought to result from disruption of normal cerebral autoregulation in the setting of hypertension, renal failure, vascular disorder, or autoimmune diseases.[200] Signal and perfusion abnormalities show a predilection for the posterior brain, namely parieto-occipital cerebrum and cerebellum. Perfusion imaging can help to characterize other vascular abnormalities, including stenoses, occlusions, and aneurysms (**Fig. 6**).[201,202]

Vascular Malformations

Vascular malformations are congenital defects of vascular morphogenesis that can be high-flow malformations (arteriovenous malformation, arteriovenous fistula) or low-flow malformations (venous, capillary, lymphatic). ASL and IVIM can help characterize the level of flow, identify regional ischemic steal, and distinguish vascular malformations from soft tissue tumors.[146,203–206] ASL can be particularly helpful in characterizing flow

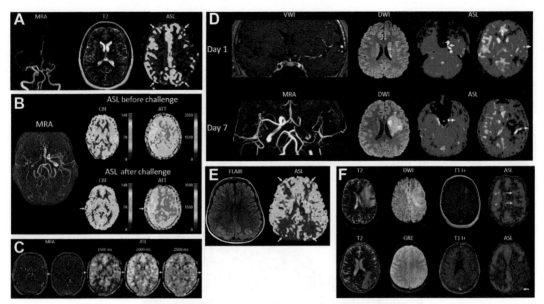

Fig. 6. Vasculopathy. (*A*) Moyamoya syndrome associated with sickle cell disease. MR arteriography (MRA) shows occluded left and stenosed right distal internal carotid artery (ICA) and branches. Multiple chronic lacunar infarcts are present. Single-delay ASL shows heterogeneous cerebral hypoperfusion, more pronounced in the left cerebral hemisphere and external vascular border zones (*arrows*). (*B*) Moyamoya disease of right ICA with external carotid artery collaterals. ASL before and after acetazolamide challenge shows increased CBF and decreased ATT in the right MCA distribution (*arrows*), indicating a degree of preserved cerebrovascular reactivity. (*C*) Moyamoya disease of left ICA after pial synangiosis. Multidelay ASL shows dynamic flow through the synangiosis (*arrows*) and into brain parenchyma. (*D*) Focal cerebral arteriopathy shows acute left basal ganglia infarct with vessel wall enhancement and narrowing of the left distal ICA and branches. ASL shows left external border-zone hypoperfusion with arterial transit artifact in the left carotid siphon and overlying leptomeningeal collaterals (*arrows*). Follow-up imaging shows blooming of the infarct core with worsening arterial stenoses. ASL shows prominent MCA territory hypoperfusion with reduction of arterial transit artifact in the left carotid siphon and leptomeningeal collaterals (*arrows*). (*E*) Posterior reversible encephalopathy syndrome. Serpiginous FLAIR-hyperintense signal involves the cortex and subcortical white matter of the external vascular border zones, posterior greater than anterior, with corresponding hypoperfusion on ASL (*arrows*). (*F*) Lupus vasculitis. (*Top row*) Acute left frontal curvilinear enhancement, restricted diffusion, and vasogenic edema with increased perfusion on ASL (*arrows*). (*Bottom row*) Chronic left parietal white matter signal with peripheral enhancement and microhemorrhages. ASL shows regional hypoperfusion with overlying arterial transit artifact (*arrows*). GRE, gradient recalled echo; VWI, vessel wall imaging.

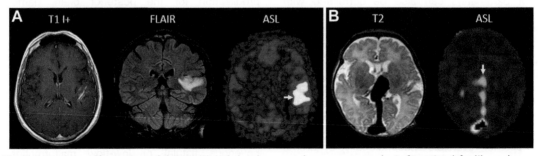

Fig. 7. Vascular malformations. (*A*) Transitional developmental venous anomaly. Left parietal fanlike enhancement with greater-than-expected surrounding vasogenic edema. Prominent increased perfusion on ASL (*arrow*) indicates a high-flow arterial component. (*B*) Vein of Galen aneurysmal malformation. Enlarged median prosencephalic vein of Markowski with diffuse white matter T2 signal. ASL shows high signal within the malformation, indicating arteriovenous shunting (*arrow*), and low flow to the surrounding brain parenchyma caused by ischemic steal.

dynamics, with the presence of bright venous signal indicating rapid arteriovenous shunting[207,208] (Fig. 7).

Epilepsy

Perfusion imaging in epilepsy can aid in seizure focus localization and/or lateralization, increasing diagnostic confidence for the epileptogenic zone. In the periictal phase of seizure, neuronal hyperexcitability leads to regional hyperperfusion of regional cortex, which can propagate to surrounding areas. Crossed cerebellar hyperperfusion can be observed in association with acute cerebral seizure. Interictal imaging often shows decreased perfusion within and surrounding the area of interest. Prominent perfusion and diffusion

abnormalities can be observed in patients with severe and chronic epilepsy[209–212] (Fig. 8).

Migraine

Migraine is neurovascular phenomenon related to cortical spreading depression with multiple characteristic phases, known as the prodrome, aura, headache, and postdrome. During the aura phase, focal neurologic symptoms can occur with regional or hemispheric hypoperfusion and vasoconstriction (hemiplegic migraine). Next occurs the headache phase with rebound hyperperfusion and vasodilation. The attack usually lasts between 4 and 72 hours if untreated, followed by a postdromal period during which symptoms gradually resolve. Perfusion imaging aids in characterization

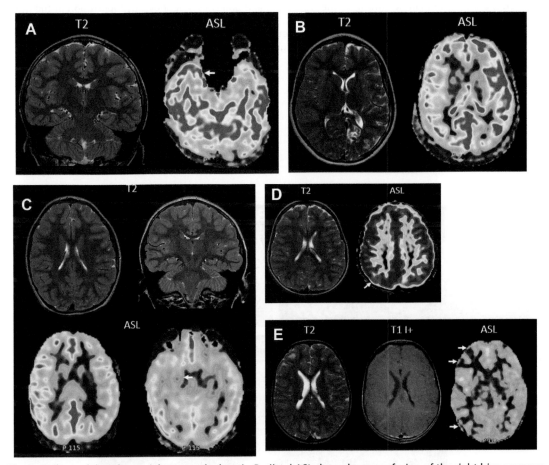

Fig. 8. Epilepsy. (*A*) Right mesial temporal sclerosis. Periictal ASL shows hyperperfusion of the right hippocampus (*arrow*) and anterior temporal lobe. (*B*) Left Rasmussen encephalitis with hemispheric volume loss and signal abnormality. Periictal ASL shows increased flow throughout the left hemispheric gray and white matter. (*C*) Perisylvian polymicrogyria, right greater than left, with lateralizing seizures and hippocampal edema. Periictal ASL shows increased flow to the right hippocampus (*arrow*) and entire cerebral hemisphere. (*D*) Right parietal focal cortical dysplasia with sulcation abnormality. Interictal ASL shows focal hypoperfusion (*arrow*). (*E*) Tuberous sclerosis with cortical/subcortical tubers and subependymal nodules. Interictal ASL shows multifocal hypoperfusion in regions of tuber involvement (*arrows*).

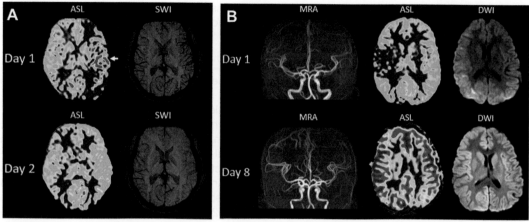

Fig. 9. Migraine. (*A*) Hemiplegic migraine on day 1, aura phase, with diffuse left hemispheric hypoperfusion and overlying arterial transit artifact (*arrow*) on ASL, and cortical venous dilation. Day 2, cephalgic phase, with diffuse left hemispheric hyperperfusion and decreased cortical venous susceptibility. (*B*) Complex hemiplegic migraine on day 1, aura phase, with mild narrowing of the right MCA and branches. ASL shows hypoperfusion in the right MCA territory, and DWI shows patchy diffusion restriction throughout the right cerebral hemisphere. Symptoms persisted on day 8 with rebound arterial dilatation, pseudonormalization of DWI abnormalities, and right hemispheric hyperperfusion on ASL. SWI, susceptibility-weighted imaging.

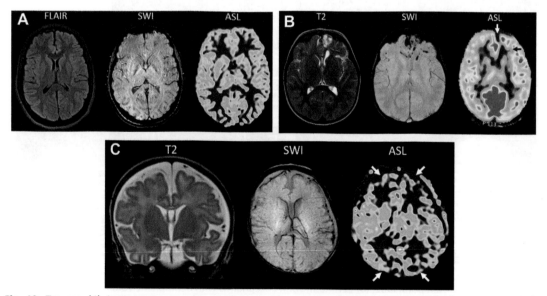

Fig. 10. Trauma. (*A*) Acute postconcussion syndrome with negative screening MR imaging, but persistent left-sided weakness. ASL shows right hemispheric hyperperfusion with decreased cortical venous susceptibility, concerning for neurovascular disruption. (*B*) Chronic TBI with left greater than right frontal lobe and callosal encephalomalacia, gray-white junctional shear injury, microhemorrhages, and superficial siderosis. ASL shows matched hypoperfusion (*arrows*). (*C*) Abusive head trauma with left greater than right subdural collections, cortical vein thrombosis, and border-zone hypoperfusion on ASL (*arrows*).

of migraine phases, distinction from acute stroke and other disorders, and response to medications[213–222] **(Fig. 9)**.

Trauma

Traumatic brain injury (TBI) is complex and depends on severity, timing, and mechanism of injury. Current anatomic imaging techniques do not correlate well with clinical course; therefore, perfusion and diffusion may aid as potential biomarkers to help evaluate cerebrovascular reactivity and microstructural integrity.[75,223,224] In children, a careful history and imaging evaluation helps to distinguish accidental from nonaccidental trauma. Accidental trauma can be associated with cerebral contusions (low impact) or diffuse axonal injury (high impact) with multifocal shear abnormalities and microhemorrhages centered in the gray-white junction, corpus callosum, and brainstem. Perfusion abnormalities that are notably asymmetric, heterogeneous, and/or excessive for clinical history raise concern for abusive head trauma. Hemispheric hypoperfusion can be observed in relation to a subdural hematoma with bridging vein disruption, or following strangulation with partial carotid occlusion[183,225] **(Fig. 10)**.

Inflammatory

Perfusion imaging of neuroinflammatory disorders can reveal hyperperfusion and restricted diffusion in the acute phase, followed by postinflammatory hypoperfusion and facilitated diffusion caused by brain gliosis. Multiple sclerosis is a common autoimmune disease that characteristically presents on imaging with leading-edge demyelination characterized by incomplete rim enhancement, restricted diffusion, and hyperperfusion[55,226–230] **(Fig. 11)**.

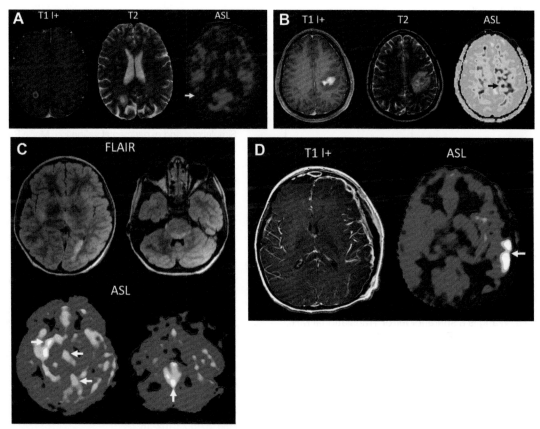

Fig. 11. Inflammation. (*A*) Multiple sclerosis with rim enhancement, susceptibility, and vasogenic edema in the right parietal lobe. ASL shows patchy peripheral hyperperfusion (*arrow*) and surrounding edema with hypoperfusion. (*B*) Tumefactive multiple sclerosis with patchy enhancement and vasogenic edema in the left centrum semiovale. ASL shows patchy rim hyperperfusion and surrounding edema with hypoperfusion (*arrow*). (*C*) Acute disseminated encephalomyelitis with multifocal flocculent FLAIR-hyperintense lesions, largest in the right insula, left thalamus, left occipital white matter, and pons with corresponding hyperperfusion on ASL (*arrows*). (*D*) Pott puffy tumor with left frontal sinusitis, meningoencephalitis, and subdural empyema. ASL shows left cerebral hypoperfusion with focal hyperperfusion (*arrow*) in the region of a developing subdural abscess.

SUMMARY

ASL and IVIM are noncontrast MR imaging perfusion techniques with multiple promising applications in children. Understanding of physical principles and parametric modeling quantitative values aids in appropriate use and interpretation of these sequences. This article highlights some current and emerging applications in children, including tumors, stroke, vasculopathies, vascular malformations, epilepsy, migraine, trauma, and inflammation.

CLINICS CARE POINTS

- Noncontrast brain perfusion techniques are very useful in children to minimize unnecessary gadolinium administration and potential deposition.

- Imaging techniques and model assumptions, as well as subject age-and physiology-dependent variations, affect quantification of cerebral perfusion.

- Arterial spin labeling magnetically labels and tracks the arrival of arterial blood water into the brain. Results are highly dependent on labeling technique and postlabel delay (PLD).

- Intravoxel incoherent motion uses diffusion imaging with multiple b-values to model both true molecular diffusion and blood microcirculation (pseudodiffusion).

- Clinical applications of noncontrast perfusion include tumors, stroke, vasculopathies, vascular malformations, epilepsy, migraine, trauma, and inflammation.

DISCLOSURE

D.J.J. Wang is a shareholder of Translational MRI, LLC. D.L. Bihan, R. Krishnamurthy, and M. Smith have no disclosures. M-L. Ho is a principal investigator on the Radiological Society of North America (RSNA) Research Scholar Grant, Society for Pediatric Radiology (SPR) Pilot Award, and American Society of Head and Neck Radiology (ASHNR) William N. Hanafee Award, for work unrelated to this article.

REFERENCES

1. Lanzman B, Heit JJ. Advanced MRI measures of cerebral perfusion and their clinical applications. Top Magn Reson Imaging 2017;26(2):83–90.

2. Zhang X, Petersen ET, Ghariq E, et al. In vivo blood T(1) measurements at 1.5 T, 3 T, and 7 T. Magn Reson Med 2013;70(4):1082–6.

3. Wong EC. An introduction to ASL labeling techniques. J Magn Reson Imaging 2014;40(1):1–10.

4. Hernandez-Garcia L, Lahiri A, Schollenberger J. Recent progress in ASL. Neuroimage 2019;187:3–16.

5. Wong EC. New developments in arterial spin labeling pulse sequences. NMR Biomed 2013;26(8):887–91.

6. Nanjappa M, Troalen T, Pfeuffer J, et al. Comparison of 2D simultaneous multi-slice and 3D GRASE readout schemes for pseudo-continuous arterial spin labeling of cerebral perfusion at 3 T. MAGMA 2021;34(3):437–50.

7. Aoike S, Sugimori H, Fujima N, et al. Three-dimensional pseudo-continuous arterial spin-labeling using turbo-spin echo with pseudo-steady state readout: a comparison with other major readout methods. Magn Reson Med Sci 2019;18(2):170–7.

8. Baas KPA, Petr J, Kuijer JPA, et al. Effects of acquisition parameter modifications and field strength on the reproducibility of brain perfusion measurements using arterial spin-labeling. AJNR Am J Neuroradiol 2021;42(1):109–15.

9. Lorenz K, Mildner T, Schlumm T, et al. Characterization of pseudo-continuous arterial spin labeling: Simulations and experimental validation. Magn Reson Med 2018;79(3):1638–49.

10. Chen Z, Zhang X, Yuan C, et al. Measuring the labeling efficiency of pseudocontinuous arterial spin labeling. Magn Reson Med 2017;77(5):1841–52.

11. Chen Y, Wang DJJ, Detre JA. Test-retest reliability of arterial spin labeling with common labeling strategies. J Magn Reson Imaging 2011a;33:940–9.

12. Hodkinson DJ, Krause K, Khawaja N, et al. Quantifying the test-retest reliability of cerebral blood flow measurements in a clinical model of on-going postsurgical pain: A study using pseudo-continuous arterial spin labelling. Neuroimage Clin 2013;3:301–10.

13. Alsop DC, Detre JA, Golay X, et al. Recommended implementation of arterial spin-labeled perfusion MRI for clinical applications: A consensus of the ISMRM perfusion study group and the European consortium for ASL in dementia. Magn Reson Med 2015;73:102–16.

14. Wang J, Licht DJ. Pediatric perfusion MR imaging using arterial spin labeling. Neuroimaging Clin 2006;16:149–67.

15. Wu C, Honarmand AR, Schnell S, et al. Age-related changes of normal cerebral and cardiac blood flow in children and adults aged 7 months to 61 years. J Am Heart Assoc 2016;5:e002657.

16. Parkes LM, Rashid W, Chard DT, et al. Normal cerebral perfusion measurements using arterial spin labeling: reproducibility, stability, and age and gender effects. Magn Reson Med 2004;51(4): 736–43.

17. Jain V, Duda J, Avants B, et al. Longitudinal reproducibility and accuracy of pseudo-continuous arterial spin–labeled perfusion MR imaging in typically developing children. Radiology 2012;263:527–36.

18. Epstein HT. Stages of increased cerebral blood flow accompany stages of rapid brain growth. Brain Dev 1999;21(8):535–9.

19. Dai W, Robson PM, Shankaranarayanan A, et al. Reduced resolution transit delay prescan for quantitative continuous arterial spin labeling perfusion imaging. Magn Reson Med 2012;67:1252–65.

20. Maccotta L, Detre JA, Alsop DC. The efficiency of adiabatic inversion for perfusion imaging by arterial spin labeling. NMR Biomed 1997;10:216–21.

21. Wang J, Licht DJ, Jahng GH, et al. Pediatric perfusion imaging using pulsed arterial spin labeling. J Magn Reson Imaging 2003;18:404–13.

22. Alsaedi A, Thomas D, Bisdas S, et al. Overview and critical appraisal of arterial spin labelling technique in brain perfusion imaging. Contrast Media Mol Imaging 2018;2018:5360375.

23. Tang S, Liu X, He L, et al. Application of postlabeling delay time in 3-Dimensional pseudocontinuous arterial spin-labeled perfusion imaging in normal children. J Comput Assist Tomogr 2019;43(5): 697–707.

24. Zaharchuk G. Arterial spin label imaging of acute ischemic stroke and transient ischemic attack. Neuroimaging Clin N Am 2011;21(2):285–301, x.

25. Di Napoli A, Cheng SF, Gregson J, et al. Arterial spin labeling MRI in carotid stenosis: arterial transit artifacts may predict symptoms. Radiology 2020; 297(3):652–60.

26. Ukai R, Mikami T, Nagahama H, et al. Arterial transit artifacts observed by arterial spin labeling in Moyamoya disease. J Stroke Cerebrovasc Dis 2020; 29(9):105058.

27. Ishida S, Kimura H, Isozaki M, et al. Robust arterial transit time and cerebral blood flow estimation using combined acquisition of Hadamard-encoded multi-delay and long-labeled long-delay pseudocontinuous arterial spin labeling: a simulation and in vivo study. NMR Biomed 2020;33:e4319.

28. Lin T, Qu J, Zuo Z, et al. Test-retest reliability and reproducibility of long-label pseudo-continuous arterial spin labeling. Magn Reson Imaging 2020; 73:111–7.

29. Qiu D, Straka M, Zun Z, et al. CBF measurements using multidelay pseudocontinuous and velocity-selective arterial spin labeling in patients with long arterial transit delays: comparison with xenon CT CBF. J Magn Reson Imaging 2012;36:110–9.

30. Hu HH, Rusin JA, Peng R, et al. Multi-phase 3D arterial spin labeling brain MRI in assessing cerebral blood perfusion and arterial transit times in children at 3T. Clin Imaging 2019;53:210–20.

31. De Vis J, Hendrikse J, Groenendaal F, et al. Impact of neonate haematocrit variability on the longitudinal relaxation time of blood: Implications for arterial spin labelling MRI. NeuroImage Clin 2014;4: 517–25.

32. Liu P, Chalak LF, Krishnamurthy LC, et al. T1 and T2 values of human neonatal blood at 3 Tesla: dependence on hematocrit, oxygenation, and temperature. Magn Reson Med 2016;75:1730–5.

33. Wu W-C, Jain V, Li C, et al. In vivo venous blood T(1) measurement using inversion recovery true-FISP in children and adults. Magn Reson Med 2010;64:1140–7.

34. Lu H, Clingman C, Golay X, et al. Determining the longitudinal relaxation time (T1) of blood at 3.0 Tesla. Magn Reson Med 2004;52:679–82.

35. Buxton RB, Frank LR, Wong EC, et al. A general kinetic model for quantitative perfusion imaging with arterial spin labeling. Magn Reson Med 1998;40: 383–96.

36. Parkes LM, Tofts PS. Improved accuracy of human cerebral blood perfusion measurements using arterial spin labeling: accounting for capillary water permeability. Magn Reson Med 2002;48:27–41.

37. St Lawrence KS, Frank JA, McLaughlin AC. Effect of restricted water exchange on cerebral blood flow values calculated with arterial spin tagging: a theoretical investigation. Magn Reson Med 2000; 44:440–9.

38. Dickie BR, Parker GJ, Parkes LM. Measuring water exchange across the blood-brain barrier using MRI. Prog Nucl Magn Reson Spectrosc 2020;116: 19–39.

39. Shao X, Ma SJ, Casey M, et al. Mapping water exchange across the blood-brain barrier using 3D diffusion-prepared arterial spin labeled perfusion MRI. Magn Reson Med 2019;81:3065–79.

40. Wang J, Fernandez-Seara MA, Wang S, et al. When perfusion meets diffusion: in vivo measurement of water permeability in human brain. J Cereb Blood Flow Metab 2007;27:839–49.

41. St Lawrence KS, Owen D, Wang DJ. A two-stage approach for measuring vascular water exchange and arterial transit time by diffusion-weighted perfusion MRI. Magn Reson Med 2012;67: 1275–84.

42. Le Bihan D, Breton E, Lallemand D, et al. Separation of diffusion and perfusion in intravoxel incoherent motion MR imaging. Radiology 1988; 168(2):497–505.

43. Vieni C, Ades-Aron B, Conti B, et al. Effect of intravoxel incoherent motion on diffusion parameters in normal brain. Neuroimage 2020;204:116228.

44. Turner R, Le Bihan D, Chesnick AS. Echo-planar imaging of diffusion and perfusion. Magn Reson Med 1991;19(2):247–53.

45. Rydhög AS, Szczepankiewicz F, Wirestam R, et al. Separating blood and water: Perfusion and free water elimination from diffusion MRI in the human brain. Neuroimage 2017;156:423–34.

46. Abdullah OM, Gomez AD, Merchant S, et al. Orientation dependence of microcirculation-induced diffusion signal in anisotropic tissues. Magn Reson Med 2016;76(4):1252–62.

47. Federau C, Hagmann P, Maeder P, et al. Dependence of brain intravoxel incoherent motion perfusion parameters on the cardiac cycle. PLoS One 2013;8(8):e72856.

48. Pavilla A, Arrigo A, Mejdoubi M, et al. Measuring cerebral hypoperfusion induced by hyperventilation challenge with intravoxel incoherent motion magnetic resonance imaging in healthy volunteers. J Comput Assist Tomogr 2018;42(1):85–91.

49. Huang HM. Reliable estimation of brain intravoxel incoherent motion parameters using denoised diffusion-weighted MRI. NMR Biomed 2020;33(4): e4249.

50. Reischauer C, Gutzeit A. Image denoising substantially improves accuracy and precision of intravoxel incoherent motion parameter estimates. PLoS One 2017;12(4):e0175106.

51. Fournet G, Li JR, Cerjanic AM, et al. A two-pool model to describe the IVIM cerebral perfusion. J Cereb Blood Flow Metab 2017;37(8): 2987–3000.

52. Le Bihan D, Turner R. The capillary network: a link between IVIM and classical perfusion. Magn Reson Med 1992;27(1):171–8.

53. Hu YC, Yan LF, Han Y, et al. Can the low and high b-value distribution influence the pseudodiffusion parameter derived from IVIM DWI in normal brain? BMC Med Imaging 2020;20(1):14.

54. Chabert S, Verdu J, Huerta G, et al. Impact of b-value sampling scheme on brain IVIM parameter estimation in healthy subjects. Magn Reson Med Sci 2020;19(3):216–26.

55. Keil VC, Mädler B, Gielen GH, et al. Intravoxel incoherent motion MRI in the brain: Impact of the fitting model on perfusion fraction and lesion differentiability. J Magn Reson Imaging 2017; 46(4):1187–99.

56. Wu WC, Chen YF, Tseng HM, et al. Caveat of measuring perfusion indexes using intravoxel incoherent motion magnetic resonance imaging in the human brain. Eur Radiol 2015;25(8):2485–92.

57. Iima M, Le Bihan D. Clinical intravoxel incoherent motion and diffusion MR imaging: past, present, and future. Radiology 2016;278:13–32.

58. Jensen JH, Helpern JA, Ramani A, et al. Diffusional kurtosis imaging: the quantification of non-gaussian water diffusion by means of magnetic resonance imaging. MRM 2005;53(6):1432–40.

59. Mulkern RV, Haker SJ, Maier SE. On high b diffusion imaging in the human brain: ruminations and experimental insights. Magn Reson Imaging 2009;27(8):1151–62.

60. Yablonskiy DA, Bretthorst GL, Ackerman JJ. Statistical model for diffusion attenuated MR signal. MRM 2003;50(4):664–9.

61. Bennett KM, Schmainda KM, Bennett RT, et al. Characterization of continuously distributed cortical water diffusion rates with a stretched-exponential model. MRM 2003;50(4):727–34.

62. Hall MG, Barrick TR. From diffusion-weighted MRI to anomalous diffusion imaging. MRM 2008;59(3): 447–55.

63. Zhou XJ, Gao Q, Abdullah O, et al. Studies of anomalous diffusion in the human brain using fractional order calculus. MRM 2010;63(3):562–9.

64. Neil JJ, Bretthorst GL. On the use of Bayesian probability theory for analysis of exponential decay data: an example taken from intravoxel incoherent motion experiments. Magn Reson Med 1993;29(5):642–7.

65. While PT. A comparative simulation study of bayesian fitting approaches to intravoxel incoherent motion modeling in diffusion-weighted MRI. Magn Reson Med 2017;78(6):2373–87.

66. Ohno N, Miyati T, Kobayashi S, et al. Modified triexponential analysis of intravoxel incoherent motion for brain perfusion and diffusion. J Magn Reson Imaging 2016;43(4):818–23.

67. Rydhög A, Pasternak O, Ståhlberg F, et al. Estimation of diffusion, perfusion and fractional volumes using a multi-compartment relaxation-compensated intravoxel incoherent motion (IVIM) signal model. Eur J Radiol Open 2019;6:198–205.

68. Federau C, Maeder P, O'Brien K, et al. Quantitative measurement of brain perfusion with intravoxel incoherent motion MR imaging. Radiology 2012; 265(3):874–81.

69. Stieb S, Boss A, Wurnig MC, et al. Non-parametric intravoxel incoherent motion analysis in patients with intracranial lesions: Test-retest reliability and correlation with arterial spin labeling. Neuroimage Clin 2016;11:780–8.

70. Le Bihan D. What can we see with IVIM MRI? Neuroimage 2019;187:56–67.

71. Le Bihan D, Ichikawa S, Motosugi U. Diffusion and intravoxel incoherent motion MR imaging-based virtual elastography: a hypothesis-generating study in the liver. Radiology 2017;285(2):609–19.

72. Kromrey ML, Le Bihan D, Ichikawa S, et al. Diffusion-weighted MRI-based virtual elastography for the assessment of liver fibrosis. Radiology 2020; 295(1):127–35.

73. Kanda T, Ishii K, Kawaguchi H, et al. High signal intensity in the dentate nucleus and globus pallidus

on unenhanced T1-weighted MR images: relationship with increasing cumulative dose of a gadolinium-based contrast material. Radiology 2014;270: 834–41.

74. Kanda T, Osawa M, Oba H, et al. High signal intensity in dentate nucleus on unenhanced T1-weighted MR Images: association with linear versus macrocyclic gadolinium chelate administration. Radiology 2015;275:803–9.

75. Haller S, Zaharchuk G, Thomas DL, et al. Arterial spin labeling perfusion of the brain: emerging clinical applications. Radiology 2016;281(2):337–56.

76. Abdel Razek AAK, Talaat M, El-Serougy L, et al. Clinical applications of arterial spin labeling in brain tumors. J Comput Assist Tomogr 2019; 43(4):525–32.

77. Wang YF, Hou B, Yang SJ, et al. Diagnostic significance of arterial spin labeling in the assessment of tumor grade in brain. J Cancer Res Ther 2016; 12(1):259–66.

78. Xi YB1, Kang XW1, Wang N1, et al. Differentiation of primary central nervous system lymphoma from high-grade glioma and brain metastasis using arterial spin labeling and dynamic contrast-enhanced magnetic resonance imaging. Eur J Radiol 2019; 112:59–64.

79. Nabavizadeh SA, Akbari H, Ware JB, et al. Arterial spin labeling and dynamic susceptibility contrast-enhanced MR Imaging for evaluation of arteriovenous shunting and tumor hypoxia in glioblastoma. Sci Rep 2019;9(1):8747.

80. Law-Ye B, Schertz M, Galanaud D, et al. Arterial spin labeling to predict brain tumor grading: limits of cutoff cerebral blood flow values. Radiology 2017;282(2):610–2.

81. Dangouloff-Ros V, Deroulers C, Foissac F, et al. Arterial spin labeling to predict brain tumor grading in children: correlations between histopathologic vascular density and perfusion MR imaging. Radiology 2016;281(2):553–66.

82. Delgado AF, De Luca F, Hanagandi P, et al. Arterial spin-labeling in children with brain tumor: a meta-analysis. AJNR Am J Neuroradiol 2018;39(8):1536–42.

83. Yeom KW, Mitchell LA, Lober RM, et al. Arterial spin-labeled perfusion of pediatric brain tumors. AJNR Am J Neuroradiol 2014;35(2):395–401.

84. Maral H, Ertekin E, Tunçyürek Ö, et al. Effects of susceptibility artifacts on perfusion MRI in patients with primary brain tumor: a comparison of arterial spin-labeling versus DSC. AJNR Am J Neuroradiol 2020;41(2):255–61.

85. Zeng Q, Jiang B, Shi F, et al. 3D Pseudocontinuous arterial spin-labeling MR imaging in the preoperative evaluation of gliomas. AJNR Am J Neuroradiol 2017;38(10):1876–83.

86. Soni N, Srindharan K, Kumar S, et al. Arterial spin labeling perfusion: Prospective MR imaging in

87. Federau C, Meuli R, O'Brien K, et al. Perfusion measurement in brain gliomas with intravoxel incoherent motion MRI. AJNR Am J Neuroradiol 2014; 35(2):256–62.

88. Lee HJ, Rha SY, Chung YE, et al. Tumor perfusion-related parameter of diffusion-weighted magnetic resonance imaging: Correlation with histological microvessel density. MRM 2014;71(4):1554–8.

89. Kim HS, Suh CH, Kim N, et al. Histogram analysis of intravoxel incoherent motion for differentiating recurrent tumor from treatment effect in patients with glioblastoma: initial clinical experience. AJNR 2014;35(3):490–7.

90. Bisdas S, Braun C, Skardelly M, et al. Correlative assessment of tumor microcirculation using contrast-enhanced perfusion MRI and intravoxel incoherent motion diffusion-weighted MRI: is there a link between them? NMR Biomed 2014;27(10): 1184–91.

91. Bisdas S, Klose U. IVIM analysis of brain tumors: an investigation of the relaxation effects of CSF, blood, and tumor tissue on the estimated perfusion fraction. MAGMA 2015;28(4):377–83.

92. Le Bihan D, Breton E, Lallemand D, et al. MR Imaging of intravoxel incoherent motions: application to diffusion and perfusion in neurologic disorders. Radiology 1986;161:401–7.

93. Hino T, Togao O, Hiwatashi A, et al. Clinical efficacy of simplified intravoxel incoherent motion imaging using three b-values for differentiating high- and low-grade gliomas. PLoS One 2018. https://doi. org/10.1371/journal.pone.0209796.

94. Fu M, Han F, Feng C, et al. Based on arterial spin labeling helps to differentiate high-grade gliomas from brain solitary metastasis: A systematic review and meta-analysis. Medicine (Baltimore) 2019; 98(19):e15580.

95. Maeda M, Kawamura Y, Tamagawa Y, et al. Intravoxel incoherent motion (IVIM) MRI in intracranial, extraaxial tumors and cysts. J Comput Assist Tomogr 1992;16(4):514–8.

96. Catanese A, Malacario F, Cirillo L, et al. Application of intravoxel incoherent motion (IVIM) magnetic resonance imaging in the evaluation of primitive brain tumours. Neuroradiol J 2018;31(1):4–9.

97. Federau C, Cerny M, Roux M, et al. IVIM perfusion fraction is prognostic for survival in brain glioma. Clin Neuroradiol 2017;27(4):485–92.

98. Hino T, Togao O, Hiwatashi A, et al. Clinical efficacy of simplified intravoxel incoherent motion imaging using three b-values for differentiating high- and low-grade gliomas. PLoS One 2018;13(12):e0209796.

99. Kikuchi K, Hiwatashi A, Togao O, et al. Intravoxel incoherent motion MR imaging of pediatric

intracranial tumors: correlation with histology and diagnostic utility. AJNR Am J Neuroradiol 2019; 40(5):878–84.

100. Minh Duc N. The diagnostic function of intravoxel incoherent motion for distinguishing between pilocytic astrocytoma and ependymoma. PLoS One 2021;16(3):e0247899.

101. Hu YC, Yan LF, Wu L, et al. Intravoxel incoherent motion diffusion-weighted MR imaging of gliomas: efficacy in preoperative grading. Sci Rep 2014;4: 7208.

102. Song S, Zhao J, Zhang P, et al. Intravoxel incoherent motion diffusion weighted imaging of high-grade gliomas and brain metastases: efficacy in preoperative differentiation. Int J Clin Exp Med 2018;11(7):7064–71.

103. Togao O, Hiwatashi A, Yamashita K, et al. Measurement of the perfusion fraction in brain tumors with intravoxel incoherent motion MR imaging: validation with histopathological vascular density in meningiomas. Br J Radiol 2018;91(1085): 20170912.

104. Shen N, Zhao L, Jiang J, et al. Intravoxel incoherent motion diffusion-weighted imaging analysis of diffusion and microperfusion in grading gliomas and comparison with arterial spin labeling for evaluation of tumor perfusion. J Magn Reson Imaging 2016;44(3):620–32.

105. Suh CH, Kim HS, Jung SC, et al. MRI as a diagnostic biomarker for differentiating primary central nervous system lymphoma from glioblastoma: A systematic review and meta-analysis. J Magn Reson Imaging 2019;50(2):560–72.

106. Lin Y, Li J, Zhang Z, et al. Comparison of intravoxel incoherent motion diffusion-weighted mr imaging and arterial spin labeling MR imaging in gliomas. Biomed Res Int 2015;2015:234245.

107. Dolgorsuren EA, Harada M, Kanazawa Y, et al. Correlation and characteristics of intravoxel incoherent motion and arterial spin labeling techniques versus multiple parameters obtained on dynamic susceptibility contrast perfusion MRI for brain tumors. J Med Invest 2019;66(3.4):308–13.

108. Wang C, Dong H. Ki-67 labeling index and the grading of cerebral gliomas by using intravoxel incoherent motion diffusion-weighted imaging and three-dimensional arterial spin labeling magnetic resonance imaging. Acta Radiol 2020;61(8): 1057–63.

109. Liu ZC, Yan LF, Hu YC, et al. Combination of IVIM-DWI and 3D-ASL for differentiating true progression from pseudoprogression of Glioblastoma multiforme after concurrent chemoradiotherapy: study protocol of a prospective diagnostic trial. BMC Med Imaging 2017;17(1):10.

110. Miyoshi F, Shinohara Y, Kambe A, et al. Utility of intravoxel incoherent motion magnetic resonance imaging and arterial spin labeling for recurrent glioma after bevacizumab treatment. Acta Radiol 2018;59(11):1372–9.

111. Hales PW, d'Arco F, Cooper J, et al. Arterial spin labelling and diffusion-weighted imaging in paediatric brain tumours. Neuroimage Clin 2019;22: 101696.

112. Zhang X, Ingo C, Teeuwisse WM, et al. Comparison of perfusion signal acquired by arterial spin labeling-prepared intravoxel incoherent motion (IVIM) MRI and conventional IVIM MRI to unravel the origin of the IVIM signal. Magn Reson Med 2018; 79(2):723–9.

113. Abdel Razek AAK, Talaat M, El-Serougy L, et al. Differentiating glioblastomas from solitary brain metastases using arterial spin labeling perfusion- and diffusion tensor imaging-derived metrics. World Neurosurg 2019;127:e593–8.

114. Wu WC, Yang SC, Chen YF, et al. Simultaneous assessment of cerebral blood volume and diffusion heterogeneity using hybrid IVIM and DK MR imaging: initial experience with brain tumors. Eur Radiol 2017;27(1):306–14.

115. Yan LF, Sun YZ, Zhao SS, et al. Perfusion, diffusion, or brain tumor barrier integrity: which represents the glioma features best? Cancer Manag Res 2019;11:9989–10000.

116. Xiao B, Wang P, Zhao Y, et al. Nasopharyngeal carcinoma perfusion MRI: Comparison of arterial spin labeling and dynamic contrast-enhanced MRI. Medicine (Baltimore) 2020;99(22):e20503.

117. Lai V, Li X, Lee VH, et al. Intravoxel incoherent motion MR imaging: comparison of diffusion and perfusion characteristics between nasopharyngeal carcinoma and post-chemoradiation fibrosis. Eur Radiol 2013;23(10):2793–801.

118. Yu XP, Hou J, Li FP, et al. Intravoxel incoherent motion diffusion weighted magnetic resonance imaging for differentiation between nasopharyngeal carcinoma and lymphoma at the primary site. J Comput Assist Tomogr 2016; 40(3):413–8.

119. Xiao B, Wang P, Zhao Y, et al. Using arterial spin labeling blood flow and its histogram analysis to distinguish early-stage nasopharyngeal carcinoma from lymphoid hyperplasia. Medicine (Baltimore) 2021;100(8):e24955.

120. Marzi S, Farneti A, Vidiri A, et al. Radiation-induced parotid changes in oropharyngeal cancer patients: the role of early functional imaging and patient-/treatment-related factors. Radiat Oncol 2018; 13(1):189.

121. Fujima N, Kameda H, Tsukahara A, et al. Diagnostic value of tumor blood flow and its histogram analysis obtained with pCASL to differentiate sinonasal malignant lymphoma from squamous cell carcinoma. Eur J Radiol 2015;84(11):2187–93.

122. Fujima N, Nakamaru Y, Sakashita T, et al. Differentiation of squamous cell carcinoma and inverted papilloma using non-invasive MR perfusion imaging. Dentomaxillofac Radiol 2015;44(9):20150074.

123. Fujima N, Shimizu Y, Yoshida D, et al. Machine-learning-based prediction of treatment outcomes using MR Imaging-derived quantitative tumor information in patients with sinonasal squamous cell carcinomas: a preliminary study. Cancers (Basel) 2019;11(6):800.

124. Xiao Z, Tang Z, Qiang J, et al. Intravoxel incoherent motion MR imaging in the differentiation of benign and malignant sinonasal lesions: comparison with conventional diffusion-weighted MR imaging. AJNR Am J Neuroradiol 2018;39(3):538–46.

125. Ryu KH, Baek HJ, Cho SB, et al. Skull metastases detecting on arterial spin labeling perfusion: Three case reports and review of literature. Medicine (Baltimore) 2017;96(44):e8432.

126. Geerts B, Leclercq D, Tezenas du Montcel S, et al. Characterization of skull base lesions using pseudo-continuous arterial spin labeling. Clin Neuroradiol 2019;29(1):75–86.

127. Kojima D, Beppu T, Saura H, et al. Apparent diffusion coefficient and arterial spin labeling perfusion of conventional chondrosarcoma in the parafalcine region: a case report. Radiol Case Rep 2017;13(1):220–4.

128. Yamamoto T, Takeuchi H, Kinoshita K, et al. Assessment of tumor blood flow and its correlation with histopathologic features in skull base meningiomas and schwannomas by using pseudo-continuous arterial spin labeling images. Eur J Radiol 2014;83(5):817–23.

129. Lin L, Chen X, Jiang R, et al. Differentiation between vestibular schwannomas and meningiomas with atypical appearance using diffusion kurtosis imaging and three-dimensional arterial spin labeling imaging. Eur J Radiol 2018;109:13–8.

130. Razek AAKA. Multi-parametric MR imaging using pseudo-continuous arterial-spin labeling and diffusion-weighted MR imaging in differentiating subtypes of parotid tumors. Magn Reson Imaging 2019;63:55–9.

131. Ma G, Xu XQ, Zhu LN, et al. Intravoxel incoherent motion magnetic resonance imaging for assessing parotid gland tumors: correlation and comparison with arterial spin labeling imaging. Korean J Radiol 2021;22(2):243–52.

132. Yamamoto T, Kimura H, Hayashi K, et al. Pseudo-continuous arterial spin labeling MR images in Warthin tumors and pleomorphic adenomas of the parotid gland: qualitative and quantitative analyses and their correlation with histopathologic and DWI and dynamic contrast enhanced MRI findings. Neuroradiology 2018;60(8):803–12.

133. Kato H, Kanematsu M, Watanabe H, et al. Perfusion imaging of parotid gland tumours: usefulness of arterial spin labeling for differentiating Warthin's tumours. Eur Radiol 2015;25(11):3247–54.

134. Khanal S, Turnbull PRK, Vaghefi E, et al. Repeatability of arterial spin labeling MRI in measuring blood perfusion in the human eye. J Magn Reson Imaging 2019;49(4):966–74.

135. Eissa L, Abdel Razek AAK, Helmy E. Arterial spin labeling and diffusion-weighted MR imaging: Utility in differentiating idiopathic orbital inflammatory pseudotumor from orbital lymphoma. Clin Imaging 2021;71:63–8.

136. Xu XQ, Hu H, Su GY, et al. Differentiation between orbital malignant and benign tumors using intravoxel incoherent motion diffusion-weighted imaging: Correlation with dynamic contrast-enhanced magnetic resonance imaging. Medicine (Baltimore) 2019;98(12):e14897.

137. Lecler A, Savatovsky J, Balvay D, et al. Repeatability of apparent diffusion coefficient and intravoxel incoherent motion parameters at 3.0 Tesla in orbital lesions. Eur Radiol 2017;27(12):5094–103.

138. Lecler A, Duron L, Zmuda M, et al. Intravoxel incoherent motion (IVIM) 3 T MRI for orbital lesion characterization. Eur Radiol 2021;31(1):14–23.

139. Jiang H, Wang S, Li Z, et al. Improving diagnostic performance of differentiating ocular adnexal lymphoma and idiopathic orbital inflammation using intravoxel incoherent motion diffusion-weighted MRI. Eur J Radiol 2020;130:109191.

140. Fujima N, Yoshida D, Sakashita T, et al. Usefulness of pseudocontinuous arterial spin-labeling for the assessment of patients with head and neck squamous cell carcinoma by measuring tumor blood flow in the pretreatment and early treatment period. AJNR Am J Neuroradiol 2016;37(2):342–8.

141. Fujima N, Kudo K, Yoshida D, et al. Arterial spin labeling to determine tumor viability in head and neck cancer before and after treatment. J Magn Reson Imaging 2014;40(4):920–8.

142. Fujima N, Kudo K, Tsukahara A, et al. Measurement of tumor blood flow in head and neck squamous cell carcinoma by pseudo-continuous arterial spin labeling: comparison with dynamic contrast-enhanced MRI. J Magn Reson Imaging 2015;41(4):983–91.

143. Abdel Razek AAK, Nada N. Arterial spin labeling perfusion-weighted MR imaging: correlation of tumor blood flow with pathological degree of tumor differentiation, clinical stage and nodal metastasis of head and neck squamous cell carcinoma. Eur Arch Otorhinolaryngol 2018;275(5):1301–7.

144. Abdel Razek AAK. Arterial spin labelling and diffusion-weighted magnetic resonance imaging in differentiation of recurrent head and neck cancer from post-radiation changes. J Laryngol Otol 2018;132(10):923–8.

145. Razek AAKA, Helmy E. Multi-parametric arterial spin labeling and diffusion-weighted imaging in differentiation of metastatic from reactive lymph nodes in head and neck squamous cell carcinoma. Eur Arch Otorhinolaryngol 2020. https://doi.org/10.1007/s00405-020-06390-0.

146. Boulouis G, Dangouloff-Ros V, Boccara O, et al. Arterial spin-labeling to discriminate pediatric cervicofacial soft-tissue vascular anomalies. AJNR Am J Neuroradiol 2017;38(3):633–8.

147. Wu B, Wang X, Guo J, et al. Collateral circulation imaging: MR perfusion territory arterial spin-labeling at 3T. AJNR Am J Neuroradiol 2008;29(10):1855–60.

148. van Osch MJ, Teeuwisse WM, Chen Z, et al. Advances in arterial spin labelling MRI methods for measuring perfusion and collateral flow. J Cereb Blood Flow Metab 2018;38(9):1461–80.

149. Morofuji Y, Horie N, Tateishi Y, et al. Arterial spin labeling magnetic resonance imaging can identify the occlusion site and collateral perfusion in patients with acute ischemic stroke: comparison with digital subtraction angiography. Cerebrovasc Dis 2019;48(1–2):70–6.

150. Okell TW, Harston GWJ, Chappell MA, et al. Measurement of collateral perfusion in acute stroke: a vessel-encoded arterial spin labeling study. Sci Rep 2019;9(1):8181.

151. Hartkamp NS, Petersen ET, Chappell MA, et al. Relationship between haemodynamic impairment and collateral blood flow in carotid artery disease. J Cereb Blood Flow Metab 2018;38(11):2021–32.

152. Lou X, Yu S, Scalzo F, et al. Multi-delay ASL can identify leptomeningeal collateral perfusion in endovascular therapy of ischemic stroke. Oncotarget 2017;8(2):2437–43.

153. Federau C, Wintermark M, Christensen S, et al. Collateral blood flow measurement with intravoxel incoherent motion perfusion imaging in hyperacute brain stroke. Neurology 2019;92(21):e2462–71.

154. Crisi G, Filice S, Scoditti U. Arterial spin labeling MRI to measure cerebral blood flow in untreated ischemic stroke. J Neuroimaging 2019;29(2):193–7.

155. Okazaki S1, Griebe M2, Gregori J2, et al. Prediction of early reperfusion from repeated arterial spin labeling perfusion magnetic resonance imaging during intravenous thrombolysis. Stroke 2016;47(1):247–50.

156. Lin T, Lai Z, Lv Y, et al. Effective collateral circulation may indicate improved perfusion territory restoration after carotid endarterectomy. Eur Radiol 2018;28(2):727–35.

157. Mirasol RV, Bokkers RP, Hernandez DA, et al. Assessing reperfusion with whole-brain arterial spin labeling: a noninvasive alternative to gadolinium. Stroke 2014;45(2):456–61.

158. Wang DJJ, Alger JR, Qiao JX, et al. Multi-delay multi-parametric arterial spin-labeled perfusion MRI in acute ischemic stroke - Comparison with dynamic susceptibility contrast enhanced perfusion imaging. Neuroimage Clin 2013;3:1–7.

159. Guo L, Zhang Q, Ding L, et al. Pseudo-continuous arterial spin labeling quantifies cerebral blood flow in patients with acute ischemic stroke and chronic lacunar stroke. Clin Neurol Neurosurg 2014;125:229–36.

160. Zhu G, Heit JJ, Martin BW, et al. Optimized combination of b-values for IVIM perfusion imaging in acute ischemic stroke patients. Clin Neuroradiol 2020;30(3):535–44.

161. Federau C, Sumer S, Becce F, et al. Intravoxel incoherent motion perfusion imaging in acute stroke: initial clinical experience. Neuroradiology 2014;56(8):629–35.

162. Suo S, Cao M, Zhu W, et al. Stroke assessment with intravoxel incoherent motion diffusion-weighted MRI. NMR Biomed 2016;29(3):320–8.

163. Yao Y, Zhang S, Tang X, et al. Intravoxel incoherent motion diffusion-weighted imaging in stroke patients: initial clinical experience. Clin Radiol 2016;71(9):938.e11–6.

164. Zhu G, Federau C, Wintermark M, et al. Comparison of MRI IVIM and MR perfusion imaging in acute ischemic stroke due to large vessel occlusion. Int J Stroke 2020;15(3):332–42.

165. Paschoal AM, Leoni RF, Dos Santos AC, et al. Intravoxel incoherent motion MRI in neurological and cerebrovascular diseases. Neuroimage Clin 2018;20:705–14.

166. Lin T, Lai Z, Zuo Z, et al. ASL perfusion features and type of circle of Willis as imaging markers for cerebral hyperperfusion after carotid revascularization: a preliminary study. Eur Radiol 2019;29(5):2651–8.

167. Okazaki S, Yamagami H, Yoshimoto T, et al. Cerebral hyperperfusion on arterial spin labeling MRI after reperfusion therapy is related to hemorrhagic transformation. J Cereb Blood Flow Metab 2017;37(9):3087–90.

168. Wang J, Pan LJ, Zhou B, et al. Crossed cerebellar diaschisis after stroke detected noninvasively by arterial spin-labeling MR imaging. BMC Neurosci 2020;21(1):46.

169. Strother MK, Buckingham C, Faraco CC, et al. Crossed cerebellar diaschisis after stroke identified noninvasively with cerebral blood flow-weighted arterial spin labeling MRI. Eur J Radiol 2016;85(1):136–42.

170. Wang J, Suo S, Zu J, et al. Detection of crossed cerebellar diaschisis by intravoxel incoherent motion MR imaging in subacute ischemic stroke. Cell Transpl 2019;28(8):1062–70.

171. Zaharchuk G, Bammer R, Straka M, et al. Arterial spin-label imaging in patients with normal bolus

perfusion-weighted MR imaging findings: pilot identification of the borderzone sign. Radiology 2009;252(3):797–807.

172. Kang JH, Yun TJ, Yoo RE, et al. Bright sinus appearance on arterial spin labeling MR imaging aids to identify cerebral venous thrombosis. Medicine (Baltimore) 2017;96(41):e8244.

173. Furuya S, Kawabori M, Fujima N, et al. Serial arterial spin labeling may be useful in assessing the therapeutic course of cerebral venous thrombosis: case reports. Neurol Med Chir (Tokyo) 2017;57(10): 557–61.

174. Huang BY, Castillo M. Hypoxic-ischemic brain injury: imaging findings from birth to adulthood. Radiographics 2008;28(2):417–39. quiz 617.

175. Kim HG, Lee JH, Choi JW, et al. Multidelay Arterial spin-labeling MRI in neonates and infants: cerebral perfusion changes during brain maturation. AJNR Am J Neuroradiol 2018;39(10):1912–8.

176. Wang JN, Li J, Liu HJ, et al. Application value of three-dimensional arterial spin labeling perfusion imaging in investigating cerebral blood flow dynamics in normal full-term neonates. BMC Pediatr 2019;19(1):495.

177. Tortora D, Severino M, Rossi A. Arterial spin labeling perfusion in neonates. Semin Fetal Neonatal Med 2020;25(5):101130.

178. Tang S, Liu X, He L, et al. Application of a 3D pseudocontinuous arterial spin-labeled perfusion MRI scan combined with a postlabeling delay value in the diagnosis of neonatal hypoxic-ischemic encephalopathy. PLoS One 2019;14(7):e0219284.

179. Watson CG, Dehaes M, Gagoski BA, et al. Arterial spin labeling perfusion magnetic resonance imaging performed in acute perinatal stroke reveals hyperperfusion associated with ischemic injury. Stroke 2016;47(6):1514–9.

180. De Vis JB, Petersen ET, Kersbergen KJ, et al. Evaluation of perinatal arterial ischemic stroke using noninvasive arterial spin labeling perfusion MRI. Pediatr Res 2013;74(3):307–13.

181. De Vis JB, Hendrikse J, Petersen ET, et al. Arterial spin-labelling perfusion MRI and outcome in neonates with hypoxic-ischemic encephalopathy. Eur Radiol 2015;25(1):113–21.

182. Pollock JM, Whitlow CT, Deibler AR, et al. Anoxic injury-associated cerebral hyperperfusion identified with arterial spin-labeled MR imaging. AJNR Am J Neuroradiol 2008;29(7):1302–7.

183. Prosser DD, Grigsby T, Pollock JM. Unilateral anoxic brain injury secondary to strangulation identified on conventional and arterial spin-labeled perfusion imaging. Radiol Case Rep 2018;13(3): 563–7.

184. Iordanova B, Li L, Clark RSB, et al. Alterations in cerebral blood flow after resuscitation from cardiac arrest. Front Pediatr 2017;5:174.

185. Li N, Wingfield MA, Nickerson JP, et al. Anoxic brain injury detection with the normalized diffusion to ASL perfusion ratio: implications for blood-brain barrier injury and permeability. AJNR Am J Neuroradiol 2020;41(4):598–606.

186. Wu B, Yang Y, Zhou S, et al. Could arterial spin labeling distinguish patients in minimally conscious state from patients in vegetative state? Front Neurol 2018;9:110.

187. Kang KM, Yun TJ, Yoon BW, et al. Clinical utility of arterial spin-labeling as a confirmatory test for suspected brain death. AJNR Am J Neuroradiol 2015 May;36(5):909–14.

188. Federau C, Nguyen A, Christensen S, et al. Cerebral perfusion measurement in brain death with intravoxel incoherent motion imaging. Neurovasc Imaging 2016;2:9.

189. Vaghefi E, Pontré B. Application of arterial spin labelling in the assessment of ocular tissues. Biomed Res Int 2016;2016:6240504.

190. Vaghefi E, Kauv K, Pan W, et al. Application of arterial spin labelling in detecting retinal ischemia. Case Rep Ophthalmol 2017;8(3):545–57.

191. Lu P, Sha Y, Wan H, et al. Assessment of nonarteritic anterior ischemic optic neuropathy with intravoxel incoherent motion diffusion-weighted imaging using readout-segmented echo-planar imaging, parallel imaging, and 2D navigator-based reacquisition. J Magn Reson Imaging 2017;46(6): 1760–6.

192. Wang R, Yu S, Alger JR, et al. Multi-delay arterial spin labeling perfusion MRI in moyamoya disease–comparison with CT perfusion imaging. Eur Radiol 2014;24(5):1135–44.

193. Fan AP, Guo J, Khalighi MM, et al. Long-delay arterial spin labeling provides more accurate cerebral blood flow measurements in moyamoya patients: a simultaneous positron emission tomography/MRI Study. Stroke 2017;48(9):2441–9.

194. Federau C, Christensen S, Zun Z, et al. Cerebral blood flow, transit time, and apparent diffusion coefficient in moyamoya disease before and after acetazolamide. Neuroradiology 2017;59(1): 5–12.

195. Kronenburg A, Bulder MMM, Bokkers RPH, et al. Cerebrovascular reactivity measured with ASL perfusion MRI, ivy sign, and regional tissue vascularization in moyamoya. World Neurosurg 2019; 125:e639–50.

196. Agarwal V, Singh P, Ahuja CK, et al. Non-invasive assessment of cerebral microvascular changes for predicting postoperative cerebral hyperperfusion after surgical revascularisation for moyamoya disease: an arterial spin labelling MRI study. Neuroradiology 2021;63(4):563–72.

197. Ha JY, Choi YH, Lee S, et al. Arterial spin labeling MRI for quantitative assessment of cerebral

perfusion before and after cerebral revascularization in children with moyamoya disease. Korean J Radiol 2019;20(6):985–96.

198. Hara S, Hori M, Ueda R, et al. Intravoxel incoherent motion perfusion in patients with Moyamoya disease: comparison with 15O-gas positron emission tomography. Acta Radiol Open 2019;8(5). 2058460119846587.

199. Bulder MM, Bokkers RP, Hendrikse J, et al. Arterial spin labeling perfusion MRI in children and young adults with previous ischemic stroke and unilateral intracranial arteriopathy. Cerebrovasc Dis 2014; 37(1):14–21.

200. Wakisaka K, Morioka T, Shimogawa T, et al. Epileptic ictal hyperperfusion on arterial spin labeling perfusion and diffusion-weighted magnetic resonance images in posterior reversible encephalopathy syndrome. J Stroke Cerebrovasc Dis 2016; 25(1):228–37.

201. Wazni W, Farooq S, Cox JA, et al. Use of arterial spin-labeling in patients with aneurysmal subarachnoid hemorrhage. J Vasc Interv Neurol 2019;10(3):10–4.

202. Heit JJ, Wintermark M, Martin BW, et al. Reduced intravoxel incoherent motion microvascular perfusion predicts delayed cerebral ischemia and vasospasm after aneurysm rupture. Stroke 2018;49(3): 741–5.

203. Fiehler J, Illies T, Piening M, et al. Territorial and microvascular perfusion impairment in brain arteriovenous malformations. AJNR Am J Neuroradiol 2009;30(2):356–61.

204. Zhang M, Telischak NA, Fischbein NJ, et al. Clinical and arterial spin labeling brain mri features of transitional venous anomalies. J Neuroimaging 2018; 28(3):289–300.

205. Iv M, Fischbein NJ, Zaharchuk G. Association of developmental venous anomalies with perfusion abnormalities on arterial spin labeling and bolus perfusion-weighted imaging. J Neuroimaging 2015;25(2):243–50.

206. Wu G, Liu X, Xiong Y, et al. Intravoxel incoherent motion and diffusion kurtosis imaging for discriminating soft tissue sarcoma from vascular anomalies. Medicine (Baltimore) 2018;97(50):e13641.

207. Iwamura M, Midorikawa H, Shibutani K, et al. High-signal venous sinuses on MR angiography: discrimination between reversal of venous flow and arteriovenous shunting using arterial spin labeling. Neuroradiology 2020. https://doi.org/10.1007/s00234-020-02588-5. Epub ahead of print.

208. Le TT, Fischbein NJ, André JB, et al. Identification of venous signal on arterial spin labeling improves diagnosis of dural arteriovenous fistulas and small arteriovenous malformations. AJNR Am J Neuroradiol 2012;33(1):61–8.

209. Lam J, Tomaszewski P, Gilbert G, et al. The utility of arterial spin labeling in the presurgical evaluation of poorly defined focal epilepsy in children. J Neurosurg Pediatr 2020;1–10.

210. Matsuura K, Maeda M, Okamoto K, et al. Usefulness of arterial spin-labeling images in periictal state diagnosis of epilepsy. J Neurol Sci 2015; 359(1–2):424–9.

211. Pizzini FB, Farace P, Manganotti P, et al. Cerebral perfusion alterations in epileptic patients during peri-ictal and post-ictal phase: PASL vs DSC-MRI. Magn Reson Imaging 2013;31(6):1001–5.

212. Schertz M, Benzakoun J, Pyatigorskaya N, et al. Specificities of arterial spin labeling (ASL) abnormalities in acute seizure. J Neuroradiol 2020; 47(1):20–6.

213. Nagesh C, Kumar S, Menon R, et al. The imaging of localization related symptomatic epilepsies: the value of arterial spin labelling based magnetic resonance perfusion. Korean J Radiol 2018;19(5): 965–77.

214. Perera T, Gaxiola-Valdez I, Singh S, et al, Calgary Comprehensive Epilepsy Program collaborators. Localizing the seizure onset zone by comparing patient postictal hypoperfusion to healthy controls. J Neurosci Res 2020;98(8):1517–31.

215. Won J, Choi DS, Hong SJ, et al. Crossed cerebellar hyperperfusion in patients with seizure-related cerebral cortical lesions: an evaluation with arterial spin labelling perfusion MR imaging. Radiol Med 2018;123(11):843–50.

216. Federau C, O'Brien K, Meuli R, et al. Measuring brain perfusion with intravoxel incoherent motion (IVIM): initial clinical experience. J Magn Reson Imaging 2014;39(3):624–32.

217. Cobb-Pitstick KM, Munjal N, Safier R, et al. Time course of cerebral perfusion changes in children with migraine with aura mimicking stroke. AJNR Am J Neuroradiol 2018;39(9):1751–5.

218. Wolf ME, Okazaki S, Eisele P, et al. Arterial spin labeling cerebral perfusion magnetic resonance imaging in migraine aura: an observational study. J Stroke Cerebrovasc Dis 2018;27(5):1262–6.

219. Cadiot D, Longuet R, Bruneau B, et al. Magnetic resonance imaging in children presenting migraine with aura: Association of hypoperfusion detected by arterial spin labelling and vasospasm on MR angiography findings. Cephalalgia 2018;38(5): 949–58.

220. Corno S, Giani L, Laganà MM, et al. The brain effect of the migraine attack: an ASL MRI study of the cerebral perfusion during a migraine attack. Neurol Sci 2018;39(Suppl 1):73–4.

221. Kato Y, Araki N, Matsuda H, et al. Arterial spin-labeled MRI study of migraine attacks treated with rizatriptan. J Headache Pain 2010;11(3):255–8.

222. Andre JB. Arterial spin labeling magnetic resonance perfusion for traumatic brain injury: technical
challenges and potentials. Top Magn Reson Imaging 2015;24(5):275–87.

223. Kenney K, Amyot F, Haber M, et al. Cerebral
vascular injury in traumatic brain injury. Exp Neurol
2016;275 Pt 3:353–66.

224. Hasan KM, Keser Z, Schulz PE, et al. Multimodal
advanced imaging for concussion. Neuroimaging
Clin N Am 2018;28(1):31–42.

225. Wong AM, Yeh CH, Liu HL, et al. Arterial spin-
labeling perfusion imaging of children with subdural
hemorrhage: Perfusion abnormalities in abusive
head trauma. J Neuroradiol 2017;44(4):281–7.

226. Koudriavtseva T, Plantone D, Renna R, et al. Brain
perfusion by arterial spin labeling MRI in multiple
sclerosis. J Neurol 2015;262(7):1769–71.

227. de la Peña MJ, Peña IC, García PG, et al. Early
perfusion changes in multiple sclerosis patients
as assessed by MRI using arterial spin labeling.
Acta Radiol Open 2019;8(12). 2058460119894214.

228. Noda T, Araki M, Yamamura T, et al. Abnormalities
of cerebral blood flow in multiple sclerosis: a pseudocontinuous arterial spin labeling MRI study.
Magn Reson Imaging 2013;31(6):990–5.

229. D'Ortenzio RM, Hojjat SP, Vitorino R, et al. Comparison of quantitative cerebral blood flow measurements performed by bookend dynamic
susceptibility contrast and arterial spin-labeling
MRI in relapsing-remitting multiple sclerosis.
AJNR Am J Neuroradiol 2016;37(12):2265–72.

230. Iwasawa T, Matoba H, Ogi A, et al. Diffusion-
weighted imaging of the human optic nerve: a
new approach to evaluate optic neuritis in multiple
sclerosis. Magn Reson Med 1997;38(3):484–91.

Contrast Pediatric Brain Perfusion
Dynamic Susceptibility Contrast and Dynamic Contrast-Enhanced MR Imaging

Mohannad Ibrahim, MD[a], Talha Ul Ghazi, BS[b], Jayapalli Rajiv Bapuraj, MD[a], Ashok Srinivasan, MD[a],*

KEYWORDS

• MR perfusion • DSC • DCE • Pediatric • Tumors • Ischemia

KEY POINTS

• MR perfusion is a noninvasive MR technique that provides insight into regional cerebral vascularity and guides the management of neoplastic and ischemic disorders.
• Relatively low relative cerebral blood volume (rCBV) is highly sensitive in excluding high-grade pediatric brain tumors. However, high rCBV values are reported in a subgroup of low-grade pediatric tumors, limiting specificity.
• MR perfusion parameters can help guide management of pediatric acute ischemic stroke by demonstrating a small core infarct and the presence of salvageable penumbra based on Tmax maps.

INTRODUCTION
Definition

Perfusion magnetic resonance (MR) imaging of the brain is a unique dynamic imaging technique that provides an insight to the perfusion of cerebral parenchyma and supplies valuable information complementary to traditional structural MRI. MR perfusion is easily implemented and is routinely used in clinical practice to diagnose and manage different brain abnormalities in adult patients. The noninvasive nature of MR perfusion, its accuracy in assessing hemodynamic alterations, and the widespread availability of MRI scanners render MR perfusion ideally suited for pediatric population, including young-age and low-weight children.[1,2] MR perfusion is a powerful imaging modality in the assessment of ischemic conditions, either by evaluating the ischemic penumbra or measuring the vascular reserve, or in the characterization of the vascularity of neoplastic lesions. Calculating the ischemic penumbra or vascular reserve provides valuable information necessary for decision making and patient management in the setting of acute infarcts or chronic ischemic conditions. Similarly, assessment of tumor vascularity can help in characterizing the biological behavior of tumors, which otherwise can appear similar on conventional imaging.

Techniques

MR perfusion uses variable imaging techniques to noninvasively evaluate a variety of hemodynamic

[a] Radiology Department, Neuroradiology Division, University of Michigan, 1500 East Medical Center Drive, Ann Arbor, MI 48109, USA; [b] Michigan State University, College of Human Medicine, 965 Fee Road A110, East Lansing, MI 48824, USA
* Corresponding author. Radiology Department, Neuroradiology Division, University of Michigan, B2-A209UH, 1500 East Medical Center Drive, Ann Arbor, MI 48109.
E-mail address: ashoks@med.umich.edu
Twitter: @AshokSrini15 (A.S.)

Magn Reson Imaging Clin N Am 29 (2021) 515–526
https://doi.org/10.1016/j.mric.2021.06.004
1064-9689/21/© 2021 Elsevier Inc. All rights reserved.

parameters that reflect regional vascularity in the brain. A commonly used technique is by tracking the first pass of an exogenous, paramagnetic, contrast agent as it passes through the tissues.[3] This technique is based on an assumption that the injected contrast agent remains restricted to the intravascular compartment without capillary permeability or diffusion into the extracellular space. Following the intravenous contrast injection and data acquisition, a set of hemodynamic parameters are generated by modeling the method of the tracer's passage or distribution in the target organ. Dynamic susceptibility contrast MR perfusion (DSC-MRP) and dynamic contrast-enhanced MR perfusion (DCE-MRP) use this technique to derive several perfusion values of the cerebral parenchyma. A less frequently used technique is arterial spin labeling, which exploits the ability of MR imaging to magnetically label arterial blood below the imaging slab without the use of externally administered intravenous gadolinium.

DYNAMIC SUSCEPTIBILITY CONTRAST MAGNETIC RESONANCE PERFUSION
Definition

DSC-MRP, or bolus-tracking MR imaging, is a commonly used technique in MR perfusion with high-quality quantitative evaluation and hemodynamic parameters in pediatric patients.[1] DSC-MRP exploits susceptibility-induced signal loss following the first pass of gadolinium-based contrast bolus through the cerebral capillary bed.[3,4] Therefore, it is probably more accurate to refer to this technique as dynamic susceptibility contrast-enhanced MR perfusion. Unfortunately, the latter name can create confusion with another perfusion MR technique, dynamic contrast-enhanced MR perfusion (DCE-MRP), which is fundamentally different as it assesses the T1 signal shortening following the intravenous administration of gadolinium-based contrast agent.

Technique

DSC technique relies on serially measuring the concentration of contrast agent in a target region of interest using ultrafast echoplanar imaging–based spin-echo or more commonly gradient-echo sequences. Gradient-echo techniques are probably more sensitive to larger vessels, whereas the capillary blood vessels are better characterized using spin-echo sequences.[5] The susceptibility effect of the contrast material is required to dominate the image contrast to generate meaningful data. Therefore, a power injector is needed to inject a narrow bolus of the contrast agent to achieve high intravascular concentrations of

gadolinium. The usage of power injector in pediatric patients is typically safe regardless of the flow rate, catheter size, or its location in the hand, arm, or foot.[1] Following the rapid intravenous injection of exogenous tracer agent and image acquisition, the region's susceptibility-induced signal loss is interrogated over the time course to generate a signal-time curve data. The signal-time curve data are then converted to a tracer tissue concentration-time curve, which can then be analyzed to determine various tissue hemodynamic parameters.

This analysis is dependent on specific features related to the contrast bolus, such as the amount of injected contrast material, injection rate, and the paramagnetic properties of the contrast agent, as well as variable factors, that is, subject-related, such as total-body vascular volume and cardiac output. Consequently, the hemodynamic parameters can differ at different times in the same subject or in-between subjects limiting its value. *Therefore, semiquantitative or relative values are typically obtained, which requires using the normal-appearing gray or white matter or an arterial input function as an internal standard of reference, allowing a reliable inter-subject and intra-subject comparison.* As the DSC-MRP technique depends on exploiting the susceptibility-induced signal loss due to small amounts of contrast, a larger susceptibility effect with significant signal loss can potentially limit the value of the collected data and the calculated hemodynamic parameters. This is typically encountered related to the presence of blood products or calcification, or due to artifact from aerated sinuses or adjacent dense bone, particularly at the skull base level. A similar limitation can be seen with prominent signal loss immediately adjacent to large vessels (**Fig. 1**).

Key Parameters

Cerebral blood volume (CBV) is defined as the volume of blood in a given region of brain tissue, most commonly measured in milliliters of blood per 100 g of brain tissue. CBV is roughly proportional to negative enhancement integral. Cerebral blood flow, measured in milliliters per minute per 100 g of brain tissue, refers to the volume of blood per unit time passing through a given region of brain tissue. Mean transit time refers to the average time it takes the bolus to pass through a given region of brain tissue, commonly measured in seconds. CBV has been the primary hemodynamic parameter used in brain tumor perfusion imaging. Calculation of CBV is performed by assessing the area under the tissue concentration-time   curve.   An   accurate

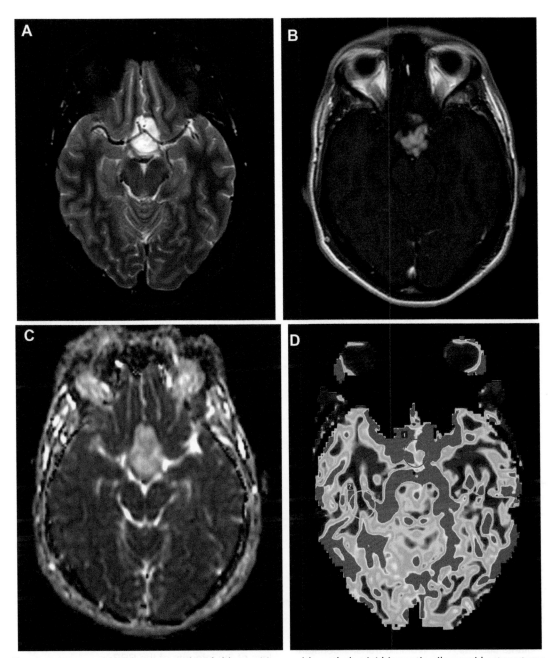

Fig. 1. A 17-year-old male presented with blurry vision and hypothalamic/chiasmatic pilomyxoid astrocytoma. Axial T2-weighted imaging demonstrated a lobulated T2 hyperintense mass (*A*), with heterogeneous enhancement (*B*). The lesion had hyperintense signal on apparent diffusion coefficient (ADC) maps (*C*) with ADC measuring 1.79×10^{-3} mm²/s (*D*). rCBV map obtained at the skull base was significantly compromised by prominent signal related to the circle of Willis vasculature.

calculation of CBV requires measuring only the first pass of contrast agent without recirculation and the lack of capillary permeability, which can vary dramatically. Therefore, the CBV is calculated relative to an internal control, such as normal white matter or an arterial input function, generating a more robust and reproducible relative CBV (rCBV), which has no unit value, as it represents a ratio. Calculation of the brain clearance, or mean transit time, is generated by deconvolution of the arterial input function from tissue concentration-time data. CBV is then divided by mean transit time to obtain cerebral blood flow. Alternatively, the cerebral blood flow can be calculated by measuring the initial height of the deconvolved tissue concentration-time curve, with the mean transit time calculated as the ratio of CBV to cerebral blood flow.

DYNAMIC CONTRAST-ENHANCED MAGNETIC RESONANCE PERFUSION
Definition and Technique

DCE-MRP or permeability MR imaging is a rapid T1-weighted MRP technique that evaluates the relaxivity effects, rather than susceptibility effect, induced by a gadolinium-based contrast bolus passing through tissue.[3,4] In contrast to the shortening of T2 or T2* relaxation times used in DSC-MRP, the relaxivity effect used in DCE-MRP refers to higher T1 signal related to shortening of the T1 relaxation time. The DCE-MRP requires a smaller amount of contrast material compared with DSC-MRP technique, as the relaxivity effects of contrast bolus are much stronger than the susceptibility effects. DCE-MRP imaging is based on a pharmacokinetic model of 2 compartments, namely the plasma space and extravascular-extracellular space. The native T1 value of the tissues typically affect the nonlinear relationship between signal intensity and concentration of the gadolinium-based contrast agent. Therefore, DCE-MRP requires a baseline T1 mapping, which is followed by acquiring MRP data, then converting the signal intensity curve to gadolinium concentration curve, and finally performing a pharmacokinetic modeling of the contrast passage and distribution. Similar to DSC-MRP technique, the use of a power injector is mandatory for bolus injection.[4]

Calculated Parameters

Various kinetic modeling of contrast movement can be calculated using this technique to assess contrast spillage and the integrity of blood brain barrier (BBB). DCE-MRP provides transfer constants such as K^{trans} (volume transfer constant between blood plasma and extravascular-extracellular space [EES]), V_e (volume of the EES per unit volume of tissue), K_{ep} (rate constant between plasma and EES, where $K_{ep} = K^{trans}/V_e$). Interpretation of K^{trans}, the most commonly calculated parameter, is variable depending on capillary permeability and blood flow. K^{trans} is dependent on plasma blood flow, vascular permeability, and capillary surface area. K^{trans} is a useful measure of permeability in instances in which the BBB is intact and the permeability is very low, whereas K^{trans} will reflect blood flow in disrupted BBB with high permeability.

CLINICAL APPLICATIONS
Pediatric Brain Tumors

Brain tumors are the second most common malignancy among children and the leading cause of death from solid tumors in pediatric patients.[5] The prognosis of pediatric brain tumors depends on the tumor's location, histology, molecular features, and genetics. Clinical and molecular stratification with recent advances in surgical techniques and adjuvant therapies have provided insights into newer therapeutic targets with improved outcome of low-grade gliomas and medulloblastomas, with the 5-year survival rate exceeding 75%.[6,7] The outcome remains discouraging for children with diffuse intrinsic pontine gliomas and high-grade gliomas despite significant advancements in chemotherapy and radiation therapy, with the 5-year survival rate remaining less than 25%.[6,7] Conventional MR imaging remains the mainstay imaging modality in the detection and characterization of pediatric brain tumors. Multiple advanced MRI techniques are typically used for evaluation of pediatric brain tumors, such as MR diffusion, MR spectroscopy (MRS), and MR perfusion, emphasizing the complementary role of these techniques.[5,7–11] MR diffusion and MRS can provide biological characterization of the tumor by assessing its cellularity and metabolism. Similarly, MR perfusion can complement structural imaging by assessing tumor vascularity, providing further insight into the tumor biological behavior. Contrast enhancement of neoplastic lesions in conventional MRI is typically related to breakdown of the BBB or vascular hyperplasia.[12] Pathologic alteration of the BBB is related to destruction of normal capillaries or neoangiogenesis with newly formed abnormal capillaries. There is, however, poor correlation between the degree of tumoral enhancement on one hand, and tumor grading and cellularity on the other,[12] with both malignant and benign tumors demonstrating variable enhancement.[5] The degree of tumor perfusion reflects its vascularity at a microscopic level regardless of the integrity of the BBB.

There are few studies assessing the utility of rCBV in pediatric brain tumors with mixed results,[7,9,11,13–16] compared with the widely accepted role of rCBV in assessing the grade of adult glial tumors.[12,17,18] In adult glial tumors, high-grade tumors are typically characterized by a higher average rCBV value compared with a significantly lower average rCBV in low-grade glioma.[12,17,18] Although rCBV values have consistently demonstrated a low rCBV value in low-grade adult glial tumors, there is considerable overlap in rCBV values of low-grade and high-grade pediatric brain

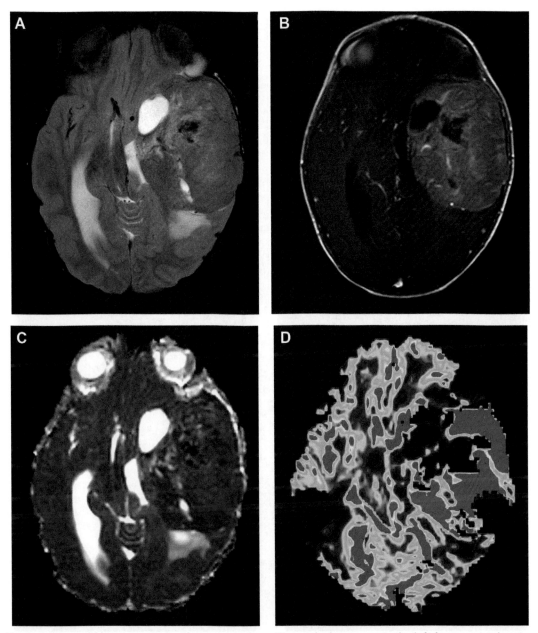

Fig. 2. A 5-year-old boy presented with nausea and vomiting and a large mass in the left frontoparietal region. Axial T2-weighted and post enhanced images demonstrated T2 isointense, heterogeneously enhancing mass (*A, B*), with hypointense signal on apparent diffusion coefficient (ADC) maps (*C*). ADC measured 0.8×10^{-3} mm^2/s (*D*). rCBV map demonstrated relative heterogeneity with extensive increased perfusion laterally and posteriorly in the lesion. Pathology confirmed anaplastic pleomorphic xanthoastrocytoma, World Health Organization grade III.

tumors.[13,19] High-grade pediatric glial tumors typically demonstrate high rCBV values (**Fig. 2**). Hence, this is valuable in excluding high-grade tumors in pediatric brain tumors when they demonstrate low rCBV values,[13] and helps to confirm the diagnosis of low-grade tumors (**Figs. 3** and **4**).[13,20] However, rCBV has a low specificity, as high

rCBV values can be seen in a subgroup of low-grade pediatric tumors.[13] Relative CBV can have an interestingly limited role in some of the pediatric brain tumors, such as pilocytic astrocytomas and medulloblastomas. Pilocytic astrocytoma, a low-grade tumor, can present with low or very high rCBV values,[5,7,16] compared with

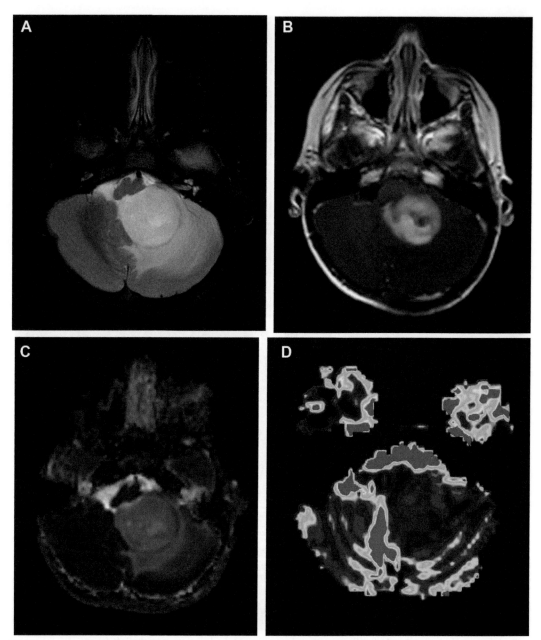

Fig. 3. A 2-year-old girl presented with headache and ataxia and a large pilocytic astrocytoma in the posterior fossa. Axial T2-weighted image demonstrated a nodular T2 hyperintense mass (*A*), with avid enhancement on postcontrast T1-weighted image (*B*). The lesion had hyperintense signal on apparent diffusion coefficient (ADC) map (*C*) with ADC measuring 1.75×10^{-3} mm^2/s (*D*). rCBV map demonstrated low signal associated with the lesion with relatively low rCBV value.

medulloblastomas, grade IV tumor, which may present with low rCBV values, particularly when presenting in older patients.[8,21]

The role of K^{trans} in the assessment of neoangiogenesis and increased leakiness of the tumor vasculature is well-documented and correlates well with tumor grade, particularly in adults.[22–24]

There is significant correlation between DCE-MRP hemodynamic parameters (K^{trans}, K_{ep}, and V_e) with tumor grade in pediatric brain tumors as well.[25,26] High-grade tumors (grade III and IV) demonstrate higher K^{trans} and K_{ep} values with a lower V_e value (**Fig. 5**), compared with low-grade tumors (grade I and II), with K_{ep} showing the

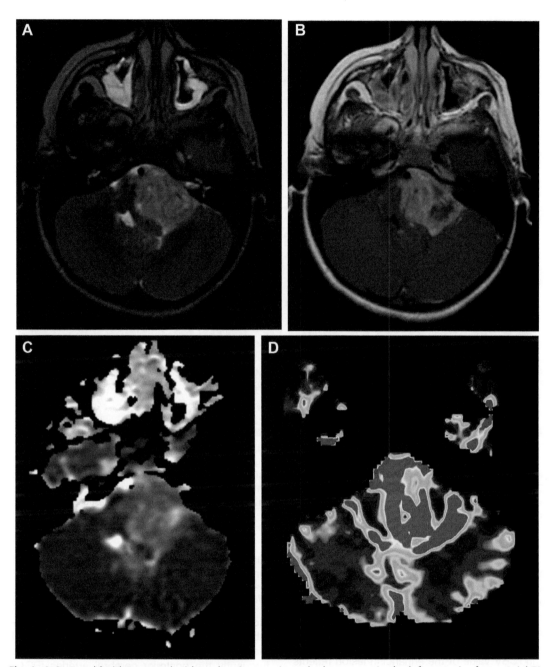

Fig. 4. A 4-year-old girl presented with neck pain, emesis, and a large mass in the left posterior fossa. Axial T2-weighted and post enhanced T1-weighted images demonstrated T2 hyperintense, heterogeneously enhancing mass (*A, B*), with slightly hyperintense signal on apparent diffusion coefficient (ADC) map (*C*). ADC measured 1.2×10^{-3} mm²/s (*D*). rCBV maps demonstrated relative heterogeneity with extensive increased perfusion. Pathology confirmed anaplastic ependymoma, World Health Organization grade III.

highest specificity for separating both grades.[25,26] Although V_e is an indicator of extracellular extravascular space, its exact role is not yet fully defined.[27] It is possible that the higher cellularity in high-grade tumors lead to decreased extracellular space with relatively packed tumor cells, and hence lower V_e.[25] Law and colleagues[18] found a strong correlation between rCBV and tumor grade; however, there is a weaker correlation of tumor grade and K^{trans}, suggesting these parameters probably reflect different tumoral characteristics.

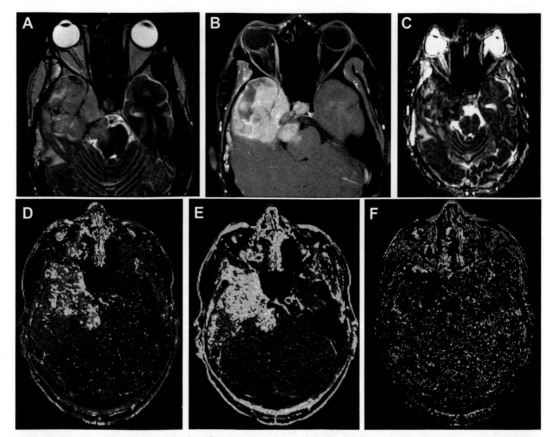

Fig. 5. An 18-year-old male individual with progressively enlarging undifferentiated sarcoma in the left middle cranial fossa. Axial T2-weighted and post enhanced T1-weighted images demonstrate mildly T2 hyperintense, heterogeneously enhancing mass (*A, B*), with hypointense signal on apparent diffusion coefficient (ADC) map (*C*). ADC measured 0.94×10^{-3} mm^2/s. (*D*) K^{trans} map demonstrates relative heterogeneity with extensive increased perfusion. There is relatively increased signal on V$_e$ map (*E*) with slightly increased signal on K$_{ep}$ map (*F*).

Distinction of posttreatment effects from recurrent or residual tumors is critical in the management of pediatric patients with malignant brain tumors. Contrast-enhanced conventional MRI is unreliable in differentiating tumor recurrence as postradiation necrosis and pseudoprogression may mimic tumor on conventional MR imaging. High rCBV value of the enhancing lesion reflects tumor recurrence in pediatric patients, compared with low rCBV value seen in radiation necrosis and postoperative granulation tissues (**Fig. 6**).[9,28,29] Ball and colleagues[19] described increased or normal perfusion patterns in recurrent tumors in children, compared with ischemia and vascular injury in radiation injury leading to regional hypoperfusion and breakdown of the BBB. The exact pathogenesis leading to radiation necrosis remains unknown. A constant pathologic features in radiation necrosis is extensive endothelial injury and fibrinoid necrosis, in contrast to vascular proliferation associated with recurrent tumor.[30]

Moyamoya Syndrome

Moyamoya syndrome (MMS) is a progressive cerebrovascular disorder resulting in occlusion of the terminal internal carotid artery (ICA), or less frequently the posterior cerebral arteries (PCA), with collateral vessels in the basal ganglia. This may be idiopathic or may occur secondary to sickle cell disease or neurofibromatosis among many other disorders.[31] Presentation is age dependent, with pediatric patients presenting with transient ischemic attacks, watershed infarcts, or hemispheric ischemic strokes, compared with cerebral hemorrhage typically seen in adults. Hemodynamically mediated perfusion abnormality typically accounts for ischemic symptoms rather than thromboembolism. Conventional MR imaging is important in identifying

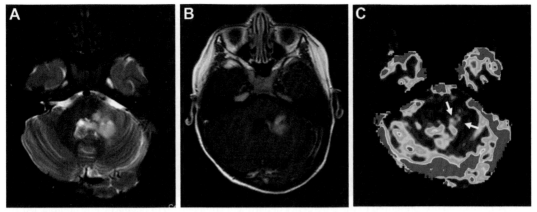

Fig. 6. A 3-year-old girl status post resection of a large cerebellar pilocytic astrocytoma. Axial T2-weighted and post enhanced T1-weighted images demonstrate irregular T2 hyperintense lesion with enhancement at the superior margin of the surgical bed (*A, B*). rCBV map overlaid on postcontrast T1-weighted image demonstrates slightly increased perfusion of the enhancing nodule, in keeping with recurrent neoplasm (*C*).

the extent of parenchymal injury and in the assessment of acute intracranial processes.

Identification of abnormal cerebral perfusion is critical in the evaluation of patients with MMS and assessing treatment response, as reperfusion using surgical cerebral revascularization is commonly performed. DSC-MRP can identify areas of diffusion-perfusion mismatch in acute ischemic strokes, believed to represent tissue "at risk," or identify hypoperfused tissue in asymptomatic patients that appear otherwise normal on conventional MR imaging. Mean transit time positively correlated with the degree of ICA and PCA stenosis reflecting abnormal cerebral perfusion.[32] In addition, prediction of postoperative revascularization outcome was directly related to the preoperative perfusion status, namely time-to-peak maps, which also facilitated the sequential monitoring of perfusion changes following treatment.[33] The value of MR perfusion can be limited by the presence of collateral vessels causing significant delays and the lack of normal internal standard of reference, particularly in bilateral ICA disease. However, MR perfusion can still provide clinically useful information in patients with MMS despite its technical limitations.[34] PET and single-photon emission computed tomography (CT) can delineate areas of cerebral hypoperfusion; however, their value is limited given the high radiation dose, thereby limiting repeated examinations and the lack of structural assessment of the hypoperfused tissue.

Stroke

Pediatric arterial ischemic stroke (AIS) is not rare, and is frequently overlooked as a possibility by caregivers and clinicians, often delaying

appropriate management. Clinical studies during the past decade, mostly in adults, have shown the ability of MR perfusion to evaluate patients presenting with acute stroke and assessing the hypoperfused volume. The combination of diffusion-weighted imaging (DWI) and perfusion is used to estimate the "mismatch" between the DWI and perfusion sequences that potentially represent the salvageable ischemic brain tissue. The DEFUSE study (Diffusion and Perfusion Imaging Evaluation for Understanding Stroke Evolution) demonstrated a favorable clinical response in patients with perfusion/diffusion mismatch. Patient selection was based on the concept of target mismatch, defined as a mismatch ratio (MMR) of at least 1.2 with minimal penumbra volume of 10 mL, in addition to severely hypoperfused tissue volume and a maximum core (time to maximum delay [Tmax] ≥8 seconds, DWI volume <100 mL).[35] The DEFUSE 2 study redefined the mismatch ratio definition to MMR greater than 1.8, penumbra greater than 15 mL, DWI volume less than 70 mL, and Tmax greater than 10 seconds, volume less than 100 mL.[36]

Few clinical studies have been performed in children for the utility of MR perfusion parameters in the management of AIS. Lee and colleagues[37] reported on the value of perfusion imaging in pediatric AIS to identify salvageable tissue in extended time windows, with Tmax >4 seconds appearing to better correlate with the National Institutes of Health Stroke Scale (NIHSS). The penumbral thresholds accepted in this unique population include evidence of a large vessel occlusion on MR or CT angiography (ICA, first or second segment of the middle cerebral artery, vertebral artery, or basilar artery), a small-core infarct

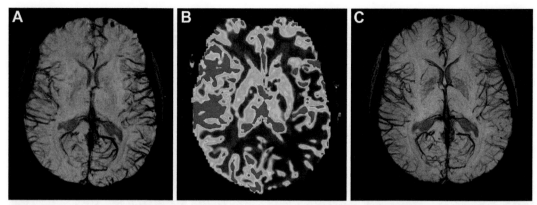

Fig. 7. A 13-year-old boy presented to the emergency department complaining of headache and aphasia. (*A*) SWI image demonstrates asymmetric prominent vessels in the left cerebral hemisphere involving mostly the parietal and occipital lobes, likely related to venous stasis. Corresponding DWI sequence (not shown) was normal. (*B*) DSC-MR perfusion (CBV) demonstrates asymmetric decreased perfusion in the left cerebral hemisphere, with involvement of the MCA and PCA territories. (*C*) Follow-up SWI image after 1 day demonstrated normalization of the SWI asymmetry.

volume (<70 mL quantified by DWI, or Alberta Stroke Programme early CT score ≥7 on noncontrast CT), presence of salvageable penumbra determined by MR or CT perfusion deficit on the Tmax maps; and abnormal neurologic examination with cortical signs, typically NIHSS ≥6. Reperfusion was achieved by thrombectomy alone (7 of 9 patients); one received intravenous (IV) alteplase and thrombectomy, and one received IV alteplase alone. Applying these criteria in patient selection for management of AIS demonstrated favorable outcome in 78% of treated patients compared with very poor outcome in untreated patients.

Hemiplegic Migraine

Hemiplegic migraine is a rare subtype of migraine associated with motor weakness, and more often seen in children. It is a subtype of complicated migraine, which refers to the association of migraine headache with neurologic deficits, such as motor disturbance, sensory impairment, or speech problems. Conversely, typical migraine typically presents with headache and aura characterized by photophobia, vertigo, nausea, and vomiting. A hemiplegic migraine can be familial (familial hemiplegic migraine) or sporadic. Although the pathogenesis of the migraine remains unclear, it is probably complex related to vasoconstriction with associated aura or neurologic symptoms, followed by vasodilation and headaches. MR perfusion typically demonstrates reduction in cerebral blood flow during the aura phase caused by vasoconstriction, which is subsequently followed by headache secondary to the vasodilation with resultant normalization of the cerebral

hemodynamics.[38,39] The perfusion abnormality is seen in multiple vascular territories of the affected hemisphere, in contrast to patients with stroke or transient ischemic attack, which typically have a perfusion abnormality localized to a specific vascular territory.[38] Susceptibility-weighted imaging (SWI) typically reveals cerebral venous prominence in the area of impaired perfusion (**Fig. 7**). This is likely related to relative increase in deoxyhemoglobin levels and decrease in oxyhemoglobin in the draining vein, probably secondary to uncoupling between oxygen supply and demand in the hypoperfused region.

Sturge-Weber Syndrome

Sturge-Weber syndrome, or encephalotrigeminal angiomatosis, is a phakomatosis characterized by leptomeningeal angiomatosis and facial naevus. MR imaging is essential in confirming the diagnosis and assessing the extent of intracranial abnormalities by demonstrating prominent leptomeningeal enhancement in the affected area and sometimes the presence of venous abnormalities. Perfusion abnormalities closely related to the area of meningeal enhancement are typically seen on MR perfusion.[40] Additional areas of decreased perfusion can be seen associated with some of the coexisting developmental venous anomalies.[40] A crossed cerebellar diaschisis with depression in the perfusion of the contralateral cerebellar hemisphere is uncommonly seen.[40]

SUMMARY

Extensive progress is being made in the understanding of brain pathologic processes in the pediatric population, including advancement in the management of acute and chronic ischemic processes, along with recent discoveries about brain tumors that have changed our understanding of tumor biology and management. MR perfusion imaging can be successfully performed in pediatric patients and has proven to expand our understanding with improving guidance for management. Although hemodynamic parameters from DSC-MRP and DCE-MRP reflect different physiologic and pathologic properties, they have been complementary to conventional MR imaging in characterizing different pathologic processes. Larger trials incorporating advanced imaging techniques, such as perfusion imaging, are crucial to further refining our understanding of their role in different diseases and help establish more quantitative metrics that can be applied in clinical practice.

CLINICS CARE POINTS

- MR perfusion provides valuable information necessary for decision making and patient management by measuring the ischemic penumbra and characterizing the vascularity of neoplastic lesions.
- Hemodynamic parameters calculated from MR perfusion techniques reflect different physiologic and pathologic properties, and more work is needed to refine their exact role.

DISCLOSURE

The authors have nothing to disclose.

REFERENCES

1. Gaudino S, Martucci M, Botto A, et al. Brain DSC MR perfusion in children: a clinical feasibility study using different technical standards of contrast administration. AJNR Am J Neuroradiol 2019; 40(2):359–65.
2. Proisy M, Mitra S, Uria-Avellana C, et al. Brain perfusion imaging in neonates: an overview. AJNR Am J Neuroradiol 2016;37(10):1766–73.
3. Petrella JR, Provenzale JM. MR perfusion imaging of the brain: techniques and applications. AJR Am J Roentgenol 2000;175(1):207–19.
4. Essig M, Nguyen TB, Shiroishi MS, et al. Perfusion MRI: the five most frequently asked clinical questions. AJR Am J Roentgenol 2013;201(3):W495–510.
5. Poussaint TY, Rodriguez D. Advanced neuroimaging of pediatric brain tumors: MR diffusion, MR perfusion, and MR spectroscopy. Neuroimaging Clin N Am 2006;16(1):169–92, ix.
6. Pollack IF. Multidisciplinary management of childhood brain tumors: a review of outcomes, recent advances, and challenges. J Neurosurg Pediatr 2011; 8(2):135–48.
7. Panigrahy A, Bluml S. Neuroimaging of pediatric brain tumors: from basic to advanced magnetic resonance imaging (MRI). J Child Neurol 2009; 24(11):1343–65.
8. Lequin M, Hendrikse J. Advanced MR imaging in pediatric brain tumors, clinical applications. Neuroimaging Clin N Am 2017;27(1):167–90.
9. Chang YW, Yoon HK, Shin HJ, et al. MR imaging of glioblastoma in children: usefulness of diffusion/perfusion-weighted MRI and MR spectroscopy. Pediatr Radiol 2003;33(12):836–42.
10. Tzika AA, Vajapeyam S, Barnes PD. Multivoxel proton MR spectroscopy and hemodynamic MR imaging of childhood brain tumors: preliminary observations. AJNR Am J Neuroradiol 1997;18(2): 203–18.
11. Tzika AA, Astrakas LG, Zarifi MK, et al. Multiparametric MR assessment of pediatric brain tumors. Neuroradiology 2003;45(1):1–10.
12. Knopp EA, Cha S, Johnson G, et al. Glial neoplasms: dynamic contrast-enhanced T2*-weighted MR imaging. Radiology 1999;211(3):791–8.
13. Ho CY, Cardinal JS, Kamer AP, et al. Relative cerebral blood volume from dynamic susceptibility contrast perfusion in the grading of pediatric primary brain tumors. Neuroradiology 2015;57(3): 299–306.
14. Dallery F, Bouzerar R, Michel D, et al. Perfusion magnetic resonance imaging in pediatric brain tumors. Neuroradiology 2017;59(11):1143–53.
15. Ho ML, Campeau NG, Ngo TD, et al. Pediatric brain MRI, Part 2: advanced techniques. Pediatr Radiol 2017;47(5):544–55.
16. Cha S. Dynamic susceptibility-weighted contrast-enhanced perfusion MR imaging in pediatric patients. Neuroimaging Clin N Am 2006;16(1): 137–47, ix.
17. Shin JH, Lee HK, Kwun BD, et al. Using relative cerebral blood flow and volume to evaluate the histopathologic grade of cerebral gliomas: preliminary results. AJR Am J Roentgenol 2002;179(3):783–9.
18. Law M, Yang S, Babb JS, et al. Comparison of cerebral blood volume and vascular permeability from dynamic susceptibility contrast-enhanced perfusion MR imaging with glioma grade. AJNR Am J Neuroradiol 2004;25(5):746–55.
19. Ball WS Jr, Holland SK. Perfusion imaging in the pediatric patient. Magn Reson Imaging Clin N Am 2001;9(1):207–30, ix.

20. Grand SD, Kremer S, Tropres IM, et al. Perfusion-sensitive MRI of pilocytic astrocytomas: initial results. Neuroradiology 2007;49(7):545–50.

21. Theillac M, Meyronet D, Savatovsky J, et al. Dynamic susceptibility contrast perfusion imaging in biopsy-proved adult medulloblastoma. J Neuroradiol 2016; 43(5):317–24.

22. Abe T, Mizobuchi Y, Nakajima K, et al. Diagnosis of brain tumors using dynamic contrast-enhanced perfusion imaging with a short acquisition time. Springerplus 2015;4:88.

23. Li X, Zhu Y, Kang H, et al. Glioma grading by microvascular permeability parameters derived from dynamic contrast-enhanced MRI and intratumoral susceptibility signal on susceptibility weighted imaging. Cancer Imaging 2015;15:4.

24. Patankar TF, Haroon HA, Mills SJ, et al. Is volume transfer coefficient (K(trans)) related to histologic grade in human gliomas? AJNR Am J Neuroradiol 2005;26(10):2455–65.

25. Vajapeyam S, Stamoulis C, Ricci K, et al. Automated processing of dynamic contrast-enhanced MRI: correlation of advanced pharmacokinetic metrics with tumor grade in pediatric brain tumors. AJNR Am J Neuroradiol 2017;38(1):170–5.

26. Gupta PK, Saini J, Sahoo P, et al. Role of dynamic contrast-enhanced perfusion magnetic resonance imaging in grading of pediatric brain tumors on 3T. Pediatr Neurosurg 2017;52(5):298–305.

27. Mills SJ, Soh C, Rose CJ, et al. Candidate biomarkers of extravascular extracellular space: a direct comparison of apparent diffusion coefficient and dynamic contrast-enhanced MR imaging–derived measurement of the volume of the extravascular extracellular space in glioblastoma multiforme. AJNR Am J Neuroradiol 2010;31(3):549–53.

28. Thompson EM, Guillaume DJ, Dósa E, et al. Dual contrast perfusion MRI in a single imaging session for assessment of pediatric brain tumors. J Neurooncol 2012;109(1):105–14.

29. Tzika AA, Astrakas LG, Zarifi MK, et al. Spectroscopic and perfusion magnetic resonance imaging predictors of progression in pediatric brain tumors. Cancer 2004;100(6):1246–56.

30. Valk PE, Dillon WP. Radiation injury of the brain. AJNR Am J Neuroradiol 1991;12(1):45–62.

31. Mugikura S, Takahashi S, Higano S, et al. The relationship between cerebral infarction and angiographic characteristics in childhood moyamoya disease. AJNR Am J Neuroradiol 1999;20(2): 336–43.

32. Togao O, Mihara F, Yoshiura T, et al. Cerebral hemodynamics in Moyamoya disease: correlation between perfusion-weighted MR imaging and cerebral angiography. AJNR Am J Neuroradiol 2006;27(2):391–7.

33. Lin YH, Kuo MF, Lu CJ, et al. Standardized MR perfusion scoring system for evaluation of sequential perfusion changes and surgical outcome of Moyamoya disease. AJNR Am J Neuroradiol 2019;40(2): 260–6.

34. Calamante F, Ganesan V, Kirkham FJ, et al. MR perfusion imaging in Moyamoya Syndrome: potential implications for clinical evaluation of occlusive cerebrovascular disease. Stroke 2001;32(12): 2810–6.

35. Albers GW, Thijs VN, Wechsler L, et al. Magnetic resonance imaging profiles predict clinical response to early reperfusion: the diffusion and perfusion imaging evaluation for understanding stroke evolution (DEFUSE) study. Ann Neurol 2006;60(5):508–17.

36. Lansberg MG, et al. MRI profile and response to endovascular reperfusion after stroke (DEFUSE 2): a prospective cohort study. Lancet Neurol 2012; 11(10):860–7.

37. Lee S, et al. Neuroimaging selection for thrombectomy in pediatric stroke: a single-center experience. J Neurointerv Surg 2019;11(9):940–6.

38. Cobb-Pitstick KM, et al. Time course of cerebral perfusion changes in children with migraine with aura mimicking stroke. AJNR Am J Neuroradiol 2018;39(9):1751–5.

39. Altinok D, et al. Pediatric hemiplegic migraine: susceptibility weighted and MR perfusion imaging abnormality. Pediatr Radiol 2010;40(12):1958–61.

40. Evans AL, et al. Cerebral perfusion abnormalities in children with Sturge-Weber syndrome shown by dynamic contrast bolus magnetic resonance perfusion imaging. Pediatrics 2006;117(6):2119–25.

Task-based and Resting State Functional MRI in Children

Mohit Maheshwari, MBBS, MD[a],*, Tejaswini Deshmukh, MBBS, MD[a],
Eric C. Leuthardt, MD[b], Joshua S. Shimony, MD, PhD[c]

KEYWORDS

• Task fMRI • Resting state fMRI • Presurgical planning • BOLD

KEY POINTS

- Functional MR imaging (fMRI) applications in children are becoming more common for presurgical planning, especially in epilepsy and brain tumors.
- Task-based fMRI needs to be customized for children accounting for age, cognitive skill, and the ability of the patient to cooperate with the task.
- Resting state fMRI is a more recent alternative method that can be used in very young children, or in children who cannot participate in a task.

INTRODUCTION
Background

Optimal surgical outcomes in patients with brain tumors involve a common dilemma for the neurosurgeon: maximal tumor resection versus minimizing functional loss. These 2 factors are often cited in the surgical literature as predictors of long-term survival.[1,2] Accurate patient-specific maps of critical areas in the brain (eloquent cortex)[3] are required for the surgeon to make informed decisions both before and during surgery. Electrical cortical stimulation mapping is considered the gold standard[4] for localization during surgery, but this method has several disadvantages and may not be possible to perform in many pediatric cases. Localization of motor and language regions using task-based functional MR imaging (fMRI) (T-fMRI) is currently considered the standard of care prior to surgical resection of brain lesions near the eloquent cortex. This information is considered critical for presurgical planning, assessing the risk for morbidity, and consultation with patients and their families. This method is used most often prior to brain tumor resection but has become common in numerous other neurosurgical procedures, such as epilepsy surgery, brain biopsies, laser ablation procedures, and others.

fMRI detects changes in the blood oxygen level–dependent (BOLD) signal that reflect the neurovascular response to neural activity. Traditionally, localization of function in the brain using fMRI has been performed by presenting stimuli or imposing tasks (such as finger tapping or object naming) to elicit a neuronal response.[5] More recently, there has been growing appreciation for the use of resting state (RS) spontaneous BOLD fluctuations, also called intrinsic brain activity, or RS-fMRI as a tool to elucidate the brain's functional organization. The idea that intrinsic brain activity could be utilized for functional localization

[a] Department of Radiology, Medical College of Wisconsin, Children's Wisconsin, MS - 721, 9000 W Wisconsin Avenue, Milwaukee, WI 53226, USA; [b] Department of Neurosurgery, Washington University, 4525 Scott Avenue Campus Box 8131, St Louis, MO 63141, USA; [c] Mallinckrodt Institute of Radiology, Washington University, 4525 Scott Avenue Campus Box 8131, St Louis, MO 63141, USA
* Corresponding author.
E-mail address: mmahesh@mcw.edu

Magn Reson Imaging Clin N Am 29 (2021) 527–541
https://doi.org/10.1016/j.mric.2021.06.005
1064-9689/21/© 2021 Elsevier Inc. All rights reserved.

was first suggested by Biswal and colleagues,[6] who demonstrated that BOLD fluctuations observed in the RS are correlated within the somatomotor system. The development of these methods has opened many new options for clinical applications, such as presurgical planning.[7–9]

The need for patient participation in the task is critical for accurate functional mapping when using T-fMRI. Customization of the T-fMRI study should consider the condition of the patient (their ability to participate in the examination and how long they can lay still in the MR imaging scanner), the location of the tumor with respect to the area of eloquent cortex, and the information that can be obtained from different specific tasks. When pediatric patients, such as very young children, cannot participate in the task, or there is a need for sedation, alternative approaches are needed. One such approach is RS-fMRI. This approach does not require patient participation and is able to extract localization maps from calculations of functional connectivity across the brain.[10,11]

The purpose of this article is to introduce readers to the methods of T-fMRI and RS-fMRI as implemented in pediatric populations. MR imaging protocols, relative advantages and disadvantages,

overview of data processing issues, and specific indications and applications are discussed.

Task-based Functional MRI

The physiologic basis of BOLD signal is the regional vasoreactive response induced by the neuronal activity (neurovascular coupling), which leads to minute changes in the deoxyhemoglobin and oxyhemoglobin in the adjacent voxels and a resultant change in the T2* signal (**Fig. 1**).[12–14]

Task-based fMRI in the setting of presurgical mapping is typically performed according to the block design, where alternating blocks of rest and task-specific activity are administered to the subject (**Fig. 2**). This boxcar-type design is advantageous in a clinical setting because the repetitive nature of the paradigm allows for signal averaging across multiple stimulus trials and, therefore, higher potential signal. Boxcar-type design is also forgiving in that if some stimuli are missed, enough data points exist to allow for accurate mapping of functional areas. The combination of an optimized acquisition protocol in conjunction with relevant task design facilitates a robust characterization of patient-specific neuronal mapping for use in

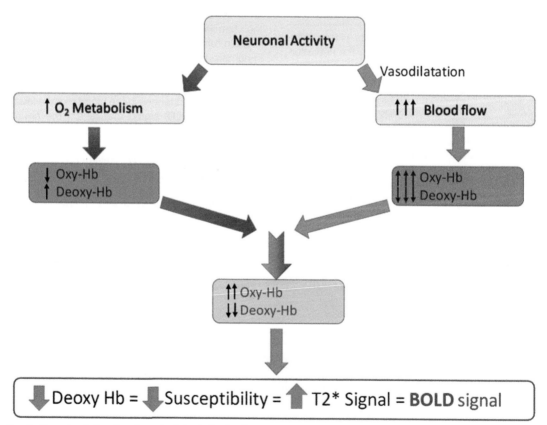

Fig. 1. Flowchart showing the physiologic basis of BOLD signal. Hb, Hemoglobin.

presurgical assessment. Throughout the task activity or control activity/rest, rapid MR images of the brain are acquired continuously. The difference between the signal of the images obtained during task activity and rest/control activity provides the fMRI signal corresponding to the task activity. For better spatial localization and clinical use of this information, fMRI signal thus obtained is coregistered with the high-resolution anatomic MR images of the brain (see **Fig. 2**).

Resting State Functional MRI

Since the earliest days of fMRI, it has been recognized that the BOLD signal exhibits spontaneous fluctuations.[15] These fluctuations initially were regarded as noise to be averaged out over many trials or task blocks.[16] More recent studies have shown that these spontaneous fluctuations reflect the brain's functional organization. Biswal and colleagues[6] first suggested that intrinsic brain activity could be utilized for functional localization and demonstrated that BOLD fluctuations observed in the RS are correlated within the somatomotor system. The development of these methods has opened many exciting possibilities for future neurocognitive research as well as clinical applications. Advantages of RS-fMRI over T-fMRI include a simpler measurement in the MR imaging scanner and no need for a patient to actively perform a task. Disadvantages of RS-fMRI are that it is less well established, and the processing of RS-fMRI data algorithmically is more complicated.

Unlike T-fMRI that identifies areas of the brain that are activated during a task, RS-fMRI identifies areas of the brain that demonstrate synchronous BOLD activity, and these areas define RS networks (RSN).[17,18] **Fig. 3** demonstrates an example of positive and negative correlations between seed regions in different regions of the brain. The most widely used measure of synchronous activity between seed regions is the Pearson product-moment. The topography of RSNs closely corresponds to responses elicited by a wide variety of sensory, motor, and cognitive tasks.[19] **Fig. 4** demonstrates the motor and language networks as identified by RS-fMRI in a group analysis. It has been established that intrinsic activity persists in a modified form during sleep[20,21] and under certain types of sedation.[22] RSNs have been identified in all mammalian species investigated to date.[23,24] This phylogenetic conservation implies that coherent intrinsic activity must be physiologically important despite its high metabolic cost.[25,26]

The use of RS-fMRI has been implemented to complement and enhance the currently established presurgical planning methods of T-fMRI and diffusion tensor imaging (DTI) tractography. The RS-fMRI information is valuable especially if the T-fMRI is of poor quality or is nonexistent,

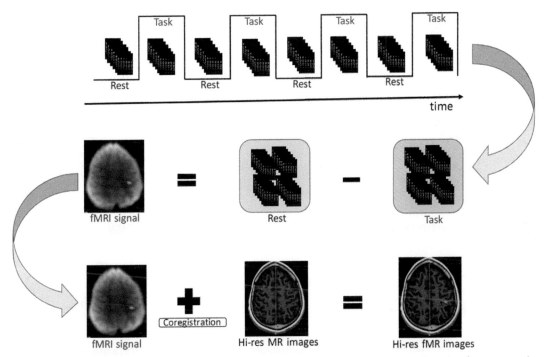

Fig. 2. Schematic representation block design for acquisition of the T-fMRI data and principle of postprocessing to generate clinical high-resolution (Hi-res) images where BOLD signal is coregistered with anatomic MR images.

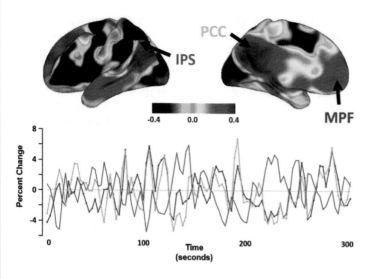

Fig. 3. BOLD time courses in the intra-parietal sulcus (IPS [blue]), the posterior cingulate cortex (PCC [yellow]), and the medial prefrontal (MPF [orange]) cortex. The IPS is correlated negatively with the PCC and MPF, which are positively correlated with each other.

such as can occur when patients are not able to cooperate with the T-fMRI requirements.

METHODS
Functional MRI Protocols

To capture the BOLD signal, an MR imaging sequence is needed which is sensitive to changes in the susceptibility (T2* signal) and fast enough to maintain the temporal resolution of this technique. Echo-planar imaging (EPI) has both these features, making it an excellent choice for fMRI. With the EPI technique, each brain slice is acquired very rapidly (entire brain can be imaged in approximately 1500 ms–3000 ms). Despite these advantages, images obtained by the EPI technique have poor spatial resolution. Therefore, to use these data for clinical purposes (presurgical mapping), signal change thus obtained with the EPI sequence is coregistered on higher-resolution MR images.

Typical parameters used for EPI are repetition time, 2000 ms to 3000 ms; echo time, 30 ms; field of view, 240 mm; flip angle = 90°; number of excitations = 1; and voxel size of between 3 mm^3 and 4 mm^3. Similar parameters can be used for RS-fMRI.

Special Considerations in Pediatric Patients

There have been several challenges in applying adult fMRI protocols and data to pediatric subjects. Some physiologic differences include higher metabolism and vascular response in the pediatric brain.[27] This in turn results in increased signal-to-noise ratio and 60% to 400% more voxel

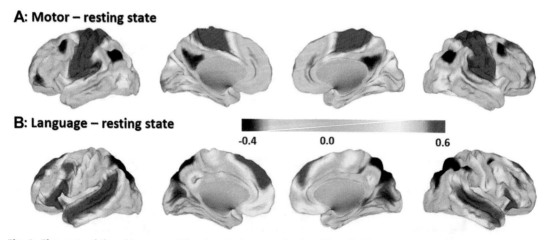

Fig. 4. The motor (A) and language (B) networks (warm colors) as identified by RS-fMRI in a group analysis. These networks are highly similar to the task identified regions with the main difference that the language network is symmetric.

activation (vs adults) with similar postprocessing techniques.[28–30]

Inability of younger children to stay still in the scanner is the biggest challenge in performing fMRI in this age group. It has been found that among younger children, boys have higher tendency to move compared with girls.[31]

A calming and child friendly environment helps in reducing patient anxiety. In the authors' experience, offering a reward of letting a child watch their favorite movie during the nonfunctional part of the scan goes a long way in improving patient compliance. Ensuring patient comfort and stabilizing the patient's head by soft cushions also mitigates head motion. In the authors' practice, a technologist observes the real-time functional activation maps and head motion plots on the scanner while the functional sequence is running. In cases of excessive head motion or lack of expected activation, the paradigm is repeated to ensure good quality data.

The patient is asked to arrive early, so that each child can be interviewed and trained by the radiologist prior to the fMRI scan. This interaction allows the radiologist to make an assessment about the maximum possible duration of the examination for each child and select suitable paradigms to be performed.

In general, for children 5 to 7 years old, typically the fMRI study is limited to 10 to 15 minutes (2–3 paradigms). For children 7 to 9 years old, the functional study is limited to 15 to 30 minutes (3–6 paradigms), and children older than 9 years are generally able to tolerate a full functional study of 45 to 60 minutes. For children younger than 5 years, passive sensory motor mapping under sedation is an option. Besides these general guidelines, the plan and duration of the functional study is individualized for each child during the interview and training with the radiologist. This is true especially for children who are developmentally delayed or have reading disabilities.

Pediatric Motor Mapping

T-fMRI motor mapping in older cooperative children does not differ greatly from that in adults. Motor mapping is typically performed for the hands, feet, and face. Standard tasks for the hands include finger tapping or squeezing a foam pad.[32–34] Typical activation is seen in the contralateral precentral gyrus in the region of the hand knob (**Fig. 5**). Activation is also seen in the bilateral supplementary motor areas (SMAs) (posterior aspects of the superior frontal gyri), ipsilateral cerebellum, and basal ganglia. Some activation may also be seen in the contralateral postcentral gyrus (due to proprioceptive and sensory input) and ipsilateral precentral gyrus.[35]

Motor mapping of the feet is elicited by repeated flexion and extension of the feet or toes. Activation is typically seen in the contralateral paracentral lobule and SMA (see **Fig. 5**). Motor mapping of the face may be performed with repeated sideways movement of the tongue or puckering of the lips. During this paradigm, activation is seen in the lateral aspects of the precentral gyri bilaterally (see **Fig. 5**). There is high concordance between localization of the motor cortex with fMRI and direct intraoperative cortical activation.[36–38]

Passive Sensorimotor Mapping

In young children or noncooperative older subjects, motor mapping may be performed under sedation. Passive manual flexion and extension of the fingers at the metacarpophalangeal joints and toes at the metatarsophalangeal joints yield good results. This is based on the principle that afferent input modulates efferent output from the primary motor cortex. Passive joint movements result in activation of corresponding efferent zones in the primary motor cortex. This phenomenon is believed to be due to corticocortical connections between the secondary sensory cortex and the primary motor cortex.[39,40] Because the BOLD signal in passive sensorimotor mapping arises

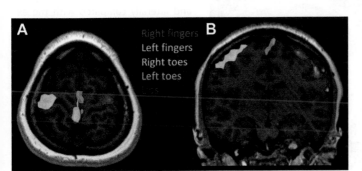

Right fingers
Left fingers
Right toes
Left toes

Fig. 5. Motor mapping in a 15-year-old girl who presented with right posterior temporal mass. fMRI activation during various motor paradigms superimposed over axial (*A*) and coronal (*B*) 3-D T1-weighted images and color coded as shown.

from both precentral and postcentral gyri (primary motor cortex and sensory cortex, respectively), the area of activation is slightly posteriorly displaced (vs active motor mapping). Kocak and colleagues[41] demonstrated high concurrence of the cortical activation between active and passive motor tasks in healthy adults. Ogg and coworkers[42] showed similar findings when they compared passive motor mapping (under sedation) with active motor mapping and direct cortical stimulation in children with focal brain lesions/masses or cortical dysplasia.

Choice of the sedative agent for passive sensorimotor mapping is important because some agents can affect vasoreactivity of the brain vessels leading to loss of BOLD signal. An ideal sedative agent should be safe, with a short induction time, short recovery time, few side effects, and minimal effect on brain vasoreactivity.[43] Various studies have shown most success with agents like propofol, dexmedetomidine and pentobarbital. Other agents such as midazolam and sevoflurane have demonstrated scattered activation and high failure rates, respectively.[43,44] Dosage of these medicines also is important because excessive sedation could lead to failure of

activation.[43,45,46] In the authors' practice, a combination of propofol and dexmedetomidine is used with very good results and few failures.

In cases of congenital malformations of the brain or chronic epilepsy, there may be cortical reorganization such that motor function maps to areas where it is not expected based on anatomic landmarks (**Fig. 6**). Motor mapping helps the neurosurgeon determine the feasibility of surgical resection and determine the risk-benefit ratio if a lesion is in close proximity to the primary motor area.[47]

Pediatric Language Mapping

fMRI is used widely for language mapping (localization and lateralization) in adults and children. Unlike adult patients where brain tumors are the most common indication for presurgical fMRI, the most common indication in children is epilepsy. A large proportion of pediatric epilepsy patients have no appreciable lesion on imaging (nonlesional epilepsy). In these patients, language lateralization is more important than precise localization of the language areas. Language laterality may be determined quantitatively with laterality index, which compares the number of activated

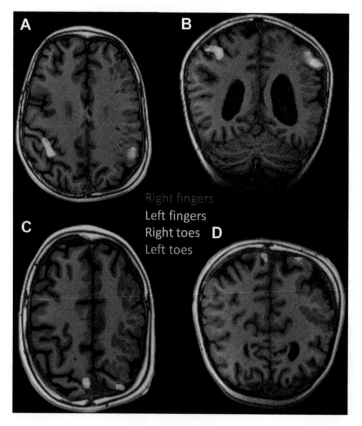

Fig. 6. Passive sensorimotor mapping in a 5-year-old boy with refractory epilepsy and extensive left frontoparietal polymicrogyria. fMRI data is superimposed in color on 3D T1 images. Axial (*A*) and coronal (*B*) show BOLD signal in the central sulcus area and during passive movement of the left fingers (*blue*) and right fingers (*red*). Activation in the left hemisphere is deranged secondary to the left frontoparietal cortical malformation. Axial (*C*) and coronal (*D*) show BOLD signal in the left paracentral lobule during passive movement of the right toe (*orange*) and left toe (*green*). Activation of the right toe movement is displaced posteriorly and laterally compared with the expected location.

Right fingers
Left fingers
Right toes
Left toes

voxels in the respective language areas in either hemisphere. In most clinical situations, however, hemispheric language dominance may be determined qualitatively with visual assessment of activated voxels.

Language mapping consists of the determination of expressive and receptive language areas. Expressive language areas include inferior frontal gyrus (pars triangularis and pars opercularis), middle frontal gyrus (dorsolateral prefrontal cortex), and anterior aspect of the superior frontal gyrus (speech SMA). Receptive language areas include the posterior third of superior and middle temporal gyri, supramarginal gyri, angular gyri, and fusiform gyri (**Fig. 7**).[35,48]

Depending on a patient's age and developmental level and the clinical question, 2 to 4 language paradigms are recommended for optimal language mapping. Use of more than 2 language paradigms increases the degree of confidence for language lateralization. Based on the expected dominant areas of activation, most common language paradigms can be divided into 3 groups:

1. Expressive and receptive
   a. Sentence completion
   b. Rhyming
2. Expressive > receptive
   a. Silent word generation
   b. Antonym generation
3. Receptive > expressive
   a. Passive story listening
   b. Auditory response naming
   c. Object naming

In a recent white paper, an American Society of Functional Neuroradiology task force proposed language mapping algorithms for paradigm selection in adult and pediatric subjects.[5] The pediatric algorithm consisted of sentence completion, rhyming, antonym generation, and passive story listening paradigms.[5] Rhyming paradigm is one of the best for lateralization and specific activation amongst various language paradigms.[49–51]

It is important to optimize the language paradigm for children. In general, cortical activation is lower if the task/paradigm is too easy or too difficult.[52,53] Most language paradigms, as they come out of the box with the standard paradigm delivery hardware and software, are optimized for adult subjects. In the authors' practice, these paradigms have been modified to have simpler and child friendly words, sentences, and auditory stimuli. Slower versions of most paradigms have also been developed, where stimulus frequency is slowed. Lastly, auditory language paradigms (where stimuli are delivered via auditory route like passive story listening or auditory naming paradigms) are helpful in younger children (5–7 years old) and those with developmental delay or reading disability. These changes have improved patient compliance and the overall success rate

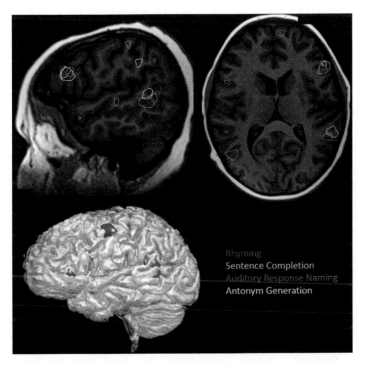

Fig. 7. Language mapping in a 10-year-old boy with solitary metastasis in the right frontoparietal region (not shown) from osteogenic sarcoma in the right femur. Activation during various language paradigms is color coded as shown. There is left hemispheric dominance for language function in this subject.

Rhyming
Sentence Completion
Auditory Response Naming
Antonym Generation

of language fMRI examinations at the authors' institute.

As with motor mapping, atypical language localization (right-sided or bilateral) can be seen with cerebral developmental malformations, chronic nonlesional epilepsy, cerebral vascular malformations, and history of stroke or supratentorial tumors. Atypical localization emphasizes the need to preoperatively map language because neither structural landmarks nor the information about handedness can reliably lateralize or localize language function.[54] Despite this, if language activation is very atypical or absent, further confirmation with repeat fMRI or Wada testing and/or intraoperative cortical mapping is always advisable before surgical decision making.[5]

Processing Resting State Data

Once the data are acquired, the investigator must choose between 2 principal modes of RS-fMRI analysis: (1) seed-based correlation (SBC) mapping and (2) spatial independent component analysis (sICA). SBC mapping is well suited to investigations of the functional connectivity of previously selected targeted regions of interest but requires extensive preprocessing to reduce the impact of artifact (discussed later). sICA provides a more direct means of separating artifact from neural signals[55] but is less well suited to investigating targeted regions of interest. Both SBC and sICA yield highly reproducible results at the group level.[56] A popular software package for sICA analysis is the MELODIC tool within the FSL package[57] (fsl.fmrib.ox.ac.uk/fsl/fslwiki).

Currently there are no push-button software packages available for SBC analysis; thus, rote analysis is not possible and the user needs to understand the sequence of analysis operations. The authors anticipate that this will change in the coming years. A new investigator may wish to use one of the freely available software packages to help process their data. The following 3 packages include all the basic operations needed to analyze RS-fMRI data: FSL,[57] AFNI,[58] and SPM (www.fil.ion.ucl.ac.uk/spm/). Each of these packages is downloadable at no cost, is documented in an easily accessible Web site, provides on-line support, and is associated with regularly scheduled training workshops. Other on-line software tools are available but are beyond the scope of this review. Basic preprocessing steps include compensation for slice-dependent time shifts, rigid body correction for head movement within and across runs, intensity scaling, atlas transformation to atlas structural images, spatial smoothing, removal of linear trends, temporal band pass filtering,

regression of nuisance variables, and removal of high motion time points. More detail on these steps is provided by Power and colleagues.[59] An advantage of SBC in comparison to sICA is that using prior information provides more robust mapping in individual patients with relatively high motion and relatively shorter scanning times that are more realistic in a population of patients with brain tumors.[60]

Similar to T-fMRI, once the networks of interest are identified, they need to be sent to the PACS system for review by the neuroradiologist and neurosurgeon and incorporated with the DTI tracking data and provided to the intraoperative navigation system for use during the surgery. As with the SBC analysis, discussed previously, the authors are not aware of any push-button systems to perform this function automatically; rather, various institutes have solved this problem individually.[61]

APPLICATIONS
Presurgical Planning

Presurgical planning prior to epilepsy surgery or resection of brain tumors are common applications of fMRI in pediatric patients. In addition, fMRI has also been used for planning prior to brain biopsies, laser ablation procedures, and placement of electrodes for stereo-electroencephalography.

The localization of eloquent cortex with respect to the tumor can also help assess the risk for morbidity and provide information for consultation with the patient and their family. During this phase, the neurosurgeon will use this data (and assessment of image quality) to inform various decisions regarding the surgery itself. These decisions may include some or all of the following: (1) location and size of the craniotomy; (2) direction and path of approach to the tumor; (3) need for a ventriculostomy catheter and where to place it; (4) need for electrocortical stimulation equipment to confirm the MR imaging findings; (5) need for an intraoperative MR imaging scan; and (6) need to vary the type of anesthesia depending on the type of anticipated stimulation mapping. Each case is different, and the MR imaging information can provide valuable help in decreasing morbidity and optimizing the tumor resection.

Alternative techniques to localizing and lateralizing these functions include intraoperative cortical mapping, which remains a gold standard, and intracarotid amobarbital (Wada) testing. Intraoperative cortical mapping is invasive, expensive, time consuming in the operating room and difficult to repeat. Wada testing has been used for many years for language lateralization, but is also invasive, expensive, and nonlocalizing and leads to unclear results if a child is oversedated or unable to respond.[62] In addition, both Wada testing and intraoperative cortical mapping are extremely challenging if not completely infeasible to perform in younger pediatric patients. Currently, Wada testing is largely replaced by fMRI, which is less expensive, noninvasive, and easily reproducible and provides localization of both language and motor function. The current clinical role of both these techniques is complementary to fMRI in cases of fMRI that is either not feasible or the results of which are equivocal.

Other clinical applications for fMRI are under investigation and include prediction of prognosis in patients with brain tumors[63] and changes related to epilepsy.[64–70]

Motor System/Network

The authors provide several case examples of fMRI localization adjacent to a brain lesion.

Case 1 is a 10-year-old boy with solitary brain metastasis from osteogenic sarcoma in the right femur. **Fig. 8** demonstrates the lesion and motor fMRI activation superimposed over axial T1 and 3-dimensional (3-D) volume-rendered images of the brain. T-fMRI activation during left finger

tapping (red) is noted to abut the posterior border of the mass.

Case 2 is an 11-year-old girl with seizures. Axial fluid-attenuated inversion recovery (FLAIR) image shows a lobulated mass in the left frontal region (**Fig. 9**). The fMRI signal from multiple language paradigms (as color coded) is superimposed over a sagittal T1 and 3-D volume-rendered image of the brain. Activation in the region of pars opercularis (expressive language area/Broca area) is seen along the posteroinferior border of the mass. This mass was partially resected and diagnosed as ganglioglioma on histopathology. Axial T1 postcontrast image of the brain performed 18 months after surgery shows interval development of recurrent enhancing mass in the surgical bed (see **Figs. 9**D and E). Repeat fMRI language mapping was performed. Language fMRI signal superimposed over sagittal T1 post contrast image again shows the same area of activation in the pars opercularis (expressive language area/Broca area), posteroinferior to the surgical bed / recurrent tumor. This example shows reliable reproducibility of the fMRI results.

Case 3 is a 16-year-old boy with intractable seizures localized to the right frontal lobe caused by cortical dysplasia and heterotopic gray matter (**Fig. 10**A). Surgery was planned and fMRI was

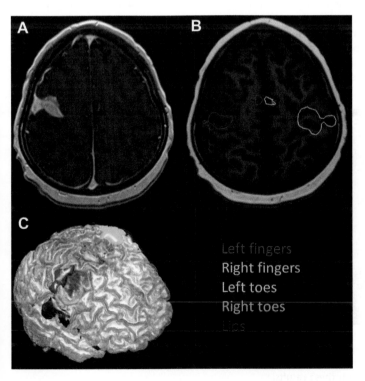

Fig. 8. Motor mapping in a 10-year-old boy with solitary brain metastasis from osteogenic sarcoma in the right femur (same patient shown in **Fig. 7**). Axial T1 postcontrast image showing enhancing lesion (metastasis) in the right frontoparietal region (*A*). Motor fMRI activation is superimposed over axial T1 (*B*) and 3-D volume-rendered images of the brain (*C*).

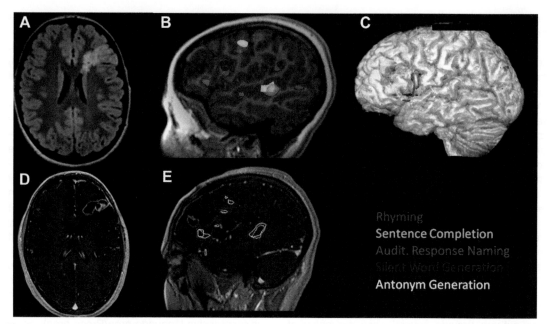

Rhyming
Sentence Completion
Audit. Response Naming
Silent Word Generation
Antonym Generation

Fig. 9. Language mapping in an 11-year-old girl with seizures due to a ganglioglioma. Axial FLAIR image shows a lobulated mass in the left frontal region (*A*). fMRI signal from multiple language paradigms (as color coded) is superimposed over a sagittal T1 (*B*) and 3-D volume-rendered image of the brain (*C*). Axial T1 postcontrast image of the brain (*D*) performed 18 months after surgery shows interval development of recurrent enhancing mass in the surgical bed. Repeat fMRI language mapping was performed. Language fMRI signal superimposed over sagittal T1 postcontrast image (*E*) again shows same area of activation in the pars opercularis (expressive language area/Broca's area), posterior inferior to the surgical bed/recurrent tumor.

performed. T-fMRI was successful only on the left side (see **Fig. 10**B). Localization of the motor system using RS-fMRI was more successful, demonstrating areas of the motor system on both sides of the brain (see **Fig. 10**C). On the right side, however, motor network extended into the areas of cortical dysplasia. Based on these results, surgery was deemed too risky and was canceled.

Other Systems/Networks

Although the motor and language systems are the most commonly localized areas of eloquent

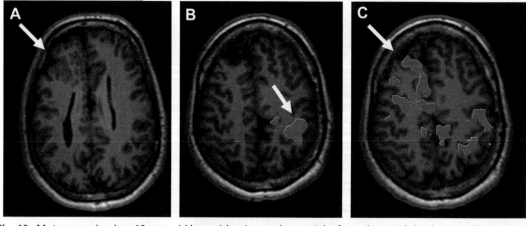

Fig. 10. Motor mapping in a 16-year-old boy with seizures due to right frontal cortical dysplasia and heterotopic gray matter (*A* [*arrow*]). T-fMRI motor mapping was successful only on the left side (*B* [*arrow*]). RS-fMRI motor localization demonstrated extension of the motor system into the frontal areas of cortical dysplasia (*C* [*arrow*]). The planned surgery was canceled based on these results.

cortex, localizing other primary sensory systems, such as the visual system, may be of great utility depending on the specific location of the lesion.

Visual cortex activation is obtained easily in older children with flashing checkerboards, which produce robust BOLD signal in the primary visual cortex (calcarine sulcus) and some of the visual association areas.[71] This information usually suffices for presurgical mapping because it identifies all or most of the components of the visual system, which need to be avoided for preservation of the visual function following surgery. Identification of the optic radiations with the help of DTI is an essential complement to visual cortex mapping with fMRI. More advanced vision mapping techniques utilizing expanding annular flashing checker box rings and rotating flashing checkered wedges may provide temporal and spatial resolution to the primary visual cortex activation (with respect to the stimulus in the visual field). With the help of this technique, functional field maps can be generated from fMRI data.[72]

Mapping of the visual cortex is also feasible in younger children under sedation. Li and colleagues[73] have performed visual cortical mapping in younger children under sedation with light stimulus provided over closed eyelids with a lot of success.

Another advantage of RS-fMRI is that a single data acquisition contains information about all RSNs in the brain; thus, other networks can be extracted from the raw data without additional scanning time. Examples of using RS-fMRI to localize other networks are available with both sICA[19] and SBC.[74]

Multiple other RSNs have been identified as association networks and include default mode,[75,76] dorsal and ventral attention,[17] frontoparietal,[77] cingulo-opercular,[18,78] salience,[79] and others. These RSNs show more variability across individuals and map onto higher-level cognitive functions; however, traditionally these regions of the brain rarely have been considered as eloquent cortex. Many of the networks are involved in essential aspects of human life, such as executive task control, forming memories, and attending to the environment. Further research on the clinical consequences of disruptions in these networks is necessary to improve patient outcomes, and these possibly will be considered eloquent in specific cases in the future.

Pitfalls

There are several pitfalls that may need consideration in all presurgical fMRI studies, but some are encountered more frequently in pediatric patients. Patient motion is the single most important issue in pediatric fMRI examinations. Real-time monitoring of the motion plots and the activation pattern (on the scanner) by an appropriately trained MR imaging technologist goes a long way to ensuring good quality data for post processing. This also ensures that if real-time data are suboptimal, then that sequence can be repeated right away to avoid patient recall later.

Presence of dental braces is a common occurrence in pediatric subjects. These braces cause extensive susceptibility artifact, which in most cases obscures fMRI information in the inferior frontal gyrus (expressive language area) (Fig. 11). All patients should be screened for braces and other hardware prior to scheduling the fMRI appointment. Susceptibility artifact from the metallic shunt hardware or vascular clips may also mask fMRI signal depending on their location.

Because the physiologic basis of BOLD signal is the regional vasoreactive response induced by the neuronal activity (neurovascular coupling), in situations where cerebrovascular reactivity is compromised, there may be underestimation of the BOLD signal (intensity and extent). This may be

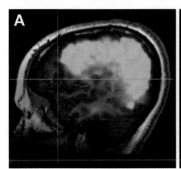 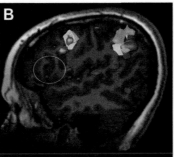 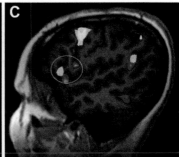

Fig. 11. Language mapping in a 12-year-old girl with dental braces. EPI signal superimposed on the 3-D T1 anatomic image showing loss of signal in the frontotemporal region due to braces (A). No signal detected in the inferior frontal gyrus (expressive language area) on language mapping because BOLD signal was masked by the susceptibility artifact (B). Repeat language mapping following removal of the braces shows robust BOLD signal in the left inferior frontal gyrus (C).

seen in cases of cerebral vascular disease, intra-cranial arteriovenous malformations and cerebral neoplasms.[80–82] In the presence of these lesions, especially if they are seen near the eloquent cortex, the possibility of underestimation of BOLD signal should be considered.

Several pediatric epilepsy patients have indwelling vagal nerve stimulators. Routine MR imaging coils are unsafe in these patients and a special transmit-receive coil is required to perform MR imaging or fMRI on these patients.

Lastly, BOLD response in language areas may be transiently diminished following a prolonged seizure episode.[83] The authors ask patients to continue their antiseizure medications when they come for fMRI examinations. If patients are admitted for long-term monitoring of seizures (where their antiseizure medication is tapered to induce and record epileptic activity), fMRI is scheduled before the antiseizure medication is tapered. Also, language fMRI is best avoided for 24 hours following a prolonged seizure episode.

SUMMARY

fMRI is a valuable tool for presurgical planning that is well established in adult patients. The use of T-fMRI is increasing in children because it provides similar benefits. This article surveys the most commonly used methods of T-fMRI, common pitfalls, and customizations to map pediatric motor, language, and other networks of interest. The more recently introduced method of RS-fMRI may provide useful information when a child cannot actively perform tasks. A current disadvantage of RS-fMRI methods, which likely will be corrected in the future, is the lack of push-button systems that can make the method easy to use in clinical practice.

CLINICS CARE POINTS

- The greatest challenge for performing fMRI in children is patient motion.
- Paradigms should be modified for the child's age and maturity.
- The family should arrive early so there is time to explain the study and train the patient with the assistance of child life specialists.
- Passive movement or resting state fMRI are additional options for patients who are mildly sedated or otherwise cannot actively perform tasks.

DISCLOSURE

Drs. Maheshwari and Deshmukh have no conflicts. Drs. Leuthardt and Shimony own shares in Sora Therapeutics.

ACKNOWLEDGMENTS

We wish to thank the National Cancer Institute of the National Institute for Health for its support via grant R01CA203861.

REFERENCES

1. Lacroix M, Abi-Said D, Fourney DR, et al. A multivariate analysis of 416 patients with glioblastoma multiforme: prognosis, extent of resection, and survival. J Neurosurg 2001;95(2):190–8.
2. McGirt MJ, Chaichana KL, Gathinji M, et al. Independent association of extent of resection with survival in patients with malignant brain astrocytoma. J Neurosurg 2009;110(1):156–62.
3. Petrella JR, Shah LM, Harris KM, et al. Preoperative functional MR imaging localization of language and motor areas: effect on therapeutic decision making in patients with potentially resectable brain tumors. Radiology 2006;240(3):793–802.
4. Ojemann GA. Functional mapping of cortical language areas in adults. Intraoperative approaches. Adv Neurol 1993;63:155–63.
5. Black DF, Vachha B, Mian A, et al. American Society of Functional Neuroradiology-Recommended fMRI Paradigm Algorithms for Presurgical Language Assessment. AJNR Am J neuroradiology 2017; 38(10):E65–73.
6. Biswal B, Yetkin FZ, Haughton VM, et al. Functional connectivity in the motor cortex of resting human brain using echo-planar MRI. Magn Reson Med : official J Soc Magn Reson Med/Soc Magn Reson Med 1995;34(4):537–41.
7. Kokkonen SM, Nikkinen J, Remes J, et al. Preoperative localization of the sensorimotor area using independent component analysis of resting-state fMRI. Magn Reson Imaging 2009;27(6):733–40.
8. Liu H, Buckner RL, Talukdar T, et al. Task-free presurgical mapping using functional magnetic resonance imaging intrinsic activity. J Neurosurg 2009; 111(4):746–54.
9. Shimony JS, Zhang D, Johnston JM, et al. Resting-state spontaneous fluctuations in brain activity: a new paradigm for presurgical planning using fMRI. Acad Radiol 2009;16(5):578–83.
10. Dierker D, Roland JL, Kamran M, et al. Resting-state Functional Magnetic Resonance Imaging in Presurgical Functional Mapping: Sensorimotor Localization. Neuroimaging Clin N Am 2017;27(4): 621–33.

11. Park KY, Lee JJ, Dierker D, et al. Mapping language function with task-based vs. resting-state functional MRI. PloS one 2020;15(7):e0236423.

12. Chen W, Ogawa S. Principles of BOLD functiona MRI. In: Moonen CTW, Bandettini PA, editors. Functional MRI. Berlin, Heidelberg, New York: Springer Verlag; 2000. p. 103–13.

13. Magistretti PJ, Pellerin L. Cellular mechanisms of brain energy metabolism and their relevance to functional brain imaging. Philosophical Trans R Soc Lond Ser B, Biol Sci 1999;354(1387):1155–63.

14. Wilke M, Holland SK, Myseros JS, et al. Functional magnetic resonance imaging in pediatrics. Neuropediatrics 2003;34(5):225–33.

15. Purdon PL, Weisskoff RM. Effect of temporal autocorrelation due to physiological noise and stimulus paradigm on voxel-level false-positive rates in fMRI. Hum Brain Mapp 1998;6(4):239–49.

16. Triantafyllou C, Hoge RD, Krueger G, et al. Comparison of physiological noise at 1.5 T, 3 T and 7 T and optimization of fMRI acquisition parameters. NeuroImage 2005;26(1):243–50.

17. Fox MD, Corbetta M, Snyder AZ, et al. Spontaneous neuronal activity distinguishes human dorsal and ventral attention systems. Proc Natl Acad Sci United States America 2006;103(26):10046–51.

18. Seeley WW, Menon V, Schatzberg AF, et al. Dissociable intrinsic connectivity networks for salience processing and executive control. J Neurosci 2007;27(9):2349–56.

19. Smith SM, Fox PT, Miller KL, et al. Correspondence of the brain's functional architecture during activation and rest. Proc Natl Acad Sci United States America 2009;106(31):13040–5.

20. Larson-Prior LJ, Zempel JM, Nolan TS, et al. Cortical network functional connectivity in the descent to sleep. Proc Natl Acad Sci United States America 2009;106(11):4489–94.

21. Samann PG, Tully C, Spoormaker VI, et al. Increased sleep pressure reduces resting state functional connectivity. MAGMA 2010;23(5–6):375–89.

22. Mhuircheartaigh RN, Rosenorn-Lanng D, Wise R, et al. Cortical and subcortical connectivity changes during decreasing levels of consciousness in humans: a functional magnetic resonance imaging study using propofol. J Neurosci 2010;30(27):9095–102.

23. Hutchison RM, Gallivan JP, Culham JC, et al. Functional connectivity of the frontal eye fields in humans and macaque monkeys investigated with resting-state fMRI. J Neurophysiol 2012;107(9):2463–74.

24. Nasrallah FA, Tay HC, Chuang KH. Detection of functional connectivity in the resting mouse brain. Neuroimage 2014;86:417–24. https://doi.org/10.1016/j.neuroimage.2013.10.025.

25. Raichle ME. A paradigm shift in functional brain imaging. J Neurosci 2009;29(41):12729–34.

26. Raichle ME. Two views of brain function. Trends Cogn Sci 2010;14(4):180–90.

27. Chugani HT, Phelps ME, Mazziotta JC. Positron emission tomography study of human brain functional development. Ann Neurol 1987;22(4):487–97.

28. D'Esposito M, Zarahn E, Aguirre GK, et al. The effect of normal aging on the coupling of neural activity to the bold hemodynamic response. NeuroImage 1999;10(1):6–14.

29. Gaillard WD, Hertz-Pannier L, Mott SH, et al. Functional anatomy of cognitive development: fMRI of verbal fluency in children and adults. Neurology 2000;54(1):180–5.

30. Huettel SA, Singerman JD, McCarthy G. The effects of aging upon the hemodynamic response measured by functional MRI. NeuroImage 2001;13(1):161–75.

31. Yuan W, Altaye M, Ret J, et al. Quantification of head motion in children during various fMRI language tasks. Hum Brain Mapp 2009;30(5):1481–9.

32. Hirsch J, Ruge MI, Kim KH, et al. An integrated functional magnetic resonance imaging procedure for preoperative mapping of cortical areas associated with tactile, motor, language, and visual functions. Neurosurgery 2000;47(3):711–21 [discussion 721-712].

33. Lee CC, Jack CR Jr, Riederer SJ. Mapping of the central sulcus with functional MR: active versus passive activation tasks. AJNR Am J neuroradiology 1998;19(5):847–52.

34. Rivkin MJ, Vajapeyam S, Hutton C, et al. A functional magnetic resonance imaging study of paced finger tapping in children. Pediatr Neurol 2003;28(2):89–95.

35. Altman NR, Bernal B. Pediatric applications of functional magnetic resonance imaging. Pediatr Radiol 2015;45(Suppl 3):S382–96.

36. Puce A. Comparative assessment of sensorimotor function using functional magnetic resonance imaging and electrophysiological methods. J Clin Neurophysiol 1995;12(5):450–9.

37. Puce A, Constable RT, Luby ML, et al. Functional magnetic resonance imaging of sensory and motor cortex: comparison with electrophysiological localization. J Neurosurg 1995;83(2):262–70.

38. Yousry T, Schmid UD, Schmidt D, et al. [The motor hand area. Noninvasive detection with functional MRI and surgical validation with cortical stimulation]. Radiologe 1995;35(4):252–5.

39. Rosen I, Asanuma H. Peripheral afferent inputs to the forelimb area of the monkey motor cortex: input-output relations. Exp Brain Res 1972;14(3):257–73.

40. Yetkin FZ, Mueller WM, Morris GL, et al. Functional MR activation correlated with intraoperative cortical mapping. AJNR Am J neuroradiology 1997;18(7):1311–5.

41. Kocak M, Ulmer JL, Sahin Ugurel M, et al. Motor homunculus: passive mapping in healthy volunteers by using functional MR imaging–initial results. Radiology 2009;251(2):485–92.

42. Ogg RJ, Laningham FH, Clarke D, et al. Passive range of motion functional magnetic resonance imaging localizing sensorimotor cortex in sedated children. J Neurosurg Pediatr 2009;4(4):317–22.

43. Bernal B, Grossman S, Gonzalez R, et al. FMRI under sedation: what is the best choice in children? J Clin Med Res 2012;4(6):363–70.

44. Gemma M, de Vitis A, Baldoli C, et al. Functional magnetic resonance imaging (fMRI) in children sedated with propofol or midazolam. J Neurosurg Anesthesiol 2009;21(3):253–8.

45. Altman NR, Bernal B. Pediatric Applications of fMRI. In: Faro SH, Mahamed FB, editors. Functional Neuroradiology. New York: Springer; 2011. p. 545–74.

46. Marcar VL, Schwarz U, Martin E, et al. How depth of anesthesia influences the blood oxygenation level-dependent signal from the visual cortex of children. AJNR Am J neuroradiology 2006;27(4):799–805.

47. De Tiege X, Connelly A, Liegeois F, et al. Influence of motor functional magnetic resonance imaging on the surgical management of children and adolescents with symptomatic focal epilepsy. Neurosurgery 2009;64(5):856–64 [discussion 864].

48. Binder JR, Frost JA, Hammeke TA, et al. Human brain language areas identified by functional magnetic resonance imaging. J Neurosci 1997;17(1): 353–62.

49. Lurito JT, Kareken DA, Lowe MJ, et al. Comparison of rhyming and word generation with FMRI. Hum Brain Mapp 2000;10(3):99–106.

50. Pillai JJ, Zaca D. Relative utility for hemispheric lateralization of different clinical fMRI activation tasks within a comprehensive language paradigm battery in brain tumor patients as assessed by both threshold-dependent and threshold-independent analysis methods. NeuroImage 2011;54(Suppl 1): S136–45.

51. Zaca D, Nickerson JP, Deib G, et al. Effectiveness of four different clinical fMRI paradigms for preoperative regional determination of language lateralization in patients with brain tumors. Neuroradiology 2012; 54(9):1015–25.

52. Bookheimer SY. Functional MRI applications in clinical epilepsy. NeuroImage 1996;4(3 Pt 3):S139–46.

53. Nagel BJ, Barlett VC, Schweinsburg AD, et al. Neuropsychological predictors of BOLD response during a spatial working memory task in adolescents: what can performance tell us about fMRI response patterns? J Clin Exp Neuropsychol 2005;27(7): 823–39.

54. Gaillard WD, Berl MM, Moore EN, et al. Atypical language in lesional and nonlesional complex partial epilepsy. Neurology 2007;69(18):1761–71.

55. McKeown MJ, Hansen LK, Sejnowsk TJ. Independent component analysis of functional MRI: what is signal and what is noise? Curr Opin Neurobiol 2003;13(5):620–9.

56. Damoiseaux JS, Rombouts SA, Barkhof F, et al. Consistent resting-state networks across healthy subjects. Proc Natl Acad Sci United States America 2006;103(37):13848–53.

57. Jenkinson M, Beckmann CF, Behrens TE, et al. Fsl Neuroimage 2012;62(2):782–90.

58. Cox RW. AFNI: what a long strange trip it's been. NeuroImage 2012;62(2):743–7.

59. Power JD, Barnes KA, Snyder AZ, et al. Spurious but systematic correlations in functional connectivity MRI networks arise from subject motion. NeuroImage 2012;59(3):2142–54.

60. Lee MH, Miller-Thomas MM, Benzinger TL, et al. Clinical Resting-state fMRI in the Preoperative Setting: Are We Ready for Prime Time? Top Magn Reson Imaging 2016;25(1):11–8.

61. Leuthardt EC, Guzman G, Bandt SK, et al. Integration of resting state functional MRI into clinical practice - A large single institution experience. PloS one 2018;13(6):e0198349.

62. Benbadis SR, Binder JR, Swanson SJ, et al. Is speech arrest during wada testing a valid method for determining hemispheric representation of language? Brain Lang 1998;65(3):441–6.

63. Daniel AGS, Park KY, Roland JL, et al. Functional connectivity within glioblastoma impacts overall survival. Neuro Oncol 2021;23(3):412–21. https://doi.org/10.1093/neuonc/noaa189.

64. Boerwinkle VL, Wilfong AA, Curry DJ. Resting-state functional connectivity by independent component analysis-based markers corresponds to areas of initial seizure propagation established by prior modalities from the hypothalamus. Brain connectivity 2016;6(8):642–51.

65. Grassia F, Poliakov AV, Poliachik SL, et al. Changes in resting-state connectivity in pediatric temporal lobe epilepsy. J Neurosurg Pediatr 2018;22(3):270–5.

66. Hunyadi B, Tousseyn S, Mijovic B, et al. ICA extracts epileptic sources from fMRI in EEG-negative patients: a retrospective validation study. PloS one 2013;8(11):e78796.

67. Pravata E, Sestieri C, Mantini D, et al. Functional connectivity MR imaging of the language network in patients with drug-resistant epilepsy. AJNR Am J neuroradiology 2011;32(3):532–40.

68. Rajpoot K, Riaz A, Majeed W, et al. Functional Connectivity Alterations in Epilepsy from Resting-State Functional MRI. PloS one 2015;10(8):e0134944.

69. Vadivelu S, Wolf VL, Bollo RJ, et al. Resting-state functional MRI in pediatric epilepsy surgery. Pediatr Neurosurg 2013;49(5):261–73.

70. Widjaja E, Zamyadi M, Raybaud C, et al. Abnormal functional network connectivity among resting-state

networks in children with frontal lobe epilepsy. AJNR Am J neuroradiology 2013;34(12):2386–92.

71. DeYoe EA, Bandettini P, Neitz J, et al. Functional magnetic resonance imaging (FMRI) of the human brain. J Neurosci Methods 1994;54(2):171–87.

72. DeYoe EA, Ulmer JL, Mueller WM. fMRI in Human Visual Pathways. In: Faro SH, Mohamed FB, editors. Functional Neuroradiology. New York: Springer; 2011. p. 485–512.

73. Li W, Wait SD, Ogg RJ, et al. Functional magnetic resonance imaging of the visual cortex performed in children under sedation to assist in presurgical planning. J Neurosurg Pediatr 2013;11(5):543–6.

74. Hacker CD, Laumann TO, Szrama NP, et al. Resting state network estimation in individual subjects. NeuroImage 2013;82:616–33.

75. Greicius MD, Krasnow B, Reiss AL, et al. Functional connectivity in the resting brain: a network analysis of the default mode hypothesis. Proc Natl Acad Sci United States America 2003;100(1):253–8.

76. Gusnard DA, Raichle ME, Raichle ME. Searching for a baseline: functional imaging and the resting human brain. Nat Rev Neurosci 2001;2(10):685–94.

77. Power JD, Petersen SE. Control-related systems in the human brain. Curr Opin Neurobiol 2013;23(2): 223–8.

78. Dosenbach NU, Visscher KM, Palmer ED, et al. A core system for the implementation of task sets. Neuron 2006;50(5):799–812.

79. Power JD, Cohen AL, Nelson SM, et al. Functional network organization of the human brain. Neuron 2011;72(4):665–78.

80. Lehericy S, Biondi A, Sourour N, et al. Arteriovenous brain malformations: is functional MR imaging reliable for studying language reorganization in patients? Initial observations. Radiology 2002;223(3): 672–82.

81. Schreiber A, Hubbe U, Ziyeh S, et al. The influence of gliomas and nonglial space-occupying lesions on blood-oxygen-level-dependent contrast enhancement. AJNR Am J neuroradiology 2000;21(6): 1055–63.

82. Ulmer JL, Hacein-Bey L, Mathews VP, et al. Lesion-induced pseudo-dominance at functional magnetic resonance imaging: implications for preoperative assessments. Neurosurgery 2004;55(3):569–79 [discussion 580-561].

83. Jayakar P, Bernal B, Santiago Medina L, et al. False lateralization of language cortex on functional MRI after a cluster of focal seizures. Neurology 2002; 58(3):490–2.

Proton and Multinuclear Spectroscopy of the Pediatric Brain

Matthew T. Whitehead, MD[a,b,c,*], Stefan Bluml, PhD[d,e]

KEYWORDS

- Spectroscopy • ^{1}H MRS • Multinuclear • Metabolism • Metabolic • Tumor

KEY POINTS

- In vivo proton magnetic resonance spectroscopy (^{1}H MRS) is a robust technique to obtain clinically relevant metabolic information about the pediatric brain in healthy and pathologic states.
- MRS has the potential to improve diagnosis, prognosticate, and guide therapeutic endeavors in patients with tumors, metabolic diseases, hypoxic-ischemic encephalopathy, stroke, epilepsy, demyelinating disease, and infection.
- Multinuclear MRS using ^{31}P, ^{13}C, and [23]Na are promising ways to evaluate cellular biochemistry and metabolism, yet to be fully explored in the clinical realm.
- Technical progress includes higher field strength magnets, faster acquisitions, improved editing techniques, and X-nuclei MRS.

INTRODUCTION

In vivo magnetic resonance spectroscopy (MRS) is a powerful and often underutilized clinical tool to evaluate the metabolic status of the pediatric brain in a direct, noninvasive manner. Technical advancements have made MRS more user friendly, both in terms of acquisition and interpretation. MRS offers complementary valuable insight into numerous central nervous system (CNS) diseases beyond structural imaging changes, with the potential to improve diagnosis and guide treatment.

MRS detects mobile protons on molecules other than water. Normal and abnormal molecules with different resonance frequencies are displayed on a frequency spectrum scale. Baseline deviations ("peaks") represent substances with different Larmor frequencies (chemical shifts), reflecting differences in molecular proton environments.

The high gyromagnetic ratio and abundance of ^{1}H in the human body makes it the most robust particle to detect and measure. Unsurprisingly, ^{1}H MRS is currently the primary technique used in current clinical practice. Less common particles can be detected using multinuclear spectroscopy.

Magnetic Resonance Spectroscopy Technique

Technical considerations largely relate to the signal-to-noise ratio (SNR), critically important for accurate interpretation. High-channel phased array head coils should be used if possible, preferably more than or equal to 32 elements.[1] Increasing field strength from 1.5 to 3 T provides roughly 50% increase in SNR, causes increased chemical dispersion, and enables more reliable quantitation.[2] Ultrahigh field strength ($\geq$7T) provides better SNR and more opportunity to use X-nuclei (multinuclear MRS).[3,4] Higher field strength is not without drawbacks, however. Although chemical dispersion/peak separation is generally valuable to distinguish overlapping

[a] Department of Radiology, Children's National Hospital, 111 Michigan Avenue NW, Washington, DC 20010, USA; [b] Prenatal Pediatrics Institute, Children's National Hospital, Washington, DC, USA; [c] The George Washington University School of Medicine and Health Sciences, Washington, DC, USA; [d] Department of Radiology, Children's Hospital Los Angeles, Keck School of Medicine, University of Southern California, 450 Sunset Boulevard, Los Angeles, CA 90027, USA; [e] Rudi Schulte Research Institute, Santa Barbara, CA, USA
* Corresponding author.
E-mail address: MWhitehe@childrensnational.org

Magn Reson Imaging Clin N Am 29 (2021) 543–555
https://doi.org/10.1016/j.mric.2021.06.006
1064-9689/21/© 2021 Elsevier Inc. All rights reserved.

proton peaks in different molecules, dispersion of summed peaks from the same molecule reduces peak visibility (eg, myoinositol).[2] Magnetic field heterogeneity and chemical shift displacement are additional challenges at higher field strengths.[1,4] Prescan shimming improves field homogeneity. Chemical shift displacement, artificial displacement of the more peripheral intravoxel resonances, can be reduced by using very selective saturation pulses and semi-LASAR for improved slice selection profile.[1] SNR scales with voxel size; therefore, voxels should be as large as possible to cover the region of interest while minimizing partial volume averaging with undesired tissue.[2] A 4x increase in acquisition time is required to double SNR; longer times mean more opportunity for patient motion artifact. Cubic voxels are better shimmed.[2,5]

Proton Magnetic Resonance Spectroscopy

^{1}H MRS is Food and Drug Administration approved and available on all modern scanners. No longer is it nor should it be considered "experimental." Lack of knowledge, apathy, throughput, and reimbursement are among the many reasons why it has not yet enjoyed universal acceptance. Generally, neuroradiologists are insufficiently exposed to MRS during training and thus feel uncomfortable performing/interpreting it, perpetuating the misconception that MRS is usually "not helpful." Although simpler and more visually pleasing, long-echo MRS is inherently lacking in data from metabolites with fast signal decay and/or low concentrations, which may lead one to the erroneous conclusion that it is nonspecific (eg, increased choline, decreased N-acetyl aspartate [NAA]). Ample data collection and accurate interpretation necessitate a high-quality spectrum with reasonable SNR at sufficiently short echo times (TEs). Extra time and effort is required to perform MRS, problematic for a busy clinical service. With the exception of brain tumors, reimbursement has been challenging. Despite these obstacles, there are many instances when clinical MRS is just "the right thing to do" for the patient.

Single voxel spectroscopy (SVS) is the most common technique. It is faster, easier, and less cognitively demanding than multivoxel (ie, chemical shift imaging) MRS. Further, SVS offers better SNR and shorter TEs than multivoxel. PRESS (point-resolved spectroscopy) and STEAM (stimulated echo acquisition mode) are the primary sequence types, PRESS being more widely used given its better SNR. However, design constraints limit PRESS minimum TEs to 30 msec, whereas with STEAM, TEs can be as short as 14 msec. Shorter TEs reduce T2 relaxation effects, decrease dephasing from J-coupling evolution, and may capture metabolites with smaller concentrations.[1] In addition, PRESS is subject to more chemical shift displacement error; J-coupling effects are also disturbed.[1]

Two or more TEs are preferred, short (<40 msec) and longer (130–288 msec); J-coupling and molecular T2 differences help identify overlapping peaks. Myoinositol (MI), glutamate (glu), glutamine (gln), and most macromolecules are undetectable at longer TEs. Repetition times (TR) must be long to reduce T1 saturation. However, excessive TR costs time, increasing patient motion potential. A TR of 1500 to 2000 msec is reasonable for most disorders at 3T.

Voxel size and location are predicated on the disease, anatomy, and lesion appearance. Sources of spectral distortion/contamination (bone, calcium, blood, vessels, scalp fat) should be avoided. Be mindful of age-related physiologic mineralization of the cerebral deep gray nuclei; in older children, cortical gray and/or white matter may be better sites to interrogate. Focal lesions of sufficient size may be evaluated by SVS or multivoxel MRS. SVS is preferred in most cases; however, multivoxel can assess `normal-appearing brain for comparison simultaneously as well as lesional margins, which may be important for preoperative/treatment planning in high-grade tumors.

Although postprocessing is preferred to quantify metabolites (eg, LCModel) and enhance sensitivity, specificity, consistency, and reproducibility, the required expertise is often unavailable. Indeed, qualitative assessment is often sufficient and robust for most diseases in the clinical setting. However, qualitative interpretation partially relies on peak ratio comparisons. Creatine (Cr) is often the denominator, as it is assumed to be stable over time, an assumption that is not always valid, especially when energetic alterations are present. Familiarity with age, location, and TE-related ratio changes can mitigate this pitfall. Nonetheless, apparently increased NAA and Cho, for instance, could be interpreted as such or alternatively be explained by decreased creatine. A potential advantage of qualitative over quantitative interpretation is that ratios are uninfluenced by intravoxel fluid alterations because all metabolites experience similar changes.

Multinuclear Magnetic Resonance Spectroscopy

Multinuclear spectroscopy (MNS) requires nonstandard equipment, special expertise, and is limited by low signal-to-noise (long scan times). This, and the general challenges of conducting studies in the pediatric population, has resulted in few MNS studies being conducted in children. With availability of high-field MR scanners, an MNS renaissance is conceivable. MNS has advantages over proton spectroscopy when studying energy metabolism, phosphorylated membrane metabolites, and measuring pH noninvasively.

MNS targets nuclei other than ^{1}H and may be more disease specific in some circumstances. Varying Larmor frequencies necessitate coil and radiofrequency pulse adjustments specific to the nuclei one wishes to assess.[3] Double-tuned coils that can capture ^{1}H and X-nuclei simultaneously are desirable because they (1) allow coregistration of brain tissue and X-nuclei data and (2) improve shimming.[3] Compressed sensing techniques improve image quality.[3]

^{31}P provides insight into brain energy metabolism, showing the state of adenosine triphosphate (ATP), nicotinamide adenine dinucleotide (NAD)+/NAD+hydrogen, phosphocreatine, and other phosphate molecules involved in oxidative phosphorylation which are of great interest in metabolic diseases, ischemia, and tumors.[4] Minshew and colleagues found abnormal phosphocreatine in autistic children and adolescents and describe a correlation between test performance and membrane phosphomonoesters and phosphodiesters.[6] ^{31}P MRS has also been used to monitor treatment of patients in whom the biosynthesis of creatine is impaired.[4] With *proton-decoupled* ^{31}P, membrane metabolites such as phosphocholine and glycerophosphocholine have been investigated in pediatric brain tumors and a rare form of leukodystrophy.[7,8]

Cellular membrane potential/ion channel abnormalities and secondary sodium shifts are the basis for ^{23}NA MRS. Potential applications in children include tumor, stroke, demyelination, and traumatic brain injury. For example, excess tissue sodium is found in irreversible cell damage during ischemic injury.[3]

^{13}C MRS, in combination with ^{13}C-labeled substrate infusion, can be used to study in vivo flux rates of fundamental metabolic pathways such as glycolysis and the glutamate/glutamine neurotransmitter cycle, but there are significant logistical challenges.[3,9] The few studies that have been performed in children have shown reduced glucose oxidation in a juvenile and premature infant with hypoxic injury, abnormal glucose metabolism in leukodystrophies and mitochondrial disorders,[9] and a reduced NAA synthesis rate in Canavan disease.[10]

Normal Brain Development

The newborn brain undergoes dramatic structural/maturational changes, including outgrowth, myelination, gliogenesis, dendritic arborization, and angiogenesis. Significant metabolic adjustments are required to provide energy and structural "building blocks" for rapid growth, neurotransmission, and synaptic function. Studying "normal" metabolic brain maturation is challenging, as completely healthy newborns rarely make it to MR scanners. Nevertheless, major metabolic trends of some selected brain regions have been studied using clinically indicated MRS from newborns who had unremarkable clinical follow-up.[11–15] Spectra that illustrate age-dependent changes in "closest-to-normal" clinical patients are shown in **Fig. 1**.

DEVELOPING BRAIN—KEY POINTS

- Most metabolic changes occur in the first 3 months of life
- Prematurity mildly influences brain maturation; however, metabolism mostly follows gestational age
- NAA (indicates adult-type neurons/axons), Cr (energy metabolite), and Glu (excitatory neurotransmitter) all increase rapidly between birth and 3 months
- Myo-inositol (phospholipid membrane precursor, osmolyte, astrocyte marker) declines rapidly
- Choline (membrane metabolite) peaks from birth until 3 months, then declines gradually
- Lactate (anaerobic metabolism): low concentrations in normal newborn brains
  ○ Pyruvate dehydrogenase activity lacking at birth

Brain Tumors

Pediatric brain tumors exhibit high biological and pathologic heterogeneity. Adult tumors mainly comprise gliomas with relatively predictable outcomes based on type, grade, and patient age. In contradistinction, pediatric tumors include embryonal types, pilocytic astrocytomas, ependymomas, germ cell tumors, and others. Furthermore, recent molecular advances have identified subtypes with significantly different outcomes. Metabolite profiles of childhood brain tumors are generally characteristic for tumor type. MR spectroscopy, added to clinical MR imaging, improves the accuracy of initial diagnosis[3,16–18] **(Fig. 2)**.

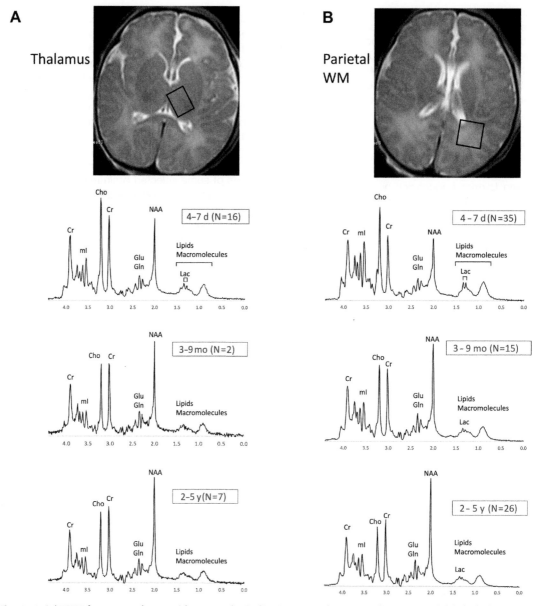

Fig. 1. Axial T2WI from a newborn, with rectangles indicating typical regions of interest in (*A*) left thalamus and (*B*) left parietal white matter. "Close-to-normal" spectra shown were acquired from pediatric patients, with normal MR examinations performed for clinically appropriate indications. Metabolic brain maturation includes increasing NAA and decreasing choline and myo-inositol. Also note that small amounts of lactate are normally detectable in the newborn brain. T2WI, T2-weighted imaging.

PEDIATRIC BRAIN TUMORS—KEY POINTS

- Diagnoses
  - Medulloblastoma: elevated taurine and glycine[18,19]
  - Diffuse intrinsic pontine gliomas/diffuse midline gliomas: citrate[20]
  - Pilocytic astrocytoma: decreased Cr; N-acetylated sugar accumulation[21]
  - Choline elevation and MI depression favors choroid plexus carcinoma over papilloma[22]
- Prognosis/stratification
  - Identifies medulloblastoma and atypical teratoid/rhabdoid tumor subtypes[18,23]
  - Citrate in grade II astrocytoma outside brainstem predicts progression[20]

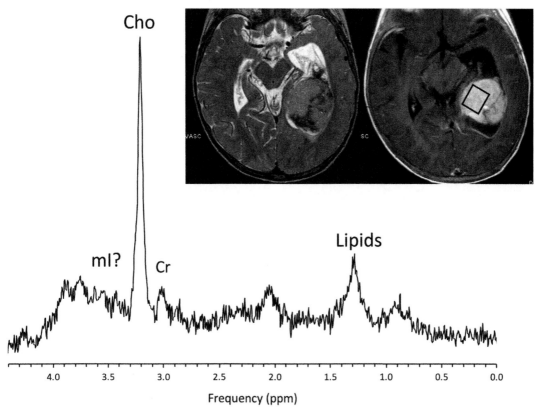

Fig. 2. Axial T2WI and postcontrast T1WI from a 12-year-old boy show a vividly enhancing mass lesion in the left lateral ventricle consistent with a choroid plexus tumor of uncertain type. MRS shows prominent Cho, whereas myo-inositol is low or absent. This strongly favors carcinoma over papilloma. Subsequent resection after enlargement and clinical worsening over 3 weeks confirmed choroid plexus carcinoma.

- Treatment/disease monitoring
  - Useful for unresectable/partially resectable tumors
  - Pediatric glioma metabolic progression similar to adults[17]
    - Increasing choline, lactate, and lipids relative to creatine
    - Decreasing myo-inositol

Genetic/Metabolic Disorders

In vivo MRS is a first-class technique to investigate brain metabolism in a direct and noninvasive manner. MRS should be performed in *all* known or suspected inborn errors of metabolism (IEM) affecting the brain, given its potential to improve diagnostic sensitivity and specificity.[5,24,25] In a study of patients who underwent MRS during childhood seizure evaluation, 40% of positive MRS cases prompted or enhanced the workup for an underlying IEM.[26] Even when the spectroscopic pattern is nonspecific, it may still be abnormal at baseline, and therefore useful for therapeutic monitoring.

GENETIC/METABOLIC DISORDERS—KEY POINTS

- Diagnosis: improves confidence; provides baseline
- Follow-up: demonstrates therapeutic response
  - Clinical, biochemical, and imaging disease severity often correlate better with *brain* than blood/CSF metabolite concentrations[5,27–29]
- Technique recommendations
  - Short-echo SVS *obligatory* to detect/evaluate metabolites with low concentrations and/or short T2 values
  - Longer TE useful to distinguish overlapping metabolites
  - Voxel location:
    - Based on suspected abnormality and brain appearance
    - Acute/active lesions: changes reflect local metabolism
    - Normal-appearing tissue useful; confirm/exclude systemic changes
    - Avoid chronic/burned out lesions

- Special acquisition/postprocessing/quantification sometimes required:
  - Metabolites in small concentrations
  - Resonances in nonstandard or populated regions
- Canavan[2,5,25]
  - NAA elevated
- Alexander[28]
  - MI elevated

- Nonketotic hyperglycinemia[5,30] (**Fig. 3**)
  - Glycine increased (3.56 ppm)
  - Longer TE eliminates overlapping MI peak
- Maple syrup urine disease[5,25]
  - Branched chain amino acids and ketoacids (0.9–1 ppm)
  - J-coupling–related peak inversion at 1.5 T intermediate TE
- Urea cycle disorders[2,25]
  - Glutamine (gln) and glutamate (glu) increased

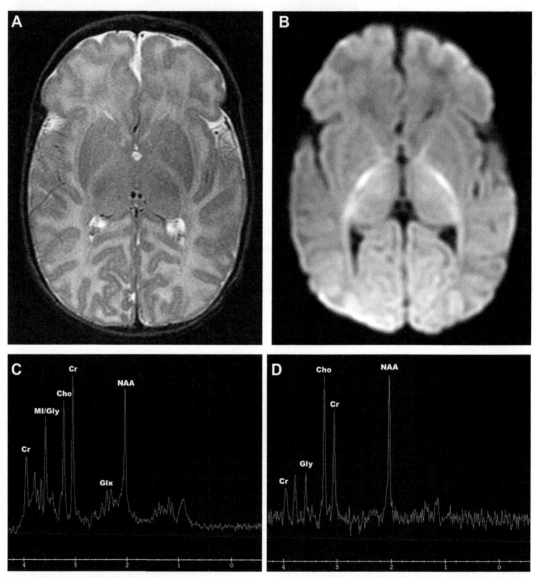

Fig. 3. (*A*) Axial T2WI and (*B*) DWI from a term 11-day-old boy with NKH presenting with seizures demonstrate lack of normal myelination-related signal in the posterior internal capsule and reduced diffusion in the thalami, internal capsules, and sagittal stratum. (*C*) SVS over the left basal ganglia (TR/TE, 1500/35) shows a large peak at 3.55 ppm attributable to myoinositol and/or glycine (MI/Gly), elevated glutamine/glutamate (glx), increased creatine (Cr), and decreased choline (Cho). (*D*) Long-echo MRS in the same region (TR/TE, 1500/35) clarifies, showing a residual peak at 3.55 ppm representing elevated glycine (Gly). DWI, diffusion-weighted imaging; NKH, nonketotic hyperglycinemia; TR/TE, repetition time/echo time.

- ○ Resonances overlap at 1.5 T from 2 to 2.4 ppm
- ○ Chemical dispersion increases peak separation at 3 T
  - ■ 2.4 ppm = gln; 2.2 ppm = glu
- ○ Alpha proton peak at 3.75 ppm important
- ○ MI depressed (osmotic buffer)
- ○ Cho reduced in chronic phase
- ○ Distal urea cycle disorder defects: hyperammonemic encephalopathy less common
  - ■ Glutamine often normal
  - ■ Arginosuccinate lyase deficiency: guanidinoacetate (3.8 ppm)[31]
  - ■ Arginase deficiency: arginine (3.87 ppm)[32]
- L-2-hydroxyglutaric aciduria: L-2-hydroxyglutaric acid (1.9, 2.2–2.5 ppm)[33]
- Glutaric aciduria type I[30,34]
  - ○ Glutaric acid (2.1–2.3 ppm)
  - ○ 3-OH-glutaric acid (2.4–2.5 ppm)
- Isovaleric acidemia: isovalerate (0.9 ppm)[24]
- Mucopolysaccharidoses: glycosaminoglycans (3.3–4.4 ppm)[24,25]
- Metachromatic leukodystrophy: MI elevation[5]
- Mitochondrial
  - ○ Lactate (1.3 ppm doublet) = hallmark; not specific, absence does not exclude
  - ○ MRS lactate improves diagnostic accuracy[5,29]
  - ○ Mitochondrial disease more closely associated with MRS than blood and cerebrospinal fluid lactate[5,27]
  - ○ Lactate detection in normal-appearing brain increases specificity for mitochondrial disease
  - ○ Beware: lactate detection unreliable with TE 144 at 3 T[35]
- Succinate dehydrogenase deficiency: succinate (2.4 ppm)[36]
- Pyruvate dehydrogenase complex deficiency: pyruvate (2.37 ppm)[37]
- Lipid metabolism: lipid elevation[24,30,38,39]
- Creatine deficiency: creatine/phosphocreatine (3, 3.9 ppm)[40]
- Galactosemia: galactitol (3.67, 3.74 ppm doublet)[41]; inverts at intermediate TE

Hypoxic-Ischemic Injury

Newborn hypoxic-ischemic encephalopathy (HIE) was the first application of MRS in the human brain—more than 3 decades ago. At that time, phosphorous (31P) was the favored methodology. Early studies demonstrated that the ATP/Pi ratio and intracerebral pH predicted outcome.[42–44] With the arrival robust ^{1}H MRS, the emphasis shifted toward NAA (neuronal/axonal injury or loss), lactate increasing proportional to the severity of injury,[45–49] and lipids (cell membrane breakdown and apoptosis).

HYPOXIC-ISCHEMIC INJURY—KEY POINTS

- Voxel locations: thalamus and/or basal ganglia and cerebral white matter
- Reduced NAA and increased lactate: indicators for extent of acute injury
- Glutamine (not glutamate): elevated in acute injury
- Lipids increase with cell death
- Regions of high-energy demand more vulnerable
- Caveat: small amounts of lactate may be normal in newborns

Demyelinating Disorders

Multiple sclerosis (MS), acute demyelinating encephalomyelitis (ADEM), and neuromyelitis optica (NMO) may cause intersecting imaging changes. The childhood MS MR imaging phenotype ranges from classic (multifocal small ovoid perivenular inflammatory demyelinating lesions in brain ± spinal cord and optic nerves) to ADEM-like (larger, amorphous lesions). Contemporary multifocal large gray and white matter demyelinating lesions characterize monophasic ADEM. Inflammatory lesions at sites of AQP4 expression typify NMO. Central periventricular/periependymal lesions increase specificity,[50] but MR imaging is often normal. MRS can help distinguish demyelinating disease subtypes. Acute MS plaques show decreased NAA and increased Cho, whereas ADEM lesions typically do not.[51,52]

DEMYELINATING DISORDERS—KEY POINTS

- MS (Fig. 4)
  - ○ *NAA reduced:* acute to chronic plaques; normal-appearing brain[52,53]
    - ■ Edema/dilution, decreased production, and/or neuronal loss
  - ○ *Cho increased:* acute lesions; normal brain[52,53]
    - ■ Cell membrane destruction; may precede focal lesions
    - ■ Normalizes after 6 months
  - ○ Lactate and macromolecules in acute plaques[52,53]
    - ■ Normalize after 3 to 6 months
  - ○ MI: increased in chronic lesions; variable, often increased in acute lesions[52,53]
  - ○ Glutamine/glutamate: increased in acute lesions, normal-appearing white matter (NAWM)[52,53]

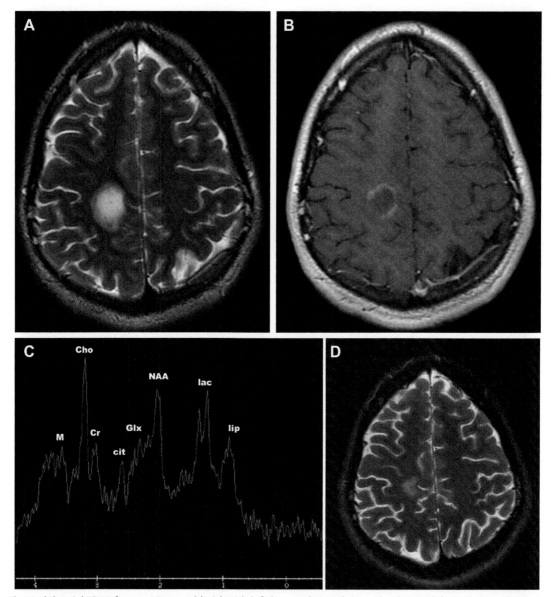

Fig. 4. (A) Axial T2WI from a 16-year-old girl with left leg weakness shows a large ovoid, hyperintense lesion in the right frontal subcortical white matter. (B) Postcontrast T1WI demonstrates discontinuous rim enhancement consistent with an actively demyelinating plaque. (C) SVS over the lesion (TR/TE msec, 1500/35) is consistent with an acute MS plaque: increased lipids (lip), citrate (cit), lactate, and glutamine and glutamate (Glx) and decreased NAA and creatine (Cr). (D) A chronic hyperintense demyelinating plaque remains 2 years later on T2WI.

- ▪ Impaired oligodendrocyte-mediated glutamate clearance[53]
  - ○ Citrate elevated[53]
    - ▪ NAWM (32%), chronic lesions (28%), acute lesions (13%)
    - ▪ Myelin instability
  - ○ Glutathione (2.95 ppm): decreased in acute plaques and gray matter at 7 T[4]
  - ○ Beware: pitfall in qualitative ratios[52]
    - ▪ [Cr] variable, negatively associated with plaque size, increases in chronic lesions

- ▪ Attributable to oligodendrocytes (gliosis vs remyelination)
- • ADEM
  - ○ Acute lesions and NAWM: Glx, macromolecules, and lactate[52,53]
    - ▪ Normal NAA and Cho
  - ○ Subacute lesions (>1 wk): decreased NAA and MI, elevated Cho[54–57]
    - ▪ NAA may normalize[58,59]
- • NMO spectrum
  - ○ Normal NAA:Cr and MI in NAWM[50]

○ Milder choline elevation in NAWM compared with MS[60]

○ Normal Cho:Cr and NAA:Cr in normal-appearing gray[50]

○ Lower MI:Cr in lesions compared with MS[50]

Infection

Childhood CNS infection may be caused by bacterial, viral, fungal, or less commonly parasitic or protozoan agents. Brain and/or spinal cord edema/swelling is common among these groups when the parenchyma is involved directly or secondarily from vascular compromise. Various additional MR imaging features help differentiate groups, although the specific agent often remains unknown even after CSF analysis. MRS can be useful to distinguish abscess from neoplasm, determine abscess type, and in some cases, suggest the infectious category or agent.

CENTRAL NERVOUS SYSTEM INFECTION—KEY POINTS

- Bacterial abscess (**Fig. 5**)
  - ○ Bacteria, byproducts, neutrophils>lymphocytes, necrosis[61]
  - ○ Cytosolic amino acids (leucine/isoleucine/valine; 0.9 ppm), alanine (1.48 ppm), lipids, lactate; no brain metabolites[2,61]
    - Cytosolic amino acids from cell membrane rupture and neutrophils
    - Lactate/lipids = necrosis
  - ○ Acetate (1.92) ± succinate (2.4 ppm) favors anerobic[62]

- ○ MRS sensitivity and specificity in culture positive cases = 100% and 75% for aerobic and 75% and 100% for anaerobic[62]
- ○ Spectral pattern changes after treatment[63]
  - Only lipid/lactate remain after 72 hours of effective antibiotics
  - MRS correlates with bacterial viability
- Viral
  - ○ Herpes simplex virus
    - Decreased NAA, increased glx and choline, ±lactate[2,64]
    - Normalization can occur following recovery[2]
  - ○ HIV: decreased NAA, increased MI
    - Nonencephalopathic[54]
      • Increased Cho, threonine, macromolecules
    - Encephalopathic[54]
      • Increased macromolecules and gamma aminobutyric acid
- Tuberculosis
  - ○ Tuberculosis, byproducts, lymphocytes > neutrophils
  - ○ Fewer proteolytic enzymes than bacterial = absent cytosolic amino acids[61]
  - ○ More lipids/lactate than bacterial[61]
    - Mycobacteria = lipid rich
- Fungal
  - ○ *Trehalose* (3.6–3.8 ppm), lactate, alanine, acetate, succinate, choline, lipids, and/or amino acids[2]
- Cestode parasites (neurocysticercosis and hydatid cysts)
  - ○ Pyruvate (2.4 ppm), acetate (1.9 ppm), lactate[55]
- Cryptococcus
  - ○ Alanine, lipids, acetate, succinate; ±lactate[61]

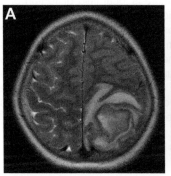 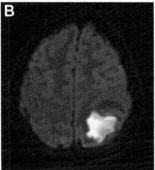 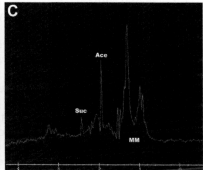

Fig. 5. (*A*) Axial T2WI and (*B*) DWI from an 11-year-old girl with right extremity weakness show a left parietal mass with central reduced diffusion, marginal T2 shortening, and marked surrounding edema consistent with abscess. (*C*) SVS (TR/TE msec, 1500/35) shows typical features of a bacterial abscess: multiple macromolecular peaks (MM) representing cytosolic amino acids (leucine, isoleucine, valine at 0.9 ppm), lipids (0.9 and 1.3 ppm), lactate (1.33 ppm), and lack of significant NAA, creatine, and choline. Acetate (1.92 ppm) and succinate (2.4 ppm) suggest anaerobic bacterial fermentation. Biopsy showed streptococcus intermedius (an aerotolerant anaerobe).

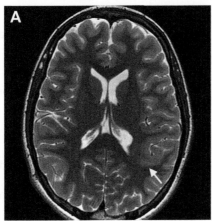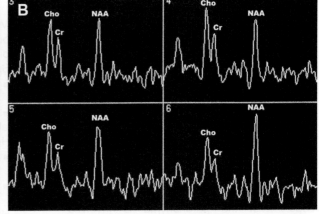

Fig. 6. (*A*) Axial T2WI from a 5-year-old woman with focal seizures shows cortical thickening/corticomedullary blurring along the left supramarginal gyrus, consistent with FCD (*arrow*). (*B*) Multivoxel MRS over the temporoparietal lobes (TR/TE msec, 1500/144) shows only mildly decreased NAA and mildly elevated choline (Cho) in the FCD (panels 3 and 4) relative to the normal right side (panels 5 and 6), suggesting dysplasia rather than neoplasia.

Epilepsy

MRS should be considered in childhood seizure evaluation. The technique has been shown to be beneficial for diagnosis, prognosis, and/or management in 43% of patients.[26] MRS can also distinguish dysplasia from tumor, prognosticate, uncover IEMs, and reveal metabolic changes in mesial temporal lobe epilepsy (MTLE).[26,56,57,65] Furthermore, MRS can monitor the status of ketosis during ketogenic diets.[66] Serum and brain β-hydroxybutyrate (1.2 ppm) levels are highly concordant, and the degree of seizure control correlates with serum β-hydroxybutyrate levels.[66] Ketones can also be found at 2.2 ppm.[2]

EPILEPSY—KEY POINTS

- MTLE
  - SVS or multivoxel[2]
  - *Decreased NAA*[56,57,65]
    - Neuronal dysfunction or injury (recent seizures) and/or loss
    - NAA can normalize if seizures resolve[2]
  - NAA/Cr + Cho lower in patients with prior febrile seizure[57]
  - NAA/Cr can localize side of seizure origin (93%)[2]
  - NAA/Cr may be reduced in both mesial temporal lobes; contralateral abnormalities resolve with successful ipsilateral surgery
  - Epileptic tissue: glutamate and MI elevated[2]
  - Lactate±
    - Seizure-related neuronal damage[2]
- Focal cortical dysplasia (FCD) (**Fig. 6**)
  - Decreased NAA ± increased Cho and/or MI (all less pronounced compared with neoplasia)[67–69]

  - Cr/NAA + Cr + Cho higher and Cho/Cr lower in FCD than ganglioglioma[70]
  - Beware: more volume averaging of normal brain = less pronounced MRS abnormalities
  - Remember: FCD and low-grade tumor can coexist
- Hypothalamic hamartomas
  - Decreased NAA, increased MI
    - Altered neuropil constituents (fewer neurons, more glial tissue)[71]

SUMMARY

MR spectroscopy is a valuable addition to the diagnostic work-up of childhood brain disease. It holds the potential to make diagnoses, narrow the differential considerations, and determine therapeutic efficacy. ^{1}H MRS should be performed at the time of initial structural MR acquisition in patients with unknown focal lesions of sufficient size, known or suspected metabolic disease, and HIE whenever possible unless there is local field distortion or a compelling clinical reason otherwise. Tumor follow-up, epilepsy, and demyelinating diseases also benefit from ^{1}H MRS. Technical challenges have impeded the dissemination of MNS into the clinical realm thus far. Future advances will pave the way for its eventual incorporation into the assessment of childhood disease, as MNS is more disease specific in some circumstances.

CLINICS CARE POINTS

- ^{1}H MRS is beneficial for diagnosis and therapeutic monitoring in tumors, IEMs, HIE, infection, demyelination, and epilepsy.

- SVS with *at least* short, but preferably short and longer TE, is recommended for most disorders.
- MNS requires nonstandard hardware and is logistically challenging.
- ^{31}P MRS is useful to evaluate energy and phosphorylated membrane metabolites with improved specificity over ^{1}H MRS.

DISCLOSURES

The authors have nothing to disclose.

REFERENCES

1. Wilson M, Andronesi O, Barker PB, et al. Methodological consensus on clinical proton MRS of the brain: review and recommendations. Magn Reson Med 2019;82(2):527–50.
2. Blüml S, Panigrahy A, editors. MR spectroscopy of pediatric brain disorders. New York: Springer-Verlag; 2013.
3. Ladd ME, Bachert P, Meyerspeer M, et al. Pros and cons of ultra-high field MRI/MRS for human application. Prog Nucl Mag Reson Spectrosc 2018;109: 1–50.
4. Henning A. Proton and multinuclear MRS in the human brain at ultra-high field strength: a review. Neuroimage 2018;168:181–98.
5. Rossi A, Biancheri R. Magnetic resonance spectroscopy in metabolic disorders. Neuroimaging Clin N Am 2013;23(3):425–48.
6. Minshew NJ, Goldstein G, Dombrowski SM, et al. A preliminary 31P MRS study of autism: evidence for undersynthesis and increased degradation of brain membranes. Biol Psychiatry 1993;33(11–12): 762–73.
7. Albers M, Krieger M, Gonzalez-Gomez I, et al. Proton-decoupled 31P MRS in untreated pediatric brain tumors. Magn Reson Med Jan 2005;53(1):22–9.
8. Bluml S, Philippart M, Schiffmann R, et al. Membrane phospholipids and high-energy metabolites in childhood ataxia with CNS hypomyelination. Neurology 2003;61(5):648–54.
9. Bluml S, Moreno A, Hwang H, et al. 1-(13)C glucose magnetic resonance spectroscopy of pediatric and adult brain disorders. NMR Biomed 2001;14(1): 19–32.
10. Moreno A, Ross B, Blüml S. Direct determination of the N-acetyl-L-aspartate synthesis rate in the human brain by (13)C MRS and [1-(13)C]glucose infusion. J Neurochem 2001;77(1):347–50.
11. Blüml S, Wisnowski JL, Nelson MD, et al. Metabolic maturation of the human brain from birth through adolescence: insights from in vivo MRS. Cereb Cortex 2013;23(12):2944–55.
12. Blüml S, Wisnowski JL, Nelson MD, et al. Metabolic maturation of white matter is altered in preterm infants. PLoS One 2014;9(1):e85829.
13. Kreis R, Ernst T, Ross BD. Development of the human brain: in vivo quantification of metabolite and water content with proton MRS. Magn Reson Med 1993;30(4):424–37.
14. Huppi PS, Posse S, Lazeyras F, et al. Magnetic resonance in preterm and term newborns: 1H-spectroscopy in developing human brain. Pediatr Res 1991; 30(6):574–8.
15. van der Knaap MS, van der Grond J, van Rijen PC, et al. Age-dependent changes in localized proton and phosphorus MR spectroscopy of the brain. Radiology 1990;176(2):509–15.
16. Shiroishi MS, Panigrahy A, Moore KR, et al. Combined MRI and MRS improves pre-therapeutic diagnoses of pediatric brain tumors over MRI alone. Neuroradiology 2015;57(9):951–6.
17. Panigrahy A, Krieger MD, Gonzalez-Gomez I, et al. Quantitative short echo time 1H-MR spectroscopy of untreated pediatric brain tumors: preoperative diagnosis and characterization. AJNR Am J Neuroradiol 2006;27(3):560–72.
18. Blüml S, Margol AS, Sposto R, et al. Molecular subgroups of medulloblastoma identification using noninvasive. MRS Neuro Oncol 2016;18(1):126–31.
19. Kovanlikaya A, Panigrahy A, Krieger M, et al. Untreated pediatric primitive neuroectodermal tumor in vivo: quantitation of taurine with MR spectroscopy. Radiology 2005;236(3):1020–5.
20. Blüml S, Panigrahy A, Laskov M, et al. Elevated citrate in pediatric astrocytomas with malignant progression. Neuro Oncol 2011;13(10):1107–17.
21. Tamrazi B, Nelson MD, Blüml S. MRS of pilocytic astrocytoma: the peak at 2 ppm may not be NAA. Magn Reson Med 2017;78(2):452–6.
22. Krieger MD, Panigrahy A, McComb JG, et al. Differentiation of choroid plexus tumors by advanced MRS. Neurosurg Focus 2005;15(6A):E4.
23. Tamrazi B, Venneti S, Margol A, et al. Pediatric atypical Teratoid/Rhabdoid tumors of the brain: identification of metabolic subgroups using InVivo MRS. AJNR Am J Neuroradiol 2019;40(5):872–7.
24. Patay Z, Blaser SI, Poretti A, et al. Neurometabolic diseases of childhood. Pediatr Radiol 2015; 45(Suppl 3):S473–84.
25. Whitehead MT, Gropman AL. Other metabolic syndromes. In: Lewis J, Keshari K, editors. Imaging and metabolism. Cham: Springer; 2018.
26. Rincon SP, Blitstein MB, Caruso PA, et al. The use of MRS in the evaluation of pediatric patients with seizures. Pediatr Neurol 2016;58:57–66.
27. Lunsing RJ, Strating K, de Koning TJ, et al. Diagnostic value of MRS-quantified brain tissue lactate level in identifying children with mitochondrial disorders. Eur Radiol 2017;27(3):976–84.

28. Sen K, Whitehead MT, Gropman AL. Multimodal imaging in urea cycle-related neurological disease - What can imaging after hyperammonemia teach us? Transl Sci Rare Dis 2020;5(1–2):87–95.

29. Mascalchi M, Montomoli M, Guerrini R. Neuroimaging in mitochondrial disorders. Essays Biochem 2018;62(3):409–21.

30. Whitehead MT, Fricke ST, Gropman AL. Structural brain defects. Clin Perinatol 2015;42(2):337–61, ix.

31. Sijens PE, Reijngoud DJ, Soorani-Lunsing RJ, et al. Cerebral 1H MRS showing elevation of brain guanidinoacetate in argininosuccinate lyase deficiency. Mol Genet Metab 2006;88(1):100–2.

32. Jichlinski A, Clarke L, Whitehead MT, et al. "Cerebral Palsy" in a patient with arginase deficiency. Semin Pediatr Neurol 2018;26:110–4.

33. Fourati H, Ellouze E, Ahmadi M, et al. MRI features in 17 patients with I2 hydroxyglutaric aciduria. Eur J Radiol Open 2016;3:245–50.

34. Harting I, Boy N, Heringer J, et al. (1)H-MRS in glutaric aciduria type 1: impact of biochemical phenotype and age on the cerebral accumulation of neurotoxic metabolites. J Inherit Metab Dis 2015; 38(5):829–38.

35. Lange T, Dydak U, Roberts TP, et al. Pitfalls in lactate measurements at 3T. AJNR Am J Neuroradiol 2006; 27(4):895–901.

36. Helman G, Caldovic L, Whitehead MT, et al. MRI spectrum of succinate dehydrogenase- related infantile leukoencephalopathy. Ann Neurol 2016; 79(3):379–86.

37. Zand DJ, Simon EM, Pulitzer SB, et al. In vivo pyruvate detected by MRS in neonatal pyruvate dehydrogenase deficiency. Am J Neuroradiol 2003; 24(7):1471–4.

38. Willemsen MA, Van Der Graaf M, Van Der Knaap MS, et al. MR imaging and proton MR spectroscopic studies in Sjögren-Larsson syndrome: characterization of the leukoencephalopathy. AJNR Am J Neuroradiol 2004;25(4):649–57.

39. Ferreira CR, Silber MH, Chang T, et al. Cerebral Lipid Accumulation Detected by MRS in a Child with Carnitine Palmitoyltransferase 2 deficiency: a case report and review of the literature on genetic etiologies of lipid peaks on MRS. JIMD Rep 2016;28:69–74.

40. Stockler-Ipsiroglu S, van Karnebeek C, Longo N, et al. Guanidinoacetate methyltransferase deficiency: outcomes in 48 individuals and recommendations for diagnosis, treatment and monitoring. Mol Genet Metab 2014;111(1):16–25.

41. Wang ZJ, Berry GT, Dreha SF, et al. Proton MRS of brain metabolites in galactosemia. Ann Neurol 2001;50(2):266–9.

42. Hamilton PA, Hope PL, Cady EB, et al. Impaired energy metabolism in brains of newborn infants with increased cerebral echodensities. Lancet 1986; 1(8492):1242–6.

43. Cady EB, Costello AM, Dawson MJ, et al. Non-invasive investigation of cerebral metabolism in newborn infants by phosphorus nuclear MRS. Lancet 1983; 1(8333):1059–62.

44. Hope PL, Costello AM, Cady EB, et al. Cerebral energy metabolism studied with phosphorus NMR spectroscopy in normal and birth-asphyxiated infants. Lancet 1984;2(8399):366–70.

45. Cheong JL, Cady EB, Penrice J, et al. Proton MRS in neonates with perinatal cerebral hypoxic-ischemic injury: metabolite peak-area ratios, relaxation times, and absolute concentrations. AJNR Am J Neuroradiol 2006;27(7):1546–54.

46. Barkovich AJ, Baranski K, Vigneron D, et al. Proton MR spectroscopy for the evaluation of brain injury in asphyxiated, term neonates. AJNR Am J Neuroradiol 1999;20(8):1399–405.

47. Shanmugalingam S, Thornton JS, Iwata O, et al. Comparative prognostic utilities of early quantitative MRI spin-spin relaxometry and proton MRS in neonatal encephalopathy. Pediatrics 2006;118(4): 1467–77.

48. Shu SK, Ashwal S, Holshouser BA, et al. Prognostic value of 1H-MRS in perinatal CNS insults. Pediatr Neurol 1997;17(4):309–18.

49. Thayyil S, Chandrasekaran M, Taylor A, et al. Cerebral magnetic resonance biomarkers in neonatal encephalopathy: a meta-analysis. Pediatrics 2010; 125(2):e382–95.

50. Kremer S, Renard F, Achard S, et al. Use of advanced MRI techniques in neuromyelitis optica spectrum disorder. JAMA Neurol 2015;72(7):815–22.

51. Mader I, Wolff M, Nägele T, et al. MRI and proton MRS in acute disseminated encephalomyelitis. Childs Nerv Syst 2005;21(7):566–72.

52. Mader I, Rauer S, Gall P, et al. (1)H MR spectroscopy of inflammation, infection and ischemia of the brain. Eur J Radiol 2008;67(2):250–7.

53. Verhey LH, Sled JG. Advanced MRI in pediatric multiple sclerosis. Neuroimaging Clin N Am 2013;23(2): 337–54.

54. Salvan AM, Lamoureux S, Michel G, et al. Localized proton MRS of the brain in children infected with HIV with and without encephalopathy. Pediatr Res 1998; 44(5):755–62.

55. Jayakumar PN, Srikanth SG, Chandrashekar HS, et al. Pyruvate: an in vivo marker of cestodal infestation of the human brain on proton MRS. J Magn Reson Imaging 2003;18(6):675–80.

56. Cohen-Gadol AA, Pan JW, Kim JH, et al. Mesial temporal lobe epilepsy: a proton MRS study and a histopathological analysis. J Neurosurg 2004;101(4):613–20.

57. Wu WC, Huang CC, Chung HW, et al. Hippocampal alterations in children with temporal lobe epilepsy with or without a history of febrile convulsions: evaluations with MR volumetry and proton MRS. AJNR Am J Neuroradiol 2005;26(5):1270–5.

58. Bizzi A, Uluğ AM, Crawford TO, et al. Quantitative proton MRS imaging in acute disseminated encephalomyelitis. AJNR Am J Neuroradiol 2001;22(6):1125–30.

59. Balasubramanya KS, Kovoor JM, Jayakumar PN, et al. Diffusion-weighted imaging and proton MRS in the characterization of acute disseminated encephalomyelitis. Neuroradiology 2007;49(2):177–83.

60. Duan Y, Liu Z, Liu Y, et al. Metabolic changes in normal-appearing white matter in patients with neuromyelitis optica and multiple sclerosis: a comparative MRS study. Acta Radiol 2017;58(9):1132–7.

61. Dusak A, Hakyemez B, Kocaeli H, et al. MRS findings of pyogenic, tuberculous, and Cryptococcus intracranial abscesses. Neurochem Res 2012;37(2):233–7.

62. Bajpai A, Prasad KN, Mishra P, et al. Multimodal approach for diagnosis of bacterial etiology in brain abscess. Magn Reson Imaging 2014;32(5):491–6.

63. Večeřa Z, Krejčí T, Krajča J, et al. Effect of antibiotic therapy on proton MR spectroscopy findings in human pyogenicbrain abscesses. J Neurosurg Sci 2019. [Epub ahead of print].

64. Triulzi F, Doneda C, Parazzini C. Neuroimaging of pediatric brain infections. Expert Rev Anti Infect Ther 2011;9(6):737–51.

65. Lopez-Acevedo ML, Martinez-Lopez M, Favila R, et al. Secondary MRI-findings, volumetric and spectroscopic measurements in mesial temporal sclerosis: a multivariate discriminant analysis. Swiss Med Wkly 2012;142:w13549.

66. Wright JN, Saneto RP, Friedman SD. β-Hydroxybutyrate detection with proton MR spectroscopy in children with drug-resistant epilepsy on the ketogenic diet. AJNR Am J Neuroradiol 2018;39(7):1336–40.

67. Tschampa HJ, Urbach H, Träber F, et al. Proton MRS in focal cortical dysplasia at 3T. Seizure 2015;32:23–9.

68. Leite CC, Lucato LT, Sato JR, et al. Multivoxel proton MRS in malformations of cortical development. AJNR Am J Neuroradiol 2007;28(6):1071–5 [discussion 1076-7].

69. Vuori K, Kankaanranta L, Häkkinen AM, et al. Low-grade gliomas and focal cortical developmental malformations: differentiation with proton MRS. Radiology 2004;230(3):703–8.

70. Fellah S, Callot V, Viout P, et al. Epileptogenic brain lesions in children: the added-value of combined diffusion imaging and proton MRS to the presurgical differential diagnosis. Childs Nerv Syst 2012;28(2):273–82.

71. Freeman JL, Coleman LT, Wellard RM, et al. MRI and spectroscopic study of epileptogenic hypothalamic hamartomas: analysis of 72 cases. AJNR Am J Neuroradiol 2004;25(3):450–62.

Fetal Neuroimaging Updates

Jeffrey N. Stout, PhD[a],[*],[1], M. Alejandra Bedoya, MD[b],[1], P. Ellen Grant, MD, MSc[a,b,c,2], Judy A. Estroff, MD[b,d,2]

KEYWORDS

- Fetus • Magnetic resonance imaging • Neuroimaging

KEY POINTS

- Fetal US and MR imaging are complementary, with US used for overall screening and MR to characterize complex anomalies in greater detail.
- MR imaging of the developing fetal brain, face/neck, and spine is complex, but crucial for optimal management to better characterize suspected abnormalities.
- Interpreting and reporting fetal MR imaging requires not only a deep understanding of embryology, normal development, and common malformations, but also a clear sense of the sequences currently available for clinical use, their strengths and limitations, as well as common artifacts.
- Significant improvements in clinical MR imaging protocols are within reach. Physiology and function are long term goals of ongoing sequence development and postacquisition analysis techniques.

INTRODUCTION

Fetal ultrasonography (US) and MR imaging provide essential information in the evaluation and management of pregnancies and have been shown to improve perinatal outcomes in cases that require antenatal or perinatal surgical and medical intervention.[1] The information provided by fetal imaging is important both to prospective parents and to the many specialists who counsel them, and it allows for more accurate diagnosis and determination of prognosis.

US and MR imaging are complementary modalities in fetal neuroimaging. US is the first-line imaging modality and thus plays an important role in the screening, identification, characterization, and follow-up of fetal and placental abnormalities. Ultrasound (US) imaging provides high spatial and temporal resolutions, color and spectral Doppler assessment, and has 3-dimensional (3D) volume rendering capabilities, important in lesion characterization. The American College of Radiology in conjunction with the American College of Obstetricians and Gynecologists and the American Institute of Ultrasound in Medicine recommend that US of the fetal head, face, and neck should routinely include images of the lateral cerebral ventricles, choroid plexus, cerebellum, cisterna magna, midline falx, cavum septum pellucidum, and upper lip.[2] A significant advantage of US in the evaluation of the fetal brain is the availability of extensive normative biometric data and the

[a] Fetal and Neonatal Neuroimaging and Developmental Science Center, Boston Children's Hospital, 300 Longwood Avenue, Boston, MA 02115, USA; [b] Department of Radiology, Boston Children's Hospital, 300 Longwood Avenue, Boston, MA 02115, USA; [c] Department of Pediatrics, Boston Children's Hospital, 300 Longwood Avenue, Boston, MA 02115, USA; [d] Maternal Fetal Care Center, Boston Children's Hospital, 300 Longwood Avenue, Boston, MA 02115, USA

[1] JNS and MAB contributed equally to this work.
[2] PEG and JAE contributed equally to this work.
* Corresponding author. Boston Children's Hospital, Neonatal Neuroimaging BCH3181, 300 Longwood Avenue, Boston, MA 02115.
E-mail address: jeffrey.stout@childrens.harvard.edu

Magn Reson Imaging Clin N Am 29 (2021) 557–581
https://doi.org/10.1016/j.mric.2021.06.007
1064-9689/21/© 2021 Elsevier Inc. All rights reserved.

reliable assessment of cranial size in cases of possible microcephaly or macrocephaly.[3] **Table 1** summarizes the advantages and disadvantages of fetal US and fetal MR.

MR can be used as a complementary modality to provide additional information when US is unable to characterize an abnormality clearly, or when the abnormality is suspected but may be sonographically occult. A fetus with a suspected brain abnormality on screening US, or with a high family risk for brain abnormalities, should undergo fetal MR imaging because it offers better contrast, higher resolution, and multiplanar capabilities, which increase the accuracy and confidence in the detection of fetal brain abnormalities.[4] This is supported by a multicenter, prospective cohort study of 570 fetuses by Griffiths and colleagues.[5] In this study, MR had a higher accuracy in the diagnosis of fetal brain abnormalities compared with US (93% vs 68%), provided additional information in 49% of the cases, changed prognostic information in 20% of cases, and led to changes in clinical management in more than 30% of the cases. A recently published meta-analysis that included 27 articles in 1184 fetuses[6] demonstrated that fetal MR was concordant with postnatal diagnosis in 80% of the cases, compared with 54% concordance with US. Nevertheless, fetal MR imaging should be performed and interpreted with same-day or concurrent US examination, because the 2 modalities provide different and complementary information, particularly in the assessment of extracranial head, neck, and spine abnormalities.

Imaging the developing brain, face, neck, and spine of the fetus is complex but crucial. Interpreting and reporting fetal MR imaging requires not only a deep understanding of embryology, normal development, and common malformations, but also a clear sense of the sequences currently available for clinical use, their strengths and limitations, and common artifacts. This article focuses on the current state-of-the-art MR sequences used in fetal neuroimaging, with a specific focus on current clinical applications, complementary contribution to US, and future directions to improve image quality.

FETAL MR: BACKGROUND
Physics

Fetal MR imaging uses hardware that has been optimized for other adult and pediatric applications (e.g., brain, heart, body, and joint imaging), which can result in poor image quality beyond the operator's control. A brief overview of MR imaging physics is necessary to understand the operator independent effects of image quality. To create an image using an MR scanner, radiofrequency (RF) waves are used to excite protons, which then resonate at a frequency determined by the magnetic field strength at that location. Gradients, spatially varying magnetic fields, are applied to encode location, which permits imaging. The series of RF and gradient pulses give rise to the common MR imaging physics phrase "pulse sequence" to describe how a specific image is acquired. The external field is known as B_0 and the fields created by the RF waves B_1. En masse, the resonating protons are detected by receive coils, and the resulting signals are processed to create an image.

Basic Imaging Setup

The unique demands of fetal MR imaging especially pressures the quality tradeoffs between signal-to-noise ratio (SNR), speed of image acquisition, and spatial resolution. The field of view for fetal imaging must typically be large enough so that all the fetal and maternal tissue can be spatially encoded, which prevents maternal tissue from being inadvertently superimposed onto the fetal tissue, an artifact called "aliasing." With a large field of view, the resolution is often coarser than desired for the fetal brain, given that a higher resolution requires more imaging time to perform the necessary spatial encoding. Ultimately, this imaging time is limited by the duration of fetal quiescence or maternal breath hold, thus fetal imaging most often consists of "single-shot" acquisitions where 1 slice from a volume is acquired at a time. The volume can be acquired over the course of seconds or minutes, but each slice can effectively "freeze" fetal and maternal motion. However, slices and even volumes can be hopelessly corrupted by unpredictable fetal motion, so it is also important to monitor images for motion artifacts and reacquire them when necessary. **Table 2** shows an example protocol from our institution conducted on Siemens 3T scanners.

Field Strength

There is a linear relationship between SNR and main magnetic field strength, such that the 3T SNR gains can be traded for greater resolution or faster scanning. Fetal scanning at 3T has been shown to be better at detecting both body and brain abnormalities.[7,8] In addition, scanning at 3T has been shown to lower RF energy exposure, known as the specific absorption rate (SAR).[8,9] However, image artifacts, particularly with steady-state free precession (SSFP) sequences, may be worse in some cases.[10] Our institution conducts fetal brain and body scanning at 3T,

Table 1
Applications, advantages and disadvantages of various fetal imaging modalities

Modality or Sequence	Applications	Advantages	Disadvantages
US	Screening for fetal brain and body abnormalities Follow-up of characterized fetal abnormalities Fetal biometry Doppler assessment of the fetus and placenta: calculation of cerebroplacental index Fetal echocardiogram	Nonionizing radiation Lower cost and higher availability High spatial resolution, good for assessment of the face (lips, nose, orbits) High temporal resolution, good for evaluation of fetal movement Extensive normative biometric data More reliable evaluation of cranial size Doppler assessment of the fetal intracranial vasculature (fetal middle cerebral artery) and placenta 3D evaluation of the face	Operator dependent Limited beam penetration and fetal assessment in cases of oligohydramniosis and anhydramnios, anterior placenta and maternal obesity Lower sensitivity in characterization of fetal central nervous system abnormalities compared with MR imaging Lower penetration of the skull with increasing gestational age owing to ossification of the skull

SS-FSE	Overall fetal body and brain anatomy
	Anatomic detail
	   Brain
	   Face
	   Lips
	   Spinal cord
	Reconstruction for high resolution brain volumes
		Single-shot (fast acquisition, freezing fetal motion)
		Volume reconstruction is possible
		High-resolution anatomic imaging
			Incoherent volume
			Contrast (blurred approximation of T2 contrast)
			Resolution/FOV tradeoff
			High SAR

bSSFP	Overall anatomy Bright blood sequence for evaluation of heart and vessels Dynamic evaluation with cine clips (extremity, fetal movement and swallowing)	High SNR Cine acquisition	Poor tissue contrast Requires very good magnetic field homogeneity to prevent banding artifacts
GRE EPI	Identification of intracranial blood products Assessing the bony components of the fetal spine	Susceptibility artifacts aid the identification of intracranial blood products Good cortical bone assessment	Extensive susceptibility artifacts Image distortion Low contrast resolution
T1-weighted 3D GRE	Mostly fetal body indications (identification of meconium, liver, thyroid) Fetal brain indications include identification of	Evaluation of structures that have intrinsic T1 shortening	Prone to motion artifacts

(continued on next page)

Table 1
(continued)

Modality or Sequence	Applications	Advantages	Disadvantages
	intracranial hemorrhage, tubers in tuberous sclerosis complex and myelination Identification of thrombosed dural venous fistulas or vein of Galen malformation		
DWI/DTI	Identification of cerebral ischemia (fetal stroke and hypoxic–ischemic injury) Identification of intracranial hemorrhage, cysts and fetal tumors DTI: potential to reveal neuroconnectivity and microstructural development	Only available sequence to identify altered diffusion	Prone to motion and susceptibility artifacts

Abbreviations: bSSFP, balanced steady-state free precession; DWI, diffusion-weighted imaging; DTI, diffusion tensor imaging; EPI, echoplanar imaging; FOV, field of view; GRE, gradient echo; SAR, specific absorption rate; SNR, signal to noise ratio; SS-FSE, single-shot fast spin echo; US, ultrasonography.

with fetal cardiac studies conducted at 1.5T. Other factors beyond B_0 strength are also important to image quality, such as patient comfort (related to bore size) and gradient and RF performance. When logistical concerns determine scanner choice, both 1.5T and 3T scanners can produce diagnostic quality images.

Dielectric Artifact

Dielectric artifacts can be a major nuisance in fetal MR imaging (**Fig. 1**). They are low spatial frequency signal intensity changes across images.[11] The brighter and darker regions are caused by the constructive and destructive interference of the RF waves used to create images—also known as B_1 inhomogeneity—that have wavelengths shorter than the object being scanned. Wavelength inversely scales with field strength, so at 1.5T wavelengths are approximately 52 cm, but decrease to approximately 26 cm at 3T, which is smaller than many pregnant abdomens. The

practical effect is that if the fetal brain is in a darker region, the lower SNR will adversely affect image interpretation or quantification. Thus, although 3T MR imaging comes with SNR advantages, dielectric effects (B_1 inhomogeneities) are a challenge.

Parallel Transmit

Parallel transmit systems can be used to decrease or eliminate dielectric effects (B_1 inhomogeneity), producing images that have a more uniform baseline signal intensity.[12] The drawback to this approach is that the total power deposited into the body as heat is no longer ultimately limited by the transmitter power, but by the geometric relationship between the transmitters and the magnitude and phase of outputted RF waves.[13,14] These additional degrees of freedom allow the design of RF pulses that obtain certain design specifications, for example, a B_1^+ field with variations of less than 5%, and heating

Table 2
Example protocol from our institution conducted on Siemens 3T scanners (Skyra and Vida, Siemens, Healthineers, Erlangen, Germany)

Sequence	TA (m:s)	FOV (cm)	TR (ms)	TE (ms)	Flip Angle (degrees)	Voxel Size (mm³)	No. of Slices	Acceleration	Other Details
SS-FSE	1:24	30 × 30	1400	103	160	1.2 × 1.2 × 2.5	60	$R_{GRAPPA} = 2$	Partial Fourier = 5/8; interleaved slice acquisition
bSSFP	0:36	32 × 32	4.16	1.77	75	1 × 1 × 2.5	40	$R_{GRAPPA} = 2$	–
GRE-EPI (motion)	2:07	30 × 30	5500	37	90	2 × 2 × 2	70	$R_{GRAPPA} = 2$	Measurements = 20; EPI factor = 150; Echo spacing = 0.65 ms; interleaved slice acquisition; partial Fourier = 7/8
GRE-EPI (high resolution)	0:09	25 × 25	8520	80	90	1 × 1 × 2	30	$R_{GRAPPA} = 2$	Measurements = 1; EPI factor = 250; Echo spacing = 1.0 ms; interleaved slice acquisition; partial Fourier = 6/8
Multi-echo SMS EPI (motion, T2* quantification)	10:00	35 × 25	8100	18/47/76	90	3.2 × 3.2 × 3.2	70	$R_{GRAPPA} = 2$, SMS = 2	Measurements = 72; EPI factor = 110; Echo spacing = 0.5 ms
T1-VIBE	0:9.2	30 × 30	3.64	1.35	9	1 × 1 × 2	40	$R_{GRAPPA} = 2$	Slab thickness = 8 cm; No fat saturation; RF spoiling; 7/8 phase partial Fourier, 6/8 slice partial Fourier; no volume interpolation in the slice direction
DWI/DTI	1:01	30 × 30	3800	57	90	2 × 2 × 4	30	$R_{GRAPPA} = 2$	12 directions, b = 0, 700 s/mm²; interleaved slice acquisition; 6/8 partial Fourier

Scans are usually conducted using the Siemens 30-channel flexible body array combined with the 18-channel spine array.
Abbreviations: DTI, diffusion tensor imaging; DWI, diffusion-weighted imaging; FOV, field of view; TA, total acquisition time; TE, echo time; TR, repetition time.

below a safety threshold (<2 W/kg local SAR), but the workflow and time to design these pulses in real time is a matter of ongoing research.[15–17] The combination of safety concerns for a vulnerable population, a lack of temperature modeling, and ongoing technical development means that each MR imaging system vendor's recommendations should be carefully followed. As of the April 2020 International Society of Magnetic Resonance in Medicine Placenta and Fetus Study Group meeting on RF Shimming, no consensus recommendation could be promulgated.

Coils

Multichannel phased-array receive coils offer significant SNR advantages because the individual coils are closer to the anatomy of interest and the spatial sensitivity of the individual coils permits accelerated image acquisition.[18,19] These advantages mean that fetal scanning should leverage the best receive coils available in terms of maternal comfort and channel count. Our institution uses the Siemens 30-channel flexible body array

combined with the 18-channel spine array for our fetal examinations, which this permits a modest parallel imaging acceleration factor of R = 2. Although there has been some work developing dedicated fetal receive coils,[20,21] the gains are modest in comparison with the latest flexible body coils that can be purchased from vendors.

Contrast

In animal models, gadolinium-based contrast agents have been shown to cross the placenta, resulting in recirculation through the amniotic fluid during a prolonged period of time.[1] The effect in the developing fetus is unknown; therefore, gadolinium-based contrast is not approved for use in pregnancy by the US Food and Drug Administration (FDA) and its use in fetal MR imaging is not recommended.

Ferumoxytol is an ultrasmall superparamagnetic iron oxide that is approved by the FDA for treating iron deficiency anemia in adults with chronic kidney disease. It has also been used off-label in nonpregnant adults as a blood pool agent owing

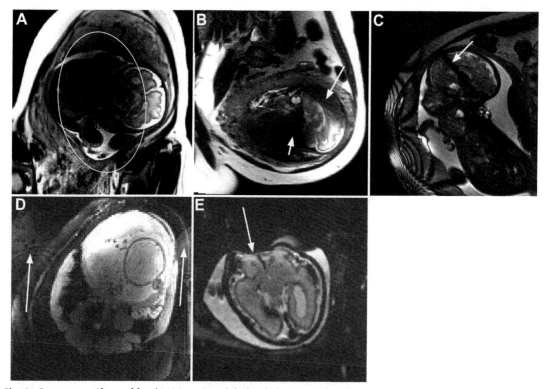

Fig. 1. Common artifacts of fetal MR imaging. (*A*) The dielectric artifact (low signal intensity in the central part of the image, *circle*) is caused by the size of the abdomen in comparison to the frequency of the RF pulses used in imaging. (*B*) SS-FSE slice corruption (low signal intensity in the anterior and inferior areas of the head, *arrows*) owing to fetal motion, and volume incoherence also causes information loss. (*C*) bSSFP banding (1 dark band crosses the brain, *arrow*) is caused by magnetic field inhomogeneities. EPI artifacts include (*D*) ghosting (image copies, *arrows*), (*E*) geometric distortion (anterior aspect of brain is distorted, *arrow*) likely caused by proximity to the maternal bowel, and susceptibility artifact as shown in **Fig. 9**.

to its long half-life and as a marker of inflammation because it is taken up by macrophages. As a result, there is interest in the use of ferumoxytol as a means to quantify perfusion and inflammation in the placenta. However, its use in pregnant women is not yet FDA approved; however, primate studies of potential diagnostic usefulness and toxicity are currently underway.[22,23]

Maternal Preparation and Positioning

Patient preparation is important for the acquisition of high-quality diagnostic images. Some centers advocate for maternal fasting and prohibition of caffeine intake before the examination in efforts to decrease fetal motion and maternal bowel motion; however, there is no evidence to support these recommendations. In 228 pregnant patients who underwent fetal MR imaging, Yen and colleagues[24] did not identify a correlation between fetal motion and food and/or caffeinated beverage intake. However, maternal comfort in the scanner is crucial, because studies can be long and maternal discomfort results in maternal anxiety and movement. Scanning is usually performed with an empty bladder and in a supine position with pillows under the knees. However, this positioning is not always possible at late gestational ages owing to compression of the inferior vena cava, requiring MR imaging to be performed in left oblique or lateral decubitus maternal positions.

Gestational Age Challenges

Technically, MR imaging can be performed at any gestational age; however, the optimal gestational age to perform fetal MR depends on the pathology suspected by US as well as maternal size. At our institution, we prefer to scan pregnant patients in the larger bore diameter (70 cm) scanners to ensure patient comfort. We have found that the smaller bore diameter systems (60 cm) are suitable before approximately 33 weeks of gestation, and when the maternal body mass index is less than approximately 30. It is important to consider that there is also a maternal weight limit for each MR scanner.

It is imperative to understand the normal rapidly evolving appearance of the developing fetal brain on MR imaging. A thorough understanding of embryology is critical for the adequate interpretation of fetal MR imaging. In general, fetal brain development occurs in a predictable pattern with structural morphologic changes in the cortical sulcation that reflect functional arealization. In addition, parenchymal signal intensity changes reflect the changes happening at the microstructural level during proliferation, cell migration, neuronal organization and maturation.[3] **Fig. 2** demonstrates the normal progressive development of cerebral sulcation in the fetal brain at different gestational ages, noting that sulcation progresses rapidly from a smooth appearance at 20 weeks gestational age to a highly folded cortex in late gestation. Brain parenchymal signal evolves in a multilayer fashion representing transient zones of brain development (**Fig. 3**).[25] In early fetal stages, between approximately 10 to 17 weeks, 5 to 6 zones can be identified across the cerebral mantle on histopathology: (1) ventricular zone, (2) subventricular zone, (3) intermediate zone, (4) presubplate zone, (5) cortical plate, and (6) marginal zone.[26,27] From about 17 weeks, 7 layers can be distinguished across the cerebral mantle on histopathology: (1) ventricular zone, (2) periventricular fiber rich zone, (3) subventricular zone, (4) intermediate zone, (5) subplate zone, (6) cortical plate, and (7) marginal zone.[26] With modern fetal MR imaging resolutions, approximately 1 mm in plane using single-shot fast spin echo (SS-FSE) imaging, the marginal zone cannot be detected and the subventricular zone is often difficult to distinguish. In general, 5 layers may be identified: (1) the ventricular zone (T2 hypointense), (2) the periventricular fiber-rich zone (T2 hyperintense), (3) the intermediate zone (mildly T2 hypointense), (4) the subplate zone (T2 hyperintense), and (5) the cortical plate (T2 hypointense).[1] The fetal cerebral mantle thickness is less than 10 mm at 20 weeks of gestation and less than approximately 15 mm by week 26 of gestation; therefore, the limited resolution and contrast of fetal brain MR imagings may result in the ventricular zone, periventricular fiber-rich zone, and subventricular zone appearing as a single entity.[28] Along the caudate nucleus, the ganglion eminence can be visualized as a T2 hypointense mass. As the fetus advances through the third trimester, the subplate, ventricular zone, and ganglionic eminence decrease in size on MR imaging and by late third trimester, the remaining zones become indistinguishable leaving only the 2 regions, white matter, and cortex.[3] The primitive lateral ventricles are seen at 13 to 14 weeks of gestation and initially seem to be large and globular in size (see **Fig. 2**). With increasing brain development, the lateral ventricles narrow, achieving an adult-like configuration by week 16 of gestation. The atrial width of the lateral ventricles is relatively independent of gestational age and therefore it is used to assess ventriculomegaly (>10 mm in atrial width) throughout gestation.[1,29]

For rare clinical indications, fetuses as young as 13 to 14 weeks may be imaged, but typically referrals for fetal neurologic concerns occur from 18 weeks onward. By this stage, early brain

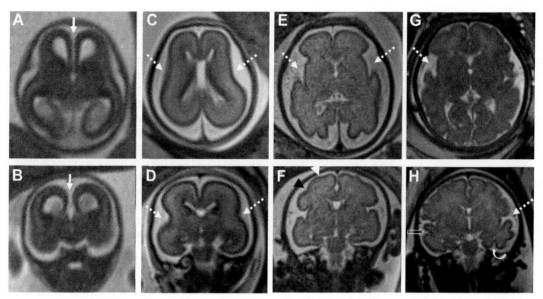

Fig. 2. Normal progressive development of cerebral sulcation in the fetal brain at different gestational ages. Axial and coronal SS-FSE images in 4 different fetuses. (*A, B*) At 15 weeks, 6 days of gestational age. (*C, D*) At 22 weeks, 2 days of gestational age. (*E, F*) At 28 weeks, 3 days of gestational age. (*G, H*) At 34 weeks, 0 days gestational age. Interhemispheric fissure (*arrow*). Sylvian fissures (*dashed arrows*), superior frontal sulcus (*white arrowhead*), inferior frontal sulcus (*black arrowhead*), inferior temporal sulcus (*curved arrow*) and superior temporal sulcus (*open arrow*).

development (hemispheric cleavage, commissuration, and neuronal proliferation) has already occurred and, therefore, abnormalities of these stages, such as holoprosencephaly (abnormality of hemispheric cleavage), can be seen. However,

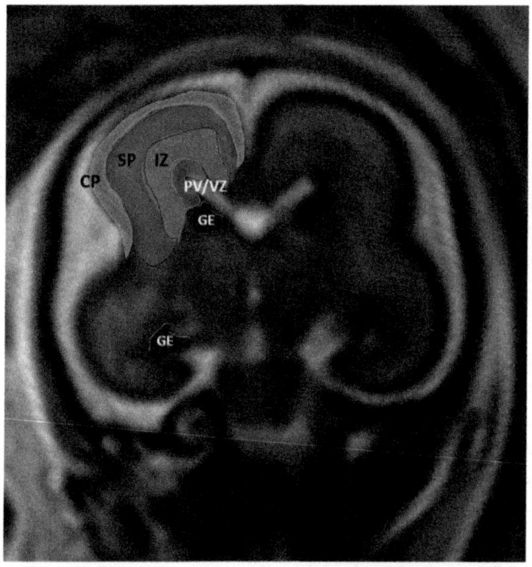

Fig. 3. Normal multilaminar appearance of the brain parenchyma in a fetus with 22 weeks of gestation. Coronal SS-FSE image. CP, cortical plate; GE, ganglionic eminences; IZ, intermediate zone; PV, periventricular fiber-rich zone; SP, subplate; VZ, ventricular zone.

cell migration, neuronal organization, and maturation are ongoing throughout fetal life, creating a risk of missing a malformation before it is structurally apparent on fetal MR imaging; for example, gray matter heterotopia are initially very small and therefore difficult to resolve, band heterotopia may be difficult to detect, and a lack of normal gyrification, as in lissencephaly/pachygyria, may be difficult to appreciate on early imaging before primary gyri appear.[3] In contrast, visible changes such as globular cavitated germinal matrix, which may seem less important, portend severe malformations that may not yet be fully apparent on imaging.[3]

Fetal Movement Challenges

Fetal movement is an inherent challenge to fetal MR imaging, particularly in early pregnancy and in the presence of polyhydramnios.[30] Owing to fetal motion, the acquisition of fetal MR imaging images becomes a dynamic process where the technician is "chasing the fetus" to acquire the necessary images for diagnosis. Strategies to minimize fetal motion-related artifacts include using the prior sequences as a scout view to prescribe the new orthogonal plane acquisition, decreasing the number of slices, and using ultrafast sequences (SS-FSE and SSFP). Motion-related artifacts can also originate from maternal breathing, where the abdominal contents shift with diaphragmatic movement; therefore, acquisitions during breath hold aim to mitigate this motion with the drawback of constraining the duration of imaging.[30]

Motion correction aims to preserve image quality by compensating for fetal motion. The 2 main categories of techniques are retrospective, where motion is corrected after the acquisition of images, and prospective, where motion is corrected during the acquisition.[31] For fetal MR imaging, retrospective motion correction algorithms are more mature. These tools enable better visualization and characterization of the posterior fossa,[32] improved performance of diffusion tensor images to enable the reconstruction of structural connectivity in the developing brain,[33] and the creation of normal reference atlases for clinical use. Gholipour and colleagues[34–37] used a robust slice-to-volume registration algorithm to reconstruct super-resolution volumetric images for each of 6 to 23 fetuses at each gestational age week that were combined into a normative spatiotemporal atlas of fetal brain development. These atlases are available online as a reference for normal fetal brain development at http://fetalmri.org. Prospective motion correction for fetal imaging is being developed and relies on the volumetric imaging capability of the scanner itself combined with machine vision technology. An automated method of slice prescription has been recently proposed for fetal brain imaging that eliminates the need for a technician to chase the fetal head during the scan.[38] Algorithms have been developed that permit head pose tracking during echo planar imaging (EPI) volume acquisitions[39] that, when combined with automated image quality assessments,[40] may soon enable fully automated fetal brain MR imaging.[41] The ultimate goal of these techniques is to make fetal MR imaging as easy as routine adult brain imaging, with automated systems obviating the training and experience requirements that limit fetal MR imaging to specialty referral hospitals. Clearly, higher quality acquired images will improve the quality of existing retrospective motion correction outputs.

SEQUENCES USED IN FETAL MR IMAGING
Single-Shot Fast Spin Echo

Technical background
The most widely used MR imaging sequences for fetal imaging are variants of SS-FSE imaging because it is fairly robust to fetal motion. This sequence is known as HASTE, SS-FSE, and single-shot TSE by Siemens, GE, and Philips respectively. SS-FSE produces an image with T2-weighted contrast. In each shot, a single RF excitation is followed by a series of RF refocusing pulses that permit readout of a single image in less than 300 ms. This approach effectively freezes any slow fetal motion, and movements in between shots do not diminish the quality of each image (see **Fig. 1**). This primary advantage comes with several current disadvantages. First, the series of shots that make up the sequential slices of a volume are often incoherent, because maternal or fetal motion affects the spatial relationship of the individual images. In the worst case, the fetal anatomy of interest has moved, such that a diagnosis is missed (**Fig. 4**). Second, T2 decay and T1 recovery during the readout RF pulse train introduces blurring and diminishes contrast. Third, the pulse train used for RF refocusing leads to power deposition in the form of tissue heating. To stay under the mandated limits for power deposition of 2 W/kg, a delay between shots is introduced by lengthening the repetition time.

Clinical applications
The SS-FSE sequence is the workhorse of fetal imaging and is the core sequence for structural assessment of the developing fetal brain. It is typically acquired in 3 standard orthogonal anatomic planes angulated to the fetal brain. T2-weighted contrast can provide a clear distinction of the multilaminar appearance of the developing cerebral mantle, and show a clear interface between brain parenchyma with extra-axial spaces and the ventricular system. Many review articles and textbooks have shown the usefulness of SS-FSE images in the detection of cerebral malformations, infections, injuries, and mass lesions.[1,3,29,42,43]

SS-FSE is a dark blood sequence and, therefore, the presence of flow voids are used to characterize hypervascular lesions such as vascular tumors (congenital hemangioma, benign hemangioendothelioma, or kaposiform hemangioendothelioma) and intracranial or extracranial vascular malformations. Congenital hemangiomas are the most common perinatal vascular tumors (**Fig. 5**),[43] characterized by increased vascular mitotic activity during the proliferative phase, which occurs before birth. In contrast, the proliferative/growth phase in infantile hemangiomas occurs postnatally. In congenital hemangioma, the involution pattern dictates the subtype, as a rapidly involuting congenital hemangioma, noninvoluting congenital hemangioma, or partially involuting type. The most common type of congenital hemangiomas in the head and neck are rapidly involuting congenital hemangioma type and, when large, can result in high-output heart failure. Locally aggressive features, such as intracranial invasion and increase in size in the postnatal

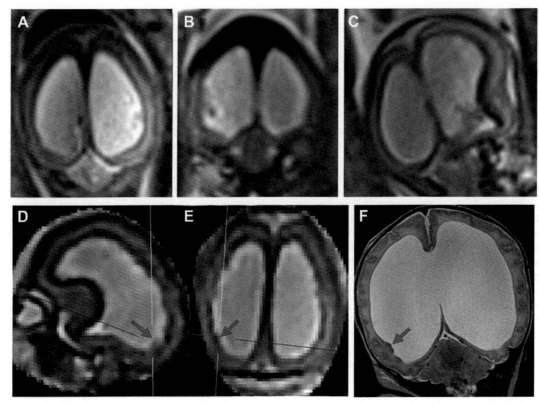

Fig. 4. Coherent fetal volumes improve identification of subependymal gray matter heterotopia in a fetus with 22 weeks of gestation. (*A–C*) Coronal images from 3 different SS-FSE stacks. No heterotopias were prospectively identified by 2 experienced fetal neuroradiologists. (*D, E*) Slice-to-volume reconstruction enables the detection of a focus of subependymal heterotopia (*red arrows*) owing to the ability to cross-reference it in a coherent volume. (*F*) Postnatal T2-weighted image confirmed the focus of heterotopia (*red arrow*). Coherent fetal volumes have the potential to improve diagnostic accuracy.

period should raise the suspicion for benign vascular or kaposiform hemangiothelioma.[43]

Future directions

Ongoing work aims to address the noted disadvantages with SS-FSE imaging. Postacquisition software tools have been created to reconstruct coherent, super-resolution volumes from multiple incoherent image stacks.[44–48] These reconstruction techniques iteratively register each slice to an estimated template volume, and then reestimate the template volume (**Fig. 6**). Eventually the 2 steps converge to a consensus volume reconstruction. These processes have been shown to improve the diagnostic usefulness of these images (see **Fig. 4**),[32,49] but integrating these techniques into the clinical workflow remains challenging mainly owing to some necessary manual steps, such as determining the initial template volume and the initial region of interest. Automated pipelines are in development that may close the loop between SS-FSE acquisitions and the availability of coherent volumes for radiologist interpretation.[50] There is also ongoing work to improve the SS-FSE acquisition itself, both by improving its motion robustness and its contrast and image quality.[38,41,51,52] One approach has designed the optimal RF pulse train for developing desired contrast between fetal tissues while minimizing SAR.[52] These acquisition improvements may decrease scan times and fetal SAR exposure, improve the resulting super-resolution reconstructions,[53] and perhaps even more important, make fetal scanning using SS-FSE available at institutions without the expertise to chase the moving fetus.

Balanced Steady-State Free Precession

Technical background

Balanced SSFP refers to a type of gradient echo sequence in which the excited magnetization is maintained in the transverse plane by the use of balanced gradient pulses. This sequence is known as TrueFISP, FIESTA, and balanced FFE by Siemens, GE, and Philips, respectively. This

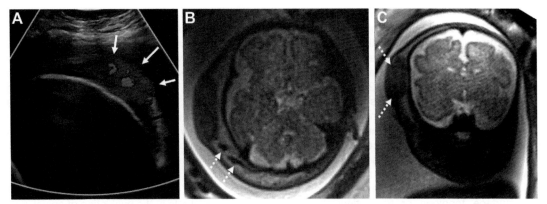

Fig. 5. Scalp congenital hemangioma in a fetus at 32 weeks of gestation. (*A*) Transverse color Doppler image of the right scalp demonstrates a well circumscribed hypoechoic subcutaneous mass with increased vascularity of color doppler interrogation (*arrows*). The mass demonstrated venous and arterial waveforms (not shown). (*B*) Axial and (*C*) coronal SS-FSE images show diffuse right-sided scalp swelling surrounding the soft tissue mass. There are multiple foci of linear low signal around and within the mass (*dashed arrows*) consistent with flow voids. There is remodeling of the skull without intracranial extension.

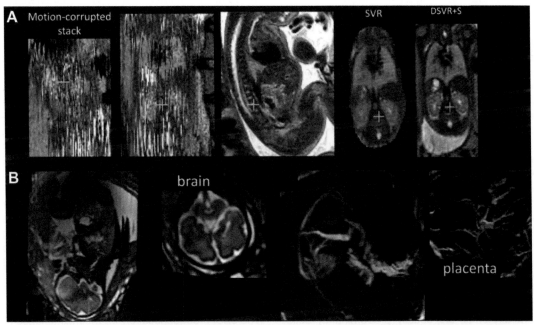

Fig. 6. Examples of 3D volume reconstructions. (*A*) A recently proposed 3D reconstruction algorithm relaxes the rigid body constraints of prior slice-to-volume registration techniques. Here a deformable slice to volume registration, super resolution reconstruction with integrated outlier removal (DSVR + S) recovers a high quality isotropic volume from the heavily motion corrupted acquisition on the left. (*B*) DSVR can be combined with novel acquisition strategies, here an excitation scheme that produces an imaging volume by continuously moving an excitation band across the volume of interest (SWEEP), to produce high quality structural (*left*) and angiographic (*right*) volumes. ([*A*] Adapted from Uus A, et al. Deformable Slice-to-Volume Registration for Motion Correction of Fetal Body and Placenta MR imaging. IEEE Trans Med Imaging. Published online February 18, 2020; with permission; and [*B*] *From* Jackson LH, et al. Motion corrected reconstruction of abdominal SWEEP data using local similarity graphs and deformable slice to volume registration. In: Proc Intl Soc Mag Reson Med.; 2020:453.; with permission.)

makes bSSFP sequences the most efficient in terms of SNR per unit time. This SNR can be used to acquire higher resolution images, or shorten the time needed to acquire images. Balanced SSFP images can be acquired quickly enough at low resolution (2.2 × 2.2 mm in plane with 30 mm thick sections permits a temporal resolution of approximately 300 ms[54]) to create movies of fetal motion. The primary disadvantage of bSSFP images is poor tissue contrast because contrast scales approximately as the ratio of T2/T1 weighting. This contrast can nevertheless be useful if the main objective is to evaluate the fetal brain surface topology or to distinguish fetal body anatomy from surrounding amniotic fluid, when observing fetal motion. Balanced SSFP acquisitions also suffer from banding artifacts that are caused by intravoxel dephasing owing to magnetic field inhomogeneities (see **Fig. 1**). This problem is lessened with modern scanners because they have improved field uniformity, but occasionally this factor impacts image quality.

Clinical applications
Balanced SSFP is a bright blood sequence used in conjunction with SS-FSE to evaluate the structural assessment of the developing fetal brain, in particular detection of gyral topology and subtle heterotopias. It is also acquired in 3 standard anatomic planes aligned to the fetal brain. Fetal motion, in particular fetal swallowing, is one of most common clinical applications of bSSFP sequences acquired as cine clips. A dynamic assessment of fetal swallowing can be evaluated after 12 weeks of gestation,[1] providing important information in fetuses with head/neck masses, micrognathia, or in cases of possible tracheoesophageal fistula. **Fig. 7** demonstrates a case of airway narrowing and swallowing impairment in a fetus at 34 weeks of gestation owing to a mass effect from a cervical teratoma. Facial/cervical teratomas are usually histologically mature and benign; however, they can result in perinatal death owing to airway compromise at birth.[43] Most teratomas demonstrate a mixed cystic and solid appearance with benign teratomas being predominantly cystic, whereas malignant teratomas are usually predominantly solid. Intratumoral hemorrhage and necrosis seen on GRE T2* sequences (as discussed elsewhere in this article) suggest an aggressive histology.[43] Fetal MR imaging plays an important role in delivery planning to include airway team availability during C-section or the ex utero intrapartum treatment procedure.

The bSSFP sequence is not only vital in the evaluation of the head and neck structures, it is also useful in the evaluation of open spinal dysraphisms, identifying the neural placode and delineating the defect level with higher spatial resolution and contrast between bone and soft tissue/fluid. Spinal dysraphisms encompass a wide spectrum of neural tube defects, based on the absence (open) or presence (closed) of overlying skin coverage.[55] The presence of skin coverage can be challenging to identify prenatally, but from a fetal surgery perspective, distinguishing an open neural tube defect is crucial because only open defects meet criteria for prenatal surgical repair.[56] Taking this caveat into account, prenatal imaging by the combination of fetal US and MR plays a crucial role in the evaluation of spinal dysraphism (**Fig. 8**). Based on the National Institutes of Health–funded Management of Myelomeningocele Study (the MOMS trial),[56] some imaging criteria exclude fetuses from prenatal repair of open spinal dysraphism. These exclusion criteria include maternal conditions (cervix <2 cm in length, multiple gestation, placenta previa and maternal Mullerian formation abnormality), fetal brain variables (intracranial abnormality not explained by open spinal dysraphism and absent hindbrain herniation), fetal spine characteristics (kyphosis of more than 30°, upper level of defect higher than T1, and inferior level of defect lower than S1), and other factors (additional fetal anomaly not explained by open spinal dysraphism). The identification of the level of the spinal defect requires the careful complementary assessment by both US and MR. US provides detail of bony structures[57] and 3D rendering can increase interpretation confidence in the level of the spinal defect. In 61 fetuses with myelomeningocele, Aaronson and colleagues[58] demonstrated that MR and US are equally accurate for the assignment of spinal defect level; however, in 20% of cases, both modalities misdiagnosed the spinal level by 2 or more segments. Using a bSSFP sequence, the level of spinal defect can be identified by detecting the L5 to S1 level (most caudal hyperintense disc space) and the L5 vertebral body (most caudal horizontal vertebral body).[55]

Future directions
The bSSFP sequences rely on the maintenance of a steady-state magnetization to produce high SNR images. One exciting extension of the bSSFP concept is to shift the imaging plane in 1 direction at a sufficiently slow rate that a front of steady state magnetization is built up that can be swept over the imaging object. This approach has been termed SWEEP, and it generates many overlapping slices with high SNR.[59] When combined with slice to volume registration methods to correct for maternal breathing, a motion corrected

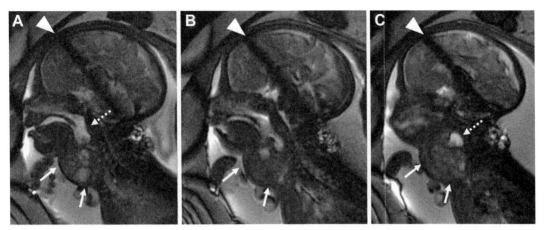

Fig. 7. Airway narrowing and swallowing impairment in a fetus at 34 weeks of gestation owing to mass effect from cervical teratoma. (*A–C*) Sagittal bSSFP cine clips show a predominantly solid mass in the anterior cervical region with macrocystic changes consistent with postnatally confirmed cervical teratoma (*arrows*). Dynamic assessment of the airways and esophagus demonstrate dilation of the hypopharynx (*dashed arrows*) and no clear visualization of the upper esophageal distention consistent with mass effect in the airway. This fetus also presented with polyhydramnios (not shown). Note the banding artifact (*arrowhead*) related to this sequence.

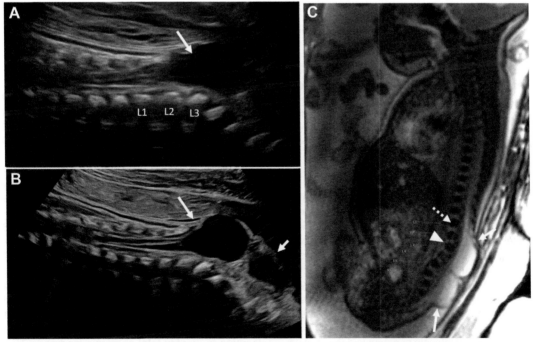

Fig. 8. Complex open neural defect in a fetus at 35 weeks of gestation. (*A, B*) Sagittal US images of the lumbosacral region shows a complex bilobed myelomeningocele (*arrows*). The exact level of spinal defect is difficult to identify on US owing to kyphosis centered at L3. (*C*) Sagittal bSSFP demonstrates spinal defect extending from about L1 (*dashed arrow*) through the sacrum (*arrows*). There is a lumbosacral kyphotic curve centered at L3 (*arrow head*). In addition, MR imaging showed moderate ventriculomegaly and mild inferior displacement of the cerebellar tonsils (not shown), consistent with a Chiari II malformation.

coherent volume can be produced (see **Fig. 6**).[60] This technique has produced impressive magnetic resonance angiograms of the uterus.[60]

Gradient Echo-Echo Planar Imaging

Technical background

EPI permits single slice readouts in less than 100 ms; therefore, EPI is very similar to SS-FSE imaging in its motion robustness. T2*-weighted imaging volumes can be obtained in approximately 6 seconds using GRE-EPI. This sequence is so universal that it does not have branded names. GRE-EPI permits the acquisition of multiple volumes with repetition times of approximately 3 seconds, that when reviewed in sequence (as a cine) can be used to evaluate fetal motion. The primary disadvantages of GRE-EPI are 4 classes of imaging artifacts (see **Fig. 1**).[61] Ghosting that appears as copies of the observed object overlaid at some interval over the main image. Often called "N/2" or "Nyquist" ghosting, it results from slight timing discrepancies in the pulse sequence that arise when gradient hardware is pushed to its maximum specifications to enable the fast switching required by EPI readouts. Geometric distortion transforms normal anatomic structures into abnormal shapes, and is caused by inhomogeneities in B_0 that lead to phase accrual over the long single shot readout. Localized susceptibility artifacts that appear as signal dropouts are caused by rapid intravoxel signal dephasing. This artifact, as discussed elsewhere in this article, can be leveraged by comparing short and long echo time (TE) acquisitions to confirm the presence of blood products or mineralization causing signal dephasing. Chemical shift artifacts can result in areas with a high fat content being displaced relative to areas with a high water content.

Clinical applications

The magnetic susceptibility artifact related to this sequence is used to advantage in the identification of calcifications or intracranial hemorrhage. Ventriculomegaly is one of the most common indications for fetal MR referral, with a wide range of prognostic outcomes ranging from no clinical implications to significant long-term neurodevelopmental sequelae.[29] The etiology of ventriculomegaly is complex and variable, with some mechanisms overlapping; however, it can be divided broadly into obstructive (subdivided into noncommunicating in cases of intrinsic or extrinsic defects of cerebrospinal fluid circulation; and communicating in cases of decreased cerebrospinal fluid resorption) and nonobstructive, which may be a result of cerebrospinal fluid overproduction in choroid plexus lesions, or malformations of brain development with

ex vacuo dilation of the ventricles.[29] Aqueductal stenosis is the classic example of noncommunicating obstructive ventriculomegaly, which could be sporadic, related to genetic or syndromic associations (such as, *L1CAM* mutations), and can be associated with additional brain malformations (such as rhombencephalic or corpus callosal agenesis) or secondary to prior hemorrhage or infection that results in webs or gliotic tissue within the cerebral aqueduct. As seen in **Fig. 9**, EPI T2* sequences play a vital role in the identification of intraventricular bleeding as one of the causes of noncommunicating obstructive ventriculomegaly.

As shown in **Fig. 10**, GRE-EPI cine clips acquired over a few minutes are a relatively new and promising tool in the assessment of subjective fetal motion. GRE-EPI provides an exquisite assessment of the bones and cartilage, with a high signal of the cartilaginous epiphyses and a low signal of the cortical diaphyseal bone. In fetuses with spinal dysraphism, lower extremity movement can yield important information about the functional defect level, important for parental counseling. Each spinal level can be assessed by the presence or absence of hip flexion (L1), hip adduction (L2), knee extension (L3), knee flexion (L4), ankle dorsiflexion (L5), and ankle plantarflexion (S1).[55] In addition, appendicular movement and fetal breathing motion are indirect markers of fetal well-being included in the fetal biophysical profile.[62]

Future directions

EPI and related artifacts have been a topic of research for more than 40 years,[63] and so there has been gradual improvement to the MR imaging hardware that enables artifact minimized EPI on modern scanners. A decrease in the EPI scan time has seen improvement by using half-Fourier, parallel imaging, and compressed sensing methods.[64–67] Recently, imaging has been greatly accelerated through the advent of simultaneous multislice imaging, and new sequences that eliminate distortion and blurring.[68,69] Multi-echo SMS EPI (see **Table 2**) is used at our site for simultaneous fetal motion monitoring, and placental T2* mapping.[70,71]

Two exciting research applications of fetal EPI data concern fetal motion and fetal brain functional MR imaging. Tools are now available that permit quantitative fetal motion evaluation using machine learning to identify fetal anatomic landmarks.[71,72] These motion trajectories may be directly relevant to clinical evaluations of fetal disease and, once calculated during the acquisition, may serve as a type of navigator for prospective motion correction of fetal MR imaging acquisitions.[41] GRE-EPI could

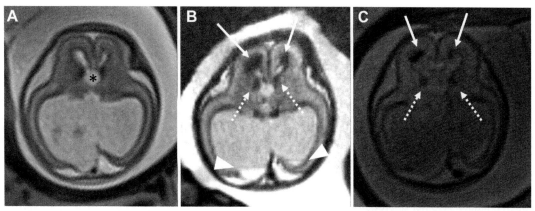

Fig. 9. Intraventricular bleeding as cause of ventriculomegaly in a fetus at 20 weeks of gestation (*A*) Axial SS-FSE image demonstrates severe lateral ventriculomegaly and moderate dilation of the third ventricle (*asterisk*). The fourth ventricle was normal in size (not shown). (*B*) EPI T2* image with high TE (80 ms) demonstrate fluid–fluid level in the lateral ventricles (*arrowheads*) and foci of susceptibility artifacts in the bilateral frontal periventricular white matter (*arrows*) and the bilateral caudothalamic grooves (*dashed arrows*) consistent with germinal matrix hemorrhage with parenchymal and intraventricular extension, and the likely cause of the ventriculomegaly. Note geometric distortion artifact of in the anterior cranium and frontal lobes. (*C*) EPI T2* image with low TE (30 ms) confirmed presence of susceptibility artifacts seen on the high TE sequence.

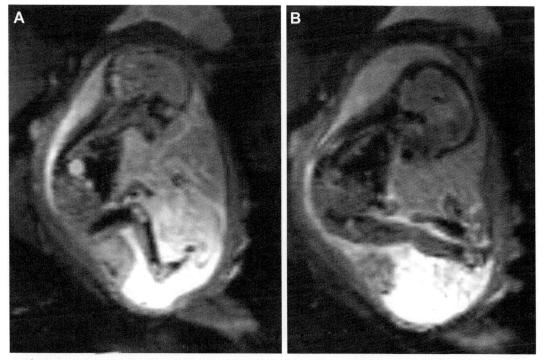

Fig. 10. Normal subjective fetal motion of the right lower extremity in a fetus with 19 weeks of gestation. (*A, B*) Sagittal GRE-EPI sequence acquired as a cine clip demonstrates flexion and extension of the left knee and ankle. Note that the cartilaginous epiphyses appear as high signal and the cortical bone of the diaphyses are low signal.

also permit fetal brain functional MR imaging, with already promising current results robustly identifying the developing major brain networks.[73,74]

T1-Weighted 3-Dimensional Gradient Echo

Technical background

T1-weighted imaging is a workhorse of mature brain imaging, but T1 contrast is difficult to achieve for fetal brain imaging. This difficulty arises from the long duration necessary to create T1 contrast by inversion methods, because waiting for about 1 second after an inversion pulse to commence image readout makes the sequence prone to fetal motion artifacts. Another approach to T1 contrast is to use a GRE sequence with appropriately selected repetition time, TE, and flip angle to achieve the desired contrast. One drawback of this approach is that typically the required flip angle is not near the Ernst angle (where the maximum SNR can be had for a certain ratio of repetition time/T1) so T1 contrast comes at the cost of SNR. To claw back some SNR, a 3D acquisition is used, and multiple acceleration schemes are also used to minimize the time for fetal motion to cause artifacts. This sequence is known as VIBE, LAVA, and THRIVE by Siemens, GE, and Philips, respectively.

Clinical applications

T1-weighted images add value in the identification of fetal organs with intrinsic high signal on T1, such as the thyroid gland, pituitary gland, and liver (**Fig. 11**), and materials that result in T1 shortening, such as meconium, hemorrhage, fat, and calcifications. In addition, T1-weighted images can be used to assess the myelination process, which begins in fetal life and continues in the postnatal period. Lipid content of the myelin demonstrates T1 shortening (high signal in T1-weighted images) in the tegmentum of the pons starting approximately at 23 weeks of gestation and in the posterior limb of the internal capsule at 31 weeks of gestation (see **Fig. 11**).[1]

Tissues that demonstrate a high signal on T1-weighted images are very limited in the head and neck; therefore, the presence of a high signal in this sequence aids in the characterization of mass lesions. For example, as shown in **Fig. 12**, fetal goiter is a rare condition with imaging findings that are characteristic. It seems to be a solid, homogeneous, usually bilobed midline mass around the trachea with increased vascularity on color Doppler interrogation and a high signal on T1-weighted images.[43] Fetal goiter can be the result of maternal thyroid disorders, such as thyroid dysfunction, medication effect, intake of iodine supplements, or endemic iodine deficiency; or it could be secondary to a primary fetal thyroid disorder, such as congenital hypothyroidism in the setting of thyroid dysmorphogenesis or owing to an error in hormone synthesis or fetal hyperthyroidism.[75] Fetal goiter usually has a benign course; however, it can result in mass effect on the upper airway and esophagus, increasing the risk of polyhydramnios, preterm delivery, hydrops, dystocia, and fetal death.[75] The management of fetal goiter depends on its etiology. Adequate management of maternal thyroid disorders can result in the resolution of fetal goiter. Profound fetal hypothyroidism, diagnosed via cordocentesis, can be treated with an intra-amniotic infusion of levothyroxine to decrease the risk of fetal high-output heart failure and fetal hydrops.[76] Because of the potential risk of airway compromise, delivery planning should include airway team availability during C-section or the ex utero intrapartum treatment procedure.

An additional important clinical application of the T1-weighted sequence is in the identification of thrombosed intracranial vascular malformations. Fetal vein of Galen aneurysmal malformation is a rare congenital malformation that forms between weeks 6 and 11 of gestation.[77] The median prosencephalic vein, a precursor of the vein of Galen, fails to regress and becomes aneurysmally dilated as a result of cerebral arteriovenous fistulas; therefore, some advocate for the term "median prosencephalic arteriovenous fistulas." As seen on **Fig. 13**, US and MR complement each other in the assessment of the vein of Galen aneurysmal malformation. On US, the malformation seems to be an anechoic structure in the midline posterior aspect of the third ventricle with increased turbulent arterial and venous flow on Doppler examination. US plays an important role in the identification of flow within the dilated malformation and in the characterization of arterial or venous waveforms in the adjacent vessels. MR imaging is used to evaluate the relationship with the adjacent brain parenchyma and the identification of potential complications, such as cerebral ischemic areas.[77] Complete or partial thrombosis of the dilated vein can be identified on T1-weighted images as an intraluminal high signal focus. High-flow cerebral shunting can result in an increased cardiac preload and high-flow congestive heart failure, which should be evaluated with fetal echocardiography.

Future directions

The challenge with 3D acquisitions for the fetal brain is unpredictable motion. GRE acquisitions that are robust to motion or have integrated motion correction are active areas of research. Non-Cartesian, radial sampling schemes can

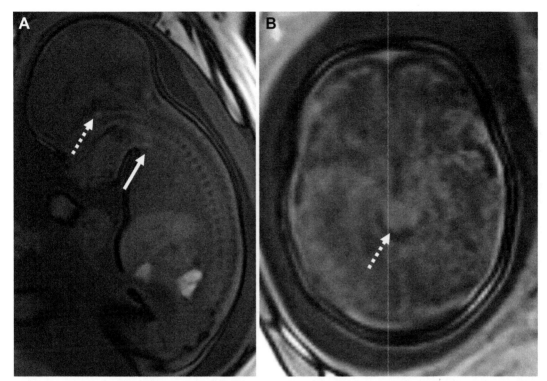

Fig. 11. Normal T1-weighted images in a fetus at 34 weeks of gestation. (*A*) Sagittal T1-weighted image shows the normal T1 hyperintense thyroid pituitary gland (*dashed arrow*) and thyroid gland (*arrow*). (*B*) Axial T1-weighted images in the same fetus show normal myelination with T1 shortening in the tegmentum of the pons (*dashed arrow*). Note the T1 contrast and lower SNR compared with the SS-FSE sequence in the fetus in **Fig. 2** (*G, H*).

dramatically improve image quality even in the presence of some motion.[78] There have been initial implementations of these approaches for fetal brain imaging, but work is needed to improve the contrast and specificity of fetal brain tracking.[79] Another approach to compensate for fetal motion is to think about fetal motion as a parameter of interest that can be estimated during the process of image reconstruction. Iterative reconstructions that jointly estimate motion parameters and images have been proposed, although they have yet to be applied to fetal imaging.[80,81] Effective fetal motion correction could even permit actual T1-weighted imaging via inversion recovery methods, which would unlock for in utero use the full set of volumetric morphometry tools that rely on T1 contrast.

Diffusion-Weighted and Diffusion Tensor Imaging

Technical background
Diffusion-weighted MR imaging provides information about the directions and magnitude of water diffusion on a voxel-wise basis. It interrogates the subvoxel environment by using magnetic

gradients to encode the magnitude and direction of spin movement in the signal intensity of the image. The amount of diffusion weighting is called the b-value and depends on gradient strength and timing. Diffusion-weighted imaging can be read on its own, but parameter maps that summarize the diffusion of water in each voxel, such as the apparent diffusion coefficient (ADC), are important clinical tools. ADC maps require at least 4 images, 3 with orthogonal diffusion directions (different b-values), and one without any diffusion weighting (b_0 image). Fetal motion proves especially challenging to parameter estimation when the component acquisitions are separated in time. Nevertheless, diffusion-weighted imaging and ADC maps are essential to determine fetal brain health in some cases; despite the typically poor quality of the maps, major shifts in the ADC can be detected.

Clinical applications
As with postnatal brain imaging, diffusion-weighted imaging plays a vital role in the detection and timing of prenatal stroke and hypoxic–ischemic injury. A particular group of fetuses that directly benefits

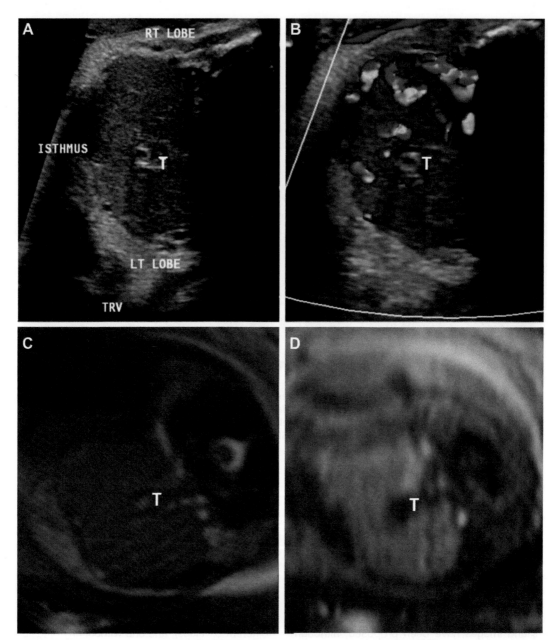

Fig. 12. Fetal goiter in a fetus at 33 weeks of gestation. (A)Transverse grayscale and (B) color Doppler US image of the neck demonstrates a solid, bilobed homogeneous midline mass around the traquea (T) with increased vascularity in color doppler interrogation. (C) Axial balanced SSFP and (D) axial T1-weighted images of the neck show that this bilobed mass demonstrate high signal of T1-weighted images consistent with thyroid tissue.

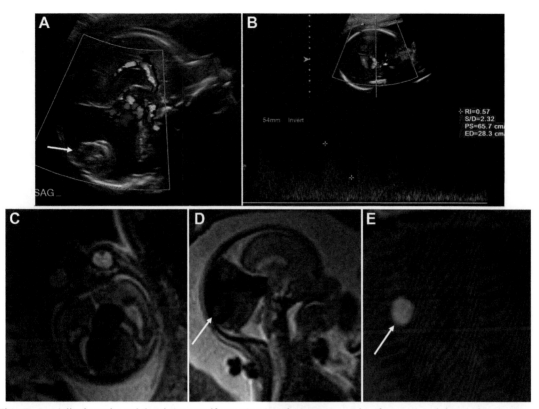

Fig. 13. Partially thrombosed dural sinus malformation in a fetus at 21 weeks of gestation. (*A*) Doppler US image in the sagittal plane shows a large midline predominantly anechoic structure at the torcula level with prominent flow in the anterior aspect, consistent with a large dural sinus malformation. There is an isoechoic round focus in the posterior margin without vascular flow (*arrow*). (*B*) Spectral Doppler image in the sagittal plane demonstrates arterial flow along the anterior margin of the malformation, suggesting presence of arteriovenous communication.[82] (*C*) Axial and (*D*) sagittal SS-FSE images demonstrate a large dural sinus malformation with predominant T2 hypointense signal. (*E*) T1-weighted sagittal image at the same level as (*D*) demonstrates a round high signal focus (*arrow*) consistent with an intralesional thrombus.

from a complementary assessment of fetal brain MR and US are fetuses with twin-to-twin transfusion syndrome (TTTS), status post laser ablation therapy. TTTS occurs in approximately 10% of monochorionic twin pregnancies and it is usually identified in the second trimester of pregnancy.[82] Fetoscopic laser-selective coagulation of placental anastomoses is a well-established first line of treatment in severe TTTS. Intracranial complications of fetoscopic laser-selective coagulation of placental anastomoses include intraventricular hemorrhage, cystic and noncystic periventricular leukomalacia, ventriculomegaly, and brain parenchymal ischemia.[82] As with the postnatal brain MR imaging evaluation, diffusion-weighted imaging sequence plays an important role in identifying cytotoxic edema/parenchymal ischemia, which appears as a decreased diffusion (high signal on high b-value images and low signal on ADC maps) that could be occult on US. US is vital in the identification of

postoperative twin anemia polycythemia sequence, which could develop after incomplete laser ablation treatment and increases the risk of prenatal fetal brain injury.[82] Twin anemia polycythemia sequence is defined as a peak systolic velocity in the middle cerebral artery higher than 1.5 times the multiple of the median of 1 twin, representing the fetus with anemia, and a multiple of the median of less than 0.8 in the other twin, representing the fetus with polycythemia.[82] In a group of 1023 cases of TTTS managed with fetoscopic laser-selective coagulation of placental anastomoses, Stirnemann and colleagues[82] identified that the overall survival rate of at least 1 twin was 81%, with both twins surviving only in 51%. As shown in **Fig. 14**, diffusion-weighted imaging sequences are helpful to confirm global decreased brain parenchymal diffusion in cases of fetal demise, which is confirmed with absent cardiac activity on US.

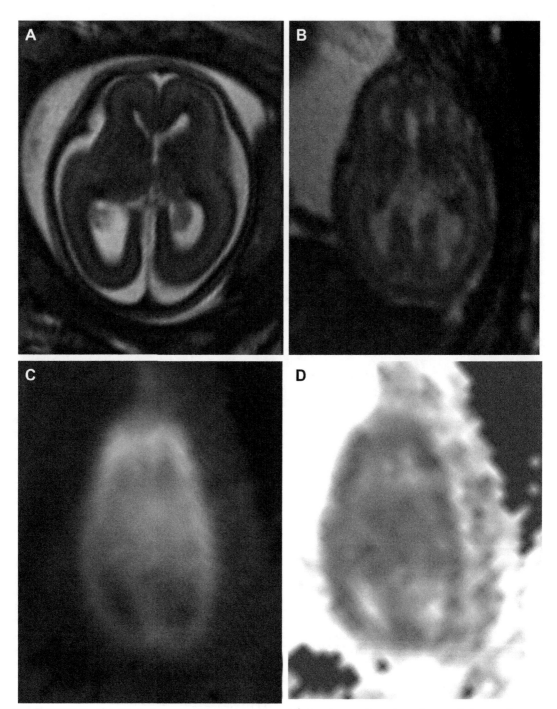

Fig. 14. Fetal demise of fetus B, status post 8 days of laser ablation therapy for twin–twin transfusion syndrome at 22 weeks of gestation. (*A*) Axial bSSFP images of fetus A shows mild right ventriculomegaly with normal appearance of the extra-axial fluid spaces for gestational age. (*B*) Axial bSSFP images of fetus B shows nonspecific diffuse decrease in extra-axial fluid spaces with normal ventricular size. The calvarium of fetus B is smaller compared with fetus A. (*C*) Axial B-500 image and (*D*) apparent diffusion coefficient (ADC) maps demonstrate global brain parenchymal diffusion restriction consistent with fetal demise.

Future directions

Ideally, diffusion MR imaging could be used to learn about the in utero development of structural brain connectivity. To understand structural connectivity, more information about the local tissue microstructure is needed, and this can be obtained with yet more diffusion weighted images. Diffusion tensor imaging uses baseline and at least 6 diffusion directions to estimate the diffusion tensor at each voxel permitting structural connectivity mapping. Fetal motion is a profound challenge when trying to perform tractography analysis. Nevertheless, techniques have been developed that permit robust motion correction and tractographic reconstruction of fetal diffusion tensor imaging with the potential to reveal fetal microstructural development and neuroconnectivity (**Fig. 15**).[33]

Quantitative Physiologic Imaging, Blood Flow, and Oxygenation

Technical background

Beyond structural imaging, MR imaging can also be used to estimate parameters related to organ perfusion and oxygen consumption. These quantitative methods include the ability to directly measure the velocity of flowing blood using phase contrast MR imaging, to measure perfusion by magnetically labeling blood to produce an endogenous tracer in a technique called arterial spin labeling, and to estimate blood oxygen saturation via relaxometry or susceptibility mapping. It is extremely difficult to apply these techniques developed for the adult brain to the fetal brain because it is much smaller, surrounded by maternal tissue that limits imaging resolution, and is freely moving. Access to the fetal heartbeat

signal, which is often used in postnatal MR imaging examinations to gate flow acquisitions, is also more difficult. Thus, recent efforts to measure fetal cerebral hemodynamics are extremely impressive given the manifold challenges.

Phase contrast MR imaging has been used to explore typical fetal hemodynamics using a retrospective approach to fetal cardiac gating called metric optimized gating, and by direct US monitoring of the fetal heartbeat using an MR imaging compatible device.[83,84] Metric optimized gating has been used to collect data showing how brain sparing physiology, that is, the preferential perfusion the brain when flow or oxygenation is limited, is associated with fetal growth restriction.[85]

Motion has largely prevented the application of arterial spin labeling to the fetal brain, given the need for numerous acquisitions to gain sufficient SNR over a small volume lower cerebral blood flow than neonates.[86] However, there have been numerous attempts to use arterial spin labeling to better understand placental perfusion.[87–89]

A combination of metric optimized gating and estimates of blood oxygenation derived from T2-mapping showed that fetal brain volume was related to ascending aorta oxygen saturation and fetal brain oxygen delivery in cases of congenital heart disease.[90] Measurements of fetal cerebral blood flow were based on the superior vena cava, assuming that this vessel mostly drains the fetal brain. The fetal brain oxygen extraction fraction was based on the ascending aorta and superior vena cava. Smaller vessels that would better represent brain perfusion alone are beyond the reach of current techniques. The larger umbilical vessels have been targeted using a similar approach to measure the oxygen delivery from the placenta to the fetus.[91] A review of the methods to monitor placental oxygenation and planning for future work in this subfield has been published recently.[92]

Future directions

Once quantitative physiologic imaging is sufficiently robust for routine application in utero, there are some immediate high impact applications. Fetal surgical interventions have been developed for a variety of congenital heart defects,[93] and are actively being developed for vein of Galen malformations.[94] As new fetal interventions are proposed, these techniques could help with risk stratification and monitoring of therapeutic effect.

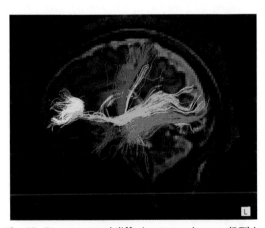

Fig. 15. Reconstructed diffusion tensor images (DTI) in a fetus at 36 weeks of gestation shows white matter fiber bundles of the brain. (Images courtesy of Camilo Jaimes Cobos, MD, and Fedel Machado, MD.)

SUMMARY

Progress in fetal neuroimaging has been challenging, but the promise of improved diagnosis, potential therapeutic benefits of appropriate fetal interventions, and improvements in our understanding of human brain development continue to drive the field forward. MR advantages as a noninvasive volumetric imaging modality with good soft tissue contrast make it a strong complement to US screening and diagnosis. However, fetal movement still severely limits practical MR imaging sequences to those that are quick enough to freeze motion. Although there has been very good progress in super-resolution volume reconstructions of the fetal brain after fast single shot image acquisition, FDA approval, and timely integration into the clinical workflow is still in progress. However, the field is undergoing rapid advancement, and both prospective and retrospective motion correction strategies promise to make other MR imaging sequences successful for fetal neuroimaging, improve the performance of existing sequences, and open new horizons to understanding in utero brain development.

CLINICS CARE POINTS

- It is imperative to understand the rapidly evolving appearance of the developing fetal brain on MR imaging. Interactive normal reference atlases are available for clinical use at http://fetalmri.org.
- The optimal gestational age to perform fetal MR depends on the pathology suspected by US, as well as maternal size.
- Radiologists must balance technical and interpretive challenges against the need for timely, efficient diagnosis and intervention.

DISCLOSURE

The authors have no commercial or financial conflicts of interest to declare.

REFERENCES

1. Coblentz AC, Teixeira SR, Mirsky DM, et al. How to read a fetal magnetic resonance image 101. Pediatr Radiol 2020;50(13):1810–29.
2. AIUM-ACR-ACOG-SMFM-SRU practice parameter for the performance of standard diagnostic obstetric ultrasound examinations. J Ultrasound Med 2018;37(11):E13–24.
3. Choi JJ, Yang E, Soul JS, et al. Fetal magnetic resonance imaging: supratentorial brain malformations. Pediatr Radiol 2020;50(13):1934–47.
4. Committee on Practice Parameters – Pediatric Radiology of the ACR Commission on Pediatric Radiology in Collaboration with the SPR. ACR–SPR practice parameter for the safe and optimal performance of fetal Magnetic Resonance Imaging (MRI). Reston, VA: The American College of Radiology; 2020. Available at: https://www.acr.org/-/media/ACR/Files/Practice-Parameters/mr-fetal.pdf. Accessed April 6, 2021.
5. Griffiths PD, Bradburn M, Campbell MJ, et al. Use of MRI in the diagnosis of fetal brain abnormalities in utero (MERIDIAN): a multicentre, prospective cohort study. Lancet 2017;389(10068):538–46.
6. van Doorn M, Oude Rengerink K, Newsum EA, et al. Added value of fetal MRI in fetuses with suspected brain abnormalities on neurosonography: a systematic review and meta-analysis. J Matern Fetal Neonatal Med 2016;29(18):2949–61.
7. Victoria T, Johnson AM, Edgar JC, et al. Comparison between 1.5-T and 3-T MRI for fetal imaging: is there an advantage to imaging with a higher field strength? AJR Am J Roentgenol 2016;206(1):195–201.
8. Krishnamurthy U, Neelavalli J, Mody S, et al. MR imaging of the fetal brain at 1.5T and 3.0T field strengths: comparing specific absorption rate (SAR) and image quality. J Perinat Med 2015;43(2):209–20.
9. Abaci Turk E, Yetisir F, Adalsteinsson E, et al. Individual variation in simulated fetal SAR assessed in multiple body models. Magn Reson Med 2020;83(4):1418–28.
10. Weisstanner C, Gruber GM, Brugger PC, et al. Fetal MRI at 3T—ready for routine use? BJR Suppl 2017;90(1069):20160362.
11. Collins CM, Liu W, Schreiber W, et al. Central brightening due to constructive interference with, without, and despite dielectric resonance. J Magn Reson Imaging 2005;21(2):192–6.
12. Webb AG, Collins CM. Parallel transmit and receive technology in high-field magnetic resonance neuroimaging. Int J Imaging Syst Technol 2010;20(1):2–13.
13. Wald LL, Adalsteinsson E. Parallel transmit technology for high field MRI. Magnetom Flash 2009;40(1):2009. Available at: https://www.magnetomworld.siemens-healthineers.com/clinical-corner/case-studies/parallel-transmit-technology-for-high-field-mri.html.
14. Wald LL, Adalsteinsson E. Specific absorption rate (SAR) in parallel transmission (pTx). Magnetom Flash 2010;65–73.
15. Yetisir F, Turk EA, Guerin B, Others. Potential of parallel transmission for fetal imaging in reducing SAR and mitigating Flip angle inhomogeneities: a simulation study at 3T. Proceedings of ISMRM Annual Meeting. Honolulu (HI), April 22-27, 2017. p. 4823. 2017.
16. Martin A, Schiavi E, Eryaman Y, et al. Parallel transmission pulse design with explicit control for the specific absorption rate in the presence of

radiofrequency errors. Magn Reson Med 2016; 75(6):2493–504. https://doi.org/10.1002/mrm.25820.

17. Murbach M, Neufeld E, Samaras T, et al. Pregnant women models analyzed for RF exposure and temperature increase in 3T RF shimmed birdcages. Magn Reson Med 2017;77(5):2048–56.

18. Blaimer M, Breuer F, Mueller M, et al. SMASH, SENSE, PILS, GRAPPA: how to choose the optimal method. Top Magn Reson Imaging 2004;15(4):223–36.

19. Gruber B, Froeling M, Leiner T, et al. RF coils: a practical guide for nonphysicists. J Magn Reson Imaging 2018;48(3):590–604. https://doi.org/10.1002/jmri.26187.

20. Chen Q, Xie G, Luo C, et al. A dedicated 36-channel receive array for fetal MRI at 3T. IEEE Trans Med Imaging 2018;37(10):2290–7.

21. Spatz M, Garcia-Polo P, Keil B, et al. A 64 channel 3T array coil for highly accelerated fetal imaging at 22 weeks of pregnancy. Proceedings of ISMRM Annual Meeting. Honolulu (HI), April 22-27, 2017. p. 1220.

22. Nguyen SM, Wiepz GJ, Schotzko M, et al. Impact of ferumoxytol magnetic resonance imaging on the rhesus macaque maternal-fetal interface. Biol Reprod 2020;102(2):434–44. https://doi.org/10.1101/699835.

23. Macdonald JA, Corrado PA, Nguyen SM, et al. Uteroplacental and fetal 4D flow MRI in the pregnant rhesus macaque. J Magn Reson Imaging 2019; 49(2):534–45.

24. Yen CJ, Mehollin-Ray AR, Bernardo F, et al. Correlation between maternal meal and fetal motion during fetal MRI. Pediatr Radiol 2019;49(1):46–50.

25. Counsell SJ, Arichi T, Arulkumaran S, et al. Fetal and neonatal neuroimaging. Handb Clin Neurol 2019; 162:67–103.

26. Kostovic I, Vasung L. Insights from in vitro fetal magnetic resonance imaging of cerebral development. Semin Perinatol 2009;33(4):220–33.

27. Kostovic I, Rakic P. Developmental history of the transient subplate zone in the visual and somatosensory cortex of the macaque monkey and human brain. J Comp Neurol 1990;297(3):441–70.

28. Vasung L, Abaci Turk E, Ferradal SL, et al. Exploring early human brain development with structural and physiological neuroimaging. Neuroimage 2019;187: 226–54.

29. Mirsky DM, Stence NV, Powers AM, et al. Imaging of fetal ventriculomegaly. Pediatr Radiol 2020;50(13): 1948–58.

30. Machado-Rivas F, Jaimes C, Kirsch JE, et al. Image-quality optimization and artifact reduction in fetal magnetic resonance imaging. Pediatr Radiol 2020; 50(13):1830–8.

31. Maclaren J, Herbst M, Speck O, et al. Prospective motion correction in brain imaging: a review. Magn Reson Med 2013;69(3):621–36.

32. Pier DB, Gholipour A, Afacan O, et al. 3D super-resolution motion-corrected MRI: validation of fetal posterior fossa measurements. J Neuroimaging 2016;26(5):539–44.

33. Marami B, Mohseni Salehi SS, Afacan O, et al. Temporal slice registration and robust diffusion-tensor reconstruction for improved fetal brain structural connectivity analysis. Neuroimage 2017;156: 475–88.

34. Gholipour A, Estroff JA, Barnewolt CE, et al. Fetal brain volumetry through MRI volumetric reconstruction and segmentation. Int J Comput Assist Radiol Surg 2011;6(3):329–39.

35. Gholipour A, Rollins CK, Velasco-Annis C, et al. A normative spatiotemporal MRI atlas of the fetal brain for automatic segmentation and analysis of early brain growth. Sci Rep 2017;7(1). https://doi.org/10.1038/s41598-017-00525-w.

36. Gholipour A, Limperopoulos C, Clancy S, et al. Construction of a deformable spatiotemporal MRI atlas of the fetal brain: evaluation of similarity metrics and deformation models. Med Image Comput Comput Assist Interv 2014;17(Pt 2):292–9.

37. Gholipour A, Akhondi-Asl A, Estroff JA, et al. Multi-atlas multi-shape segmentation of fetal brain MRI for volumetric and morphometric analysis of ventriculomegaly. Neuroimage 2012;60(3):1819–31.

38. Hoffmann M, Abaci Turk E, Gagoski B, et al. Rapid head-pose detection for automated slice prescription of fetal-brain MRI. Int J Imaging Syst Technol 2021. https://doi.org/10.1002/ima.22563.

39. Moyer D, Turk EA, Ellen Grant P, et al. Equivariant filters for efficient tracking in 3d Imaging. arXiv [csCV]. 2021. Available at: http://arxiv.org/abs/2103.10255. Accessed April 2, 2021.

40. Xu J, Lala S, Gagoski B, et al. Semi-supervised learning for fetal brain MRI quality assessment with ROI consistency. In: Martel AL, Abolmaesumi P, Stoyanov D, et al, editors. Medical image computing and computer assisted intervention – MICCAI 2020. MICCAI 2020. Lecture Notes in Computer Science, vol 12266. Cham: Springer; 2020. p. 386–95. https://doi.org/10.1007/978-3-030-59725-2_37.

41. Gagoski B, Xu J, Wighton P, et al. Automatic detection and reacquisition of motion degraded images in fetal HASTE imaging at 3T. Proceedings of ISMRM Annual Meeting. Virtual, August 8-14, 2020. p. 98.

42. Mirsky DM, Shekdar KV, Bilaniuk LT. Fetal MRI: head and neck. Magn Reson Imaging Clin N Am 2012; 20(3):605–18.

43. Feygin T, Khalek N, Moldenhauer JS. Fetal brain, head, and neck tumors: prenatal imaging and management. Prenat Diagn 2020;40(10):1203–19.

44. Gholipour A, Estroff Ja, Warfield SK. Robust super-resolution volume reconstruction from slice acquisitions: application to fetal brain MRI. IEEE Trans Med Imaging 2010;29(10):1739–58.

45. Kuklisova-Murgasova M, Quaghebeur G, Rutherford MA, et al. Reconstruction of fetal brain MRI with intensity matching and complete outlier removal. Med Image Anal 2012;16(8):1550–64.

46. Kim K, Habas Pa, Rousseau F, et al. Intersection based motion correction of multislice MRI for 3-D in utero fetal brain image formation. IEEE Trans Med Imaging 2010;29(1):146–58.

47. Uus A, Zhang T, Jackson LH, et al. Deformable slice-to-volume registration for motion correction of fetal body and placenta MRI. IEEE Trans Med Imaging 2020;39(9):2750–9. https://doi.org/10.1109/TMI.2020.2974844.

48. Kainz B, Steinberger M, Wein W, et al. Fast volume reconstruction from motion corrupted stacks of 2D slices. IEEE Trans Med Imaging 2015;34(9):1901–13.

49. Lloyd DFA, Pushparajah K, Simpson JM, et al. Three-dimensional visualisation of the fetal heart using prenatal MRI with motion corrected slice-volume registration. Lancet 2018;(18):1–10.

50. Ebner M, Wang G, Li W, et al. An automated framework for localization, segmentation and super-resolution reconstruction of fetal brain MRI. Neuroimage 2020;206:116324.

51. Arefeen Y, Arango N, Iyer S, et al. Refined-subspaces for two iteration single shot T2-Shuffling using dictionary matching. Proceedings of ISMRM Annual Meeting. Montreal, Canada, May 11-16, 2019. p. 2406.

52. Arefeen Y, Gagoski B, Turk E, et al. Single-shot T2-weighted Fetal MRI with variable flip angles, full k-space sampling, and nonlinear inversion: towards improved SAR and sharpness. Proceedings of ISMRM Annual Meeting. Virtual, August 8-14, 2020. p. 2574.

53. Singh A, Salehi SSM, Gholipour A. Deep predictive motion tracking in magnetic resonance imaging: application to fetal imaging. IEEE Trans Med Imaging 2020;39(11):3523–34.

54. Hayat TTA, Nihat A, Martinez-Biarge M, et al. Optimization and initial experience of a multisection balanced steady-state free precession cine sequence for the assessment of fetal behavior in utero. AJNR Am J Neuroradiol 2011;32(2):331–8.

55. Nagaraj UD, Kline-Fath BM. Imaging of open spinal dysraphisms in the era of prenatal surgery. Pediatr Radiol 2020;50(13):1988–98.

56. Adzick NS, Thom EA, Spong CY, et al. A randomized trial of prenatal versus postnatal repair of myelomeningocele. N Engl J Med 2011;364(11):993–1004.

57. Coleman BG, Langer JE, Horii SC. The diagnostic features of spina bifida: the role of ultrasound. Fetal Diagn Ther 2015;37(3):179–96.

58. Aaronson OS, Hernanz-Schulman M, Bruner JP, et al. Myelomeningocele: prenatal evaluation—Comparison between transabdominal US and MR imaging. Radiology 2003;227(3):839–43.

59. Jackson LH, Price AN, Hutter J, et al. Respiration resolved imaging with continuous stable state 2D acquisition using linear frequency SWEEP. Magn Reson Med 2019;82(5):1631–45.

60. Jackson LH, Uus A, Batalle D, et al. Motion corrected reconstruction of abdominal SWEEP data using local similarity graphs and deformable slice to volume registration. Proceedings of ISMRM Annual Meeting. Virtual, 2020. p. 453.

61. Afacan O, Estroff JA, Yang E, et al. Fetal echoplanar imaging: promises and challenges. Top Magn Reson Imaging 2019;28(5):245–54.

62. Lees CC, Stampalija T, Baschat A, et al. ISUOG practice guidelines: diagnosis and management of small-for-gestational-age fetus and fetal growth restriction. Ultrasound Obstet Gynecol 2020;56(2):298–312.

63. Poustchi-Amin M, Mirowitz SA, Brown JJ, et al. Principles and applications of echo-planar imaging: a review for the general radiologist. Radiographics 2001;21(3):767–79.

64. Lustig M, Donoho D, Pauly JM. Sparse MRI: the application of compressed sensing for rapid MR imaging. Magn Reson Med 2007;58(6):1182–95.

65. Feinberg DA, Hale JD, Watts JC, et al. Halving MR imaging time by conjugation: demonstration at 3.5 kG. Radiology 1986;161(2):527–31.

66. Pruessmann KP, Weiger M, Scheidegger MB, et al. SENSE: sensitivity encoding for fast MRI. Magn Reson Med 1999;42(5):952–62.

67. Griswold MA, Jakob PM, Heidemann RM, et al. Generalized autocalibrating partially parallel acquisitions (GRAPPA). Magn Reson Med 2002;47(6):1202–10.

68. Wang F, Dong Z, Reese TG, et al. Echo planar time-resolved imaging (EPTI). Magn Reson Med 2019;81(6):3599–615.

69. Feinberg DA, Setsompop K. Ultra-fast MRI of the human brain with simultaneous multi-slice imaging. J Magn Reson 2013;229:90–100.

70. Turk EA, Abulnaga SM, Luo J, et al. Placental MRI: effect of maternal position and uterine contractions on placental BOLD MRI measurements. Placenta 2020;95:69–77.

71. Xu J, Zhang M, Turk EA, et al. 3D Fetal pose estimation with adaptive variance and conditional generative adversarial network. In: Hu Y, Licandro R, Noble JA, et al, editors. Medical Ultrasound, and Preterm, Perinatal and Paediatric Image Analysis. ASMUS 2020, PIPPI 2020. Lecture Notes in Computer Science, vol 12437. Cham: Springer; 2020. p. 201-10. https://doi.org/10.1007/978-3-030-60334-2_20.

72. Zhang M, Xu J, Abaci Turk E, et al. Enhanced detection of fetal pose in 3D MRI by deep reinforcement learning with physical structure priors on anatomy. In: Martel AL, Abolmaesumi P, Stoyanov D, et al, editors. Medical image computing and computer assisted intervention – MICCAI 2020. MICCAI 2020. Lecture Notes in Computer Science, vol 12266.

Cham: Springer; 2020. p. 396–405. https://doi.org/10.1007/978-3-030-59725-2_38.

73. Sobotka D, Licandro R, Ebner M, et al. Reproducibility of Functional Connectivity Estimates in Motion Corrected Fetal fMRI. In: Wang Q, Gomez A, Hutter J, et al, editors. Smart Ultrasound Imaging and Perinatal, Preterm and Paediatric Image Analysis. PIPPI 2019, SUSI 2019. Lecture Notes in Computer Science, vol 11798. Cham: Springer; 2019. p. 123–32. https://doi.org/10.1007/978-3-030-32875-7_14.

74. Turk E, van den Heuvel MI, Benders MJ, et al. Functional connectome of the fetal brain. J Neurosci 2019;39(49):9716–24.

75. Figueiredo CM, Falcão I, Vilaverde J, et al. Prenatal diagnosis and management of a fetal goiter hypothyroidism due to dyshormonogenesis. Case Rep Endocrinol 2018;2018:9564737.

76. Machado CM, Castro JM, Campos RA, et al. Graves' disease complicated by fetal goitrous hypothyroidism treated with intra-amniotic administration of levothyroxine. BMJ Case Rep 2019;12(8). https://doi.org/10.1136/bcr-2019-230457.

77. Li T-G, Zhang Y-Y, Nie F, et al. Diagnosis of foetal vein of galen aneurysmal malformation by ultrasound combined with magnetic resonance imaging: a case series. BMC Med Imaging 2020;20(1):63.

78. Block KT, Chandarana H, Fatterpekar G, et al. Improving the robustness of clinical T1-weighted MRI using radial VIBE. Magnetom Flash 2013;5:6–11.

79. Morgan L. Development of a 3D radial MR Imaging sequence to be used for (self) navigation during the scanning of the fetal brain in utero. 2016. Available at: https://open.uct.ac.za/handle/11427/22735. Accessed April 2, 2021.

80. Haskell MW, Cauley SF, Wald LL. TArgeted Motion Estimation and Reduction (TAMER): data consistency based motion mitigation for MRI using a reduced model joint optimization. IEEE Trans Med Imaging 2018;37(5):1253–65.

81. Haskell MW, Cauley SF, Bilgic B, et al. Network Accelerated Motion Estimation and Reduction (NAMER): convolutional neural network guided retrospective motion correction using a separable motion model. Magn Reson Med 2019;82(4):1452–61.

82. Stirnemann J, Chalouhi G, Essaoui M, et al. Fetal brain imaging following laser surgery in twin-to-twin surgery. BJOG 2018;125(9):1186–91.

83. Prsa M, Sun L, van Amerom J, et al. Reference ranges of blood flow in the major vessels of the normal human fetal circulation at term by phase contrast magnetic resonance imaging. Circ Cardiovasc Imaging 2014;7(4):663–70. https://doi.org/10.1161/CIRCIMAGING.113.001859.

84. Salehi D, Sun L, Steding-Ehrenborg K, et al. Quantification of blood flow in the fetus with cardiovascular magnetic resonance imaging using Doppler ultrasound gating: validation against metric optimized gating. J Cardiovasc Magn Reson 2019;21(1):1–15.

85. Zhu MY, Milligan N, Keating S, et al. The hemodynamics of late onset intrauterine growth restriction by MRI. Am J Obstet Gynecol 2015;7:195–225.

86. Grevent D, Taso M, Millischer A, et al. OC07.07: SS-FSE FAIR ASL parameters for non-invasive measurement of fetal brain perfusion in vivo. Ultrasound Obstet Gynecol 2019;54(S1):18.

87. Francis ST, Duncan KR, Moore RJ, et al. Non-invasive mapping of placental perfusion. Lancet 1998;351(9113):1397–9.

88. Harteveld AA, Hutter J, Franklin SL, et al. Systematic evaluation of velocity-selective arterial spin labeling settings for placental perfusion measurement. Magn Reson Med 2020;84(4):1828–43.

89. Zun Z, Zaharchuk G, Andescavage NN, et al. Non-invasive placental perfusion imaging in pregnancies complicated by fetal heart disease using velocity-selective arterial spin labeled MRI. Sci Rep 2017;7(1):16126.

90. Sun L, Macgowan CK, Sled JG, et al. Reduced fetal cerebral oxygen consumption is associated with smaller brain size in fetuses with congenital heart disease. Circulation 2015;131(15):1313–23.

91. Rodríguez-Soto AE, Langham MC, Abdulmalik O, et al. MRI quantification of human fetal O2delivery rate in the second and third trimesters of pregnancy. Magn Reson Med 2018;80(3):1148–57.

92. Abaci Turk E, Stout JN, Ha C, et al. Placental MRI: developing accurate quantitative measures of oxygenation. Top Magn Reson Imaging 2019;28(5):285–97. https://doi.org/10.1097/RMR.0000000000000221.

93. Freud LR, Tworetzky W. Fetal interventions for congenital heart disease. Curr Opin Pediatr 2016;28(2):156–62.

94. Orbach D. Fetal treatment for vein of Galen malformations. 2019. Available at: https://discoveries.childrenshospital.org/fetal-treatment-vein-of-galen-malformations/. Accessed February 19, 2021.

Ultrashort Echo-Time MR Imaging of the Pediatric Head and Neck

Naoharu Kobayashi, PhD[a], Sven Bambach, PhD[b], Mai-Lan Ho, MD[c],*

KEYWORDS

- Bone MRI • Pediatric • Synthetic CT • Ultrashort echo time • Zero echo time

KEY POINTS

- Bone MR imaging uses ultrashort echo-time or zero echo-time techniques to maximize detection of short T2 tissues with low water concentrations.
- Synthetic CT generation is feasible using atlas-based, voxel-based, and deep learning approaches.
- Major clinical applications in the pediatric head and neck include evaluation for craniosynostosis and cranial vault abnormalities, sinonasal and jaw imaging, trauma, interventional planning, and postoperative follow-up.

INTRODUCTION

MR imaging is the workhorse for pediatric neuroradiology, providing excellent soft tissue contrast with various image weightings (e.g. T1, T2, diffusion) to visualize multiple tissue properties without the need for ionizing radiation. With most conventional MR imaging sequences, the echo time (TE) between radiofrequency signal excitation and reception is at least a few milliseconds. This poses major limitations for detection of short-T2 tissues with low water concentrations and extremely rapidly decaying signal, such as cortical bone, meninges, cartilage, tendons, ligaments, calcified tissues, and lungs. To increase MR imaging sensitivity to short-lived signals, various MR imaging techniques have been developed over the last few decades, of which the most promising include ultrashort TE (UTE), zero TE (ZTE), and sweep imaging with Fourier transformation (SWIFT). These techniques achieve extremely short TE (nearly zero to approximately 100 microseconds) to maximize sensitivity to fast-decaying MR imaging signals. Initially available only on research MR

imaging systems owing to the demands on high-performance hardware, these techniques have become available for routine clinical use thanks to recent technical hardware and software developments. In this article, we review the technical background and clinical applications of bone MR imaging techniques in pediatric neuroimaging.

BONE MR IMAGING TECHNIQUES

UTE MR imaging techniques begin data acquisition immediately after signal excitation to capture spin signals from tissues with T_2/T_2^* shorter than a few milliseconds. There are 2 types of UTE techniques: (1) phase encoding and (2) radial frequency encoding. The phase encoding based techniques, including constant time imaging (CTI)[1] and single point imaging (SPI),[2,3] perform spatial encoding with pure phase encoding such that data acquisition is point-by-point in the k-space domain (**Fig. 1**A and B). CTI excites spin signals without a gradient field and then applies phase encoding gradients. In SPI, a gradient field is turned on before spin excitation, and the

a Center for Magnetic Resonance Research, Department of Radiology, University of Minnesota, 2021 6th Street SE, Minneapolis, MN 55455, USA; b Abigail Wexner Research Institute at Nationwide Children's Hospital, 575 Children's Crossroad, Columbus, OH 43215, USA; c Department of Radiology, Nationwide Children's Hospital, 700 Children's Dr – ED4, Columbus, OH 43205, USA
* Corresponding author.
E-mail address: mai-lan.ho@nationwidechildrens.org

Magn Reson Imaging Clin N Am 29 (2021) 583–593
https://doi.org/10.1016/j.mric.2021.06.008
1064-9689/21/© 2021 Elsevier Inc. All rights reserved.

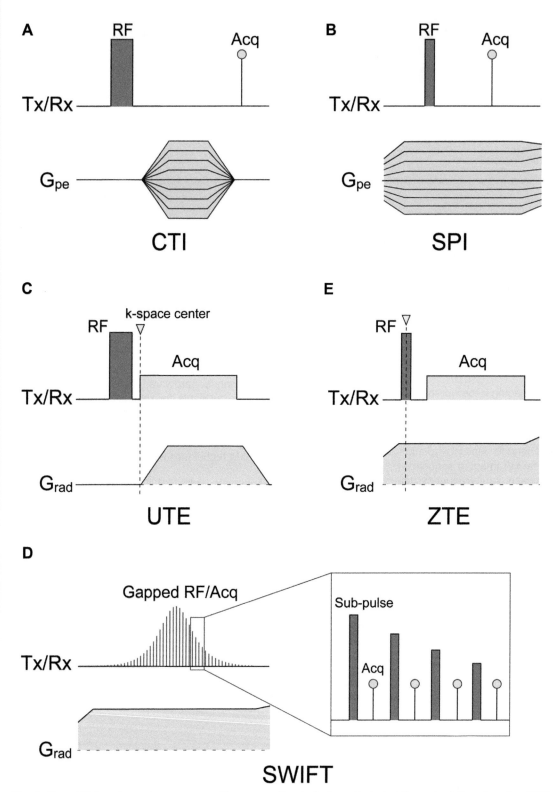

Fig. 1. Bone MR imaging pulse sequences. Phase-encoding techniques include (*A*) constant time imaging (CTI) and (*B*) single point imaging (SPI). Radial encoding techniques include (*C*) ultrashort echo-time (UTE), (*D*) sweep imaging with Fourier transformation (SWIFT), and (*E*) zero echo-time (ZTE). Tx/Rx, transmit/receive.

gradient field strength during excitation is changed from one repetition time period to the next to reach the k-space point sampled. With phase encoding based techniques, because all k-space points are sampled with a common delay time from excitation to data sampling, reconstructed images are free from image blurring associated with off-resonance frequencies and T_2* signal decay. However, there is low time efficiency of data sampling owing to point-by-point k-space acquisition, resulting in a longer scan time and/or limited image resolution.

Radial encoding techniques include most imaging sequences used in clinical diagnostics such as UTE[4,5] and ZTE imaging.[6,7] In these techniques, the k-space is sampled radially from the center out with a frequency encoding/readout gradient. The sampling of one radial k-space line in every repetition time period significantly accelerates data acquisition as compared with point-by-point acquisition in the phase encoding based techniques. In UTE, the signal acquisition starts with the readout gradient ramping up after nonselective excitation with a hard pulse (see **Fig. 1**C). Ramp sampling in UTE makes it sensitive to imperfections of gradient performance, such as gradient group delay and eddy currents. To correct image reconstruction errors associated with gradient eddy currents, various strategies are introduced including pre-emphasis correction, gradient measurement and gradient impulse response function.[8,9] Although most UTE techniques use 3-dimensional nonselective excitation with a short hard pulse, UTE has an option of slab-selective excitation at the expense of slightly longer TE. This goal is achieved with a minimum phase radiofrequency pulse[10] and variable rate selective excitation[11] to achieve slab selection while keeping a short TE.[12,13]

SWIFT is another UTE sequence with radial center-out frequency encoding.[14] In SWIFT, signal excitation and data acquisition are performed in a time shared manner using a gapped frequency-modulated radiofrequency pulse (see **Fig. 1**D). During the gapped frequency-modulated pulse, the transmit and receive mode are switched back and forth repeatedly. Therefore, fast T/R switching is essential especially for high bandwidth SWIFT acquisition. Gradient modulation can mitigate the requirements on fast T/R switching.[15–17]

ZTE, which was originally introduced as back-projection low angle shot[18] and rotating ultrafast imaging sequence,[19] has gained renewed attention in the last decade.[6,7] ZTE is similar to UTE, but the gradient field is present during signal excitation with a short hard pulse (see **Fig. 1**E). Because the gradient field does not change

from signal excitation to data acquisition, ZTE is highly insensitive to gradient imperfections (group delay and eddy currents). Moreover, ZTE generates much less acoustic noise than UTE owing to the smoothly changing gradient waveforms over time. However, because the gradient field is turned on before signal excitation, the k-space center matching the center of the excitation hard pulse cannot be sampled. When the missing k-space center area is small (up to a few points in radius), it can be estimated/recovered with algebraic reconstruction.[20,21] The size of the missing center area is determined depending on the switching time of transmit and receive mode and bandwidth in data acquisition. With hardware available in standard clinical MR imaging systems, the transmit and receive switching time is typically 20 to 30 ms, which makes the missing k-space center area too large for algebraic reconstruction or significantly limits available bandwidths. To acquire k-space data in the missing center area with the clinical MR imaging hardware, 2 strategies have been introduced. One is water- and fat-suppressed proton projection imaging (WASPI),[22] where the k-space center area is radially sampled with a low readout bandwidth (ie, reduced gradient amplitude). WASPI can acquire the missing k-space center area in a time-efficient manner, but introduces phase inconsistency for off-resonance signals (eg, chemical shift, magnetic susceptibility, and B_0 inhomogeneity) at the boundary between the missing center and outer area, which may result in artifacts in reconstructed images. The other solution is pointwise encoding time reduction with radial acquisition (PETRA),[23] a hybrid acquisition method of ZTE and SPI, in which the missing k-space center area is sampled with SPI. In PETRA, there is no phase discontinuity at the boundary of the missing center area for off-resonance signals, but SPI acquisition is time consuming when the missing center area is large. To decrease the missing k-space center area while keeping higher bandwidth in data acquisition, gradient modulation was introduced in PETRA.[24] In gradient-modulated PETRA, the gradient amplitude is set to low during excitation and then ramps up to a high amplitude after excitation to increase the readout bandwidth, similar to SWIFT.

IMAGE CONTRAST AND ARTIFACTS

Steady-state magnetization in UTE techniques is represented by the Ernst equation.[25] Using very short TE values, T_2/T_2* contrast is minimal. With short repetition time (<5 ms), the Ernst flip angle that provides an optimal signal-to-noise ratio is typically less than 5° and produces proton density or mildly T_1-weighted images. Magnetization preparation (MP) can be used to modify image contrast and is usually implemented with segmented data acquisition, where multiple radial k-space lines are acquired per MP. Inversion recovery is the most widely used MP strategy and can be used to achieve T_1-weighted contrast, fat suppression, and long T_2 suppression.[26,27] Clinical applications include myelin imaging with T_1 weighting,[28] measurement of magnetization transfer rate,[29,30] blood oxygen level-dependent functional MR imaging with T_2 preparation,[31] and dual echo acquisition with T_2^* weighting.

Radial acquisition techniques are relatively resistant to motion and flow artifacts, owing to repeated sampling of the k-space center.[32] Motion during scans results in image blurring rather than ghosting artifacts as in Cartesian MR imaging. Sparse sampling of high-frequency components in the k-space also requires more data acquisition to satisfy Nyquist sampling, but the aliasing signals are less coherent and so radial techniques remain more immune to undersampling artifacts. Image blurring can result from chemical shift, magnetic susceptibility differences, and B_0 field inhomogeneity. These effects are worse at higher field strengths owing to the increasing chemical shift frequencies and stronger magnetic susceptibility effects. A high readout bandwidth is one solution to decreasing off-resonance blurring, but requires faster transmit and receive switching in some of the UTE techniques. For fat–water chemical shift, the k-space decomposition method was introduced to differentiate fat and water images and avoid off-resonance blurring.[33] Recently, similar k-space decomposition has been used to separate in-phase and out-of-phase components in ZTE.[34]

SYNTHETIC COMPUTED TOMOGRAPHY GENERATION
Conventional Image Processing

Conversion of bone MR to synthetic CT (sCT), also known as pseudo CT or substitute CT, is desirable for greater clinical diagnostic applicability. A major challenge for sCT is the lack of consistent mathematical relationships between MR signal intensity and CT attenuation. Most approaches to sCT generation use either atlas-based or voxel-based techniques. Atlas-based techniques use co-registered pairs of MR and CT images from patients as templates for sCT generation. MR images from the template dataset are registered to MR images from a new patient.

The same deformation is applied to CT images in the template dataset, and the final sCT image is calculated by combining the deformed CT images, using various combination methods such as patch-based pattern recognition[35] and weighted average of voxel intensities.[36]

Voxel-based sCT generation techniques convert MR signal intensities to Hounsfield units in CT, based on a model trained to represent the relationship between MR signal intensity and Hounsfield units. Voxel-based techniques do not require image registration, but cortical bone on MR is mathematically difficult to distinguish from other short-T2 structures, including connective tissue and air. As a result, voxel-based techniques often require additional manual processing and are impractical for clinical workflows. In some cases, UTE pulse sequences can be combined with other standard MR weightings such as magnetization prepared rapid acquisition gradient echo[37] and T_2-SPACE[38] to achieve more automated bone classification.[39,40] Voxel-based sCT generation using ZTE with proton density weighting has achieved accurate attenuation correction in positron emission tomography (PET)/MR and MR-based radiation therapy planning.[41] For adult patients with relatively normative osseous anatomy, the signal intensity is mainly affected by spatial B_1 field variation. This issue can be addressed using methods such as histogram-based bias correction,[42] bias field estimation with polynomial fitting,[41] or nonparametric bias correction algorithms.[43] The corrected ZTE image shows a flattened soft tissue contrast and bone signal intensity distinguishable from air. Because ZTE signal intensities of bone and soft tissue are linearly and negatively correlated with Hounsfield units in CT, the intensity-inverted ZTE image shows a similar image contrast to CT, except for air. Tissue segmentation can then be performed using intensity threshold cutoffs to distinguish bone from air, with correction of partial volume effects at air–tissue interfaces. Therefore, the intensity-inverted ZTE image with constant scaling and offset can be mathematically converted to a sCT image. This approach works in adults with normal osseous anatomy, but performs less well in children with immature bone, as well as patients with complex osseous pathology and multiple tissue interfaces.[44]

Deep Learning Approaches

Deep learning is a more promising approach for sCT generation and is often used for tissue classification and image mapping purposes. In contrast with traditional point-based operations, deep learning algorithms use several layers of

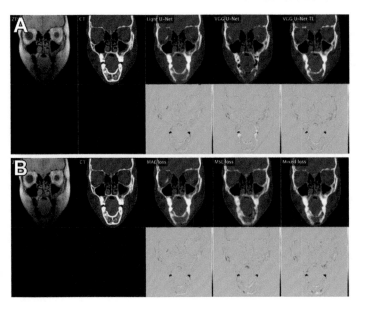

Fig. 2. Synthetic CT generation using deep learning. (*A*) Example ZTE and CT with synthetic CT generated using light U-Net, VGG-16 U-Net, and VGG-16 U-Net with transfer learning (TL). Bottom row shows color-coded subtraction maps of pixel-level differences between a CT and a synthetic CT. (*B*) Example ZTE and CT with with synthetic CT generated using light U-Net with loss functions of mean absolute error (MAE), mean squared error (MSE), and a weighted mixture of MAE and MSE. Synthetic CT models trained on MAE loss produce sharper-appearing images with fewer overall white pixels, resulting in better precision or positive predictive value for bone. Models trained on MSE loss produce smoother appearing images with more overall white pixels, enabling better bone sensitivity or recall. The mixture loss provides a weighted average of the two contributions, balancing bone precision and recall.

neighborhood-based operations to derive complex information from diverse image inputs. These approaches have shown some success in adults for radiation therapy planning and PET/MR attenuation correction.[45–49]

We have optimized a convolutional neural network for bone MR conversion to sCT, using our unique dataset of paired bone MR and CT studies in pediatric and adult patients with various pathologic diagnoses of the head and neck.[50] We trained three different encoder–decoder models based on the U-Net architecture: light U-Net[51] (2,161,361 parameters) and VGG-16 U-Net[52] (28,845,505 parameters), without and with transfer learning from Image-Net.[53] The light U-Net architecture quantitatively outperformed the VGG-16 models without and with transfer learning. Defining a loss function based on the mean absolute error resulted in better bone precision (positive predictive value), whereas the mean squared error provided better bone recall (sensitivity or true positive rate). Because our image database contained diverse training data, we also ran multiple experiments to evaluate model generalizability. The performance metrics for a given model decreased when using training data captured only in a different environment, and increased when local training data were augmented with that from different hospitals, vendors, or MR techniques (**Fig. 2**). Generative adversarial networks can also be applied for image-to-image translation

tasks, more so for unpaired sets of images from the source and target domains.[54–58]

CLINICAL APPLICATIONS

Bone MR is a useful alternative to CT for imaging various head and neck pathologies. Minimization of exposure to ionizing radiation is important in the vulnerable pediatric population, particularly for patients who may require follow-up imaging. Bone MR sequences can be used as part of a rapid screening protocol, or in combination with other sequences as a "one-stop-shop" examination.

Cranial Sutures

When evaluating an abnormal pediatric head shape, imaging helps to distinguish positional plagiocephaly from single suture and multisuture craniosynostosis. Because unossified fibrocartilage has longer T2 values than bone, open sutures appear relatively bright in signal, whereas closed sutures are dark on bone MR[59–61] (**Fig. 3**).

Cranial Vault

Cranial vault imaging is useful for evaluating calvarial remodeling secondary to intracranial masses and increased intracranial pressure.[61] Bone MR can function as an alternative to CT for interventional procedures, such as radiation therapy planning and intraoperative neuronavigation, without the complexities of CT-to-MR coregistration[62–64] (**Fig. 4**).

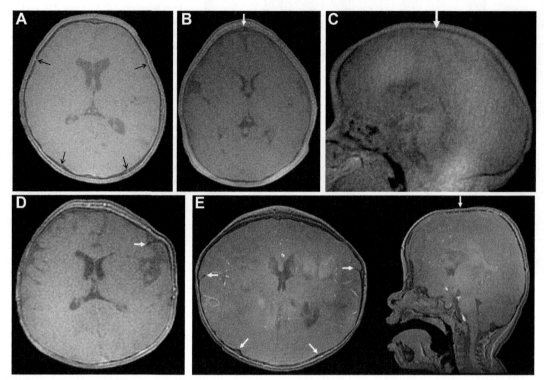

Fig. 3. Cranial sutures. (*A*) Plagiocephaly with patent coronal and lambdoid sutures (*arrows*). (*B*) Metopic synostosis with trigonocephaly, ectocranial ridging (*arrow*) and endocranial notching. (*C*) Sagittal synostosis with dolichocephaly and ectocranial ridging (*arrow*). (*D*) Left coronal synostosis (*arrow*) with anterior plagiocephaly and brachycephaly. (*E*) Apert syndrome with turribrachycephaly due to bilateral coronal, lambdoid, and sagittal synostosis (*arrows*).

Craniofacial Imaging

Craniofacial bone MR assists in evaluation of the sinonasal cavity, orbits, skull base, and jaw. Bone MR is commonly used in dentistry to achieve excellent visualization of tooth structure, jaw landmarks, and osseous remodeling. UTE minimizes MR susceptibility artifact typically associated with dental amalgam and hardware[65–68] (**Fig. 5**).

Trauma

Clinical bone MR sequences can achieve a spatial resolution of approximately 1 mm, which is satisfactory for characterizing the majority of traumatic fractures. False negatives may include microfractures and nondisplaced fractures. In the setting of accidental or nonaccidental head trauma, MR is often ordered to increase sensitivity for

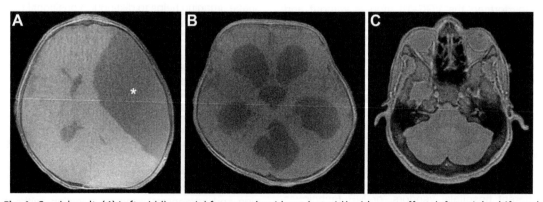

Fig. 4. Cranial vault. (*A*) Left middle cranial fossa arachnoid cyst (*asterisk*) with mass effect, left-to-right shift, and calvarial remodeling. (*B*) Tetraventricular hydrocephalus with diastatic cranial sutures. (*C*) Chronic epilepsy with hyperostosis secondary to anticonvulsant therapy.

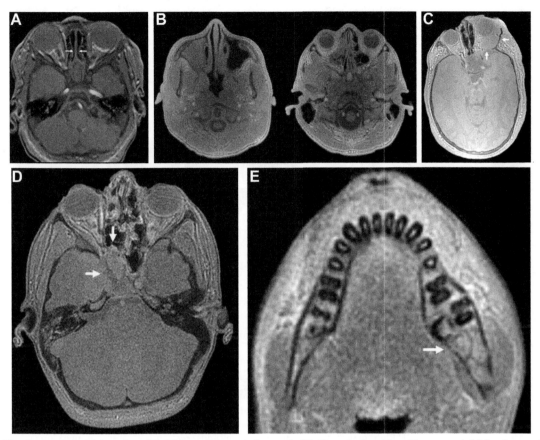

Fig. 5. Craniofacial imaging. (*A*) Midnasal stenosis (*arrows*). (*B*) Chronic sinusitis with mucosal thickening and right maxillary sinus hyperostosis. (*C*) Neurofibromatosis type 1 with left orbitotemporal neurofibroma, remodeled bony orbit, and sphenoid wing dysplasia (*arrows*). (*D*) Right skull base rhabdomyosarcoma with tumoral bone erosions (*arrows*). (*E*) Mandibular tumor with multilobulated expansile mass and dental erosions (*arrow*).

parenchymal and vascular injury. MR with the addition of a bone sequence offers a one-stop shop approach with comparable diagnostic performance to combined CT and MR imaging[69–71] (**Fig. 6**).

Postoperative Imaging

UTE MR demonstrates advantages for postoperative imaging by minimizing susceptibility artifact from surgical hardware, including shunts, clips, screws, plates, and other surgical materials[61] (**Fig. 7**).

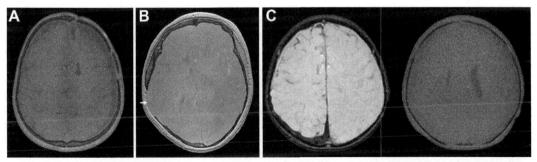

Fig. 6. Trauma. (*A*) Comminuted left frontal calvarial fractures. (*B*) Right parietal growing fracture or leptomeningeal cyst (*arrow*). (*C*) Abusive head trauma with right subdural hematoma, bridging vein injury, and diastatic sutures.

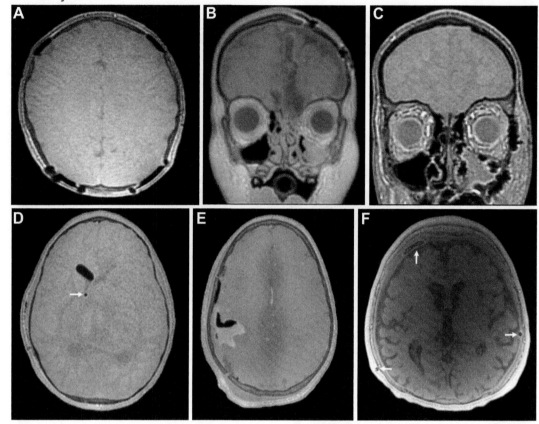

Fig. 7. Postoperative imaging. (*A*) Follow-up cranioplasty. (*B*) Left frontal calvarial fracture with fixation plate and screws. (*C*) Repaired left zygomaticomaxillary fracture. (*D*) Bithalamic glioma after shunt placement (*arrow*) with intraventricular pneumocephalus. (*E*) Right parietal tumor after craniotomy and resection, with postoperative blood products and pneumocephalus. (*F*) Chronic shunting (*arrow*) with volume loss, subdural hematomas, and hyperostosis.

SUMMARY

Bone MR uses UTE or ZTE techniques to maximize detection of short-T2 tissues with low water concentrations. Synthetic CT generation is feasible using atlas-based, voxel-based, and deep learning approaches. Major clinical applications in the pediatric head and neck include evaluation for craniosynostosis and cranial vault abnormalities, sinonasal and jaw imaging, trauma, interventional planning, and postoperative follow-up.

CLINICS CARE POINT

- Ultrashort echo-time and zero echo-time MR imaging enable visualization of short-T2 tissues such as cortical bone. These provide the opportunity for rapid screening or "one-stop-shop" imaging without the need for ionizing radiation.
- Synthetic CT reconstruction algorithms are in development and may provide improved clinical translation of bone MRI. Deep learning approaches are the most promising for pediatric applications and results depend on training data, network architecture, and problem-specific loss function selection.

- Major applications in the pediatric head and neck include craniosynostosis and cranial vault abnormalities, sinonasal and jaw imaging, trauma, interventional planning, and postoperative follow-up.

DISCLOSURE

Dr Kobayashi is funded by NIH grant P41EB027061.

Dr Bambach received the 2nd Place Research Award at the ASFNR Artificial Intelligence Workshop for part of the work presented in this article. Dr Ho is a principal investigator on the RSNA Research Scholar Grant, SPR Pilot Award, and ASHNR William N. Hanafee Award, which help support the data presented in this article. She also received the 2nd Place Research Award at the ASFNR Artificial Intelligence Workshop for part of the work presented in this article.

REFERENCES

1. Choi SM, Tang XW, Cory DG. Constant time imaging approaches to NMR microscopy. Int J Imag Syst Tech 1997;8(3):263–76.

2. Emid S, Creyghton JHN. High-resolution NMR imaging in solids. Physica B & C 1985;128(1):81–3.

3. Balcom BJ, Macgregor RP, Beyea SD, et al. Single-point ramped imaging with T1 enhancement (SPRITE). J Magn Reson Ser A 1996;123(1): 131–4.

4. Glover GH, Pauly JM, Bradshaw KM. Boron-11 imaging with a three-dimensional reconstruction method. J Magn Reson Imaging 1992;2(1):47–52.

5. Robson MD, Bydder GM. Clinical ultrashort echo time imaging of bone and other connective tissues. Nmr Biomed 2006;19(7):765–80.

6. Weiger M, Pruessmann KP, Hennel F. MRI with zero echo time: hard versus sweep pulse excitation. Magn Reson Med 2011;66(2):379–89.

7. Weiger M, Brunner DO, Dietrich BE, et al. ZTE imaging in humans. Magn Reson Med 2013;70(2):328–32.

8. Addy NO, Wu HH, Nishimura DG. Simple method for MR gradient system characterization and k-space trajectory estimation. Magn Reson Med 2012;68(1): 120–9.

9. Vannesjo SJ, Haeberlin M, Kasper L, et al. Gradient system characterization by impulse response measurements with a dynamic field camera. Magn Reson Med 2013;69(2):583–93.

10. Pauly J, Le Roux P, Nishimura D, et al. Parameter relations for the Shinnar-Le Roux selective excitation pulse design algorithm [NMR imaging]. IEEE Trans Med Imaging 1991;10(1):53–65.

11. Hargreaves BA, Cunningham CH, Nishimura DG, et al. Variable-rate selective excitation for rapid MRI sequences. Magn Reson Med 2004;52(3): 590–7.

12. Johnson KM, Fain SB, Schiebler ML, et al. Optimized 3D ultrashort echo time pulmonary MRI. Magn Reson Med 2013;70(5):1241–50.

13. Kobayashi N, Begnaud A, Allen T, et al. Robust retrospective respiratory gating for detection of small pulmonary nodules with UTE MRI. ISMRM 2018;26:4350.

14. Idiyatullin D, Corum C, Park JY, et al. Fast and quiet MRI using a swept radiofrequency. J Magn Reson 2006;181(2):342–9.

15. Zhang J, Idiyatullin D, Corum CA, et al. Gradient-modulated SWIFT. Magn Reson Med 2016;75(2): 537–46.

16. Kobayashi N, Lei J, Utecht L, et al. 3D cine magnetic resonance imaging of rat lung ARDS using gradient-modulated SWIFT with retrospective respiratory gating. Proc SPIE Int Soc Opt Eng 2015;9417: 941718.

17. Lagore R, Auerbach E, Kobayashi N, et al. Fast transmit/receive switch for SWIFT imaging at 7T. ISMRM 2019;27:573.

18. Hafner S. Fast imaging in liquids and solids with the Back-projection Low Angle ShoT (BLAST) technique. Magn Reson Imaging 1994;12(7):1047–51.

19. Madio DP, Lowe IJ. Ultra-fast imaging using low flip angles and FIDs. Magn Reson Med 1995;34(4): 525–9.

20. Kuethe DO, Caprihan A, Lowe IJ, et al. Transforming NMR data despite missing points. J Magn Reson 1999;139(1):18–25.

21. Weiger M, Brunner DO, Tabbert M, et al. Exploring the bandwidth limits of ZTE imaging: spatial response, out-of-band signals, and noise propagation. Magn Reson Med 2015;74(5):1236–47.

22. Wu Y, Dai G, Ackerman JL, et al. Water- and fat-suppressed proton projection MRI (WASPI) of rat femur bone. Magn Reson Med 2007;57(3):554–67.

23. Grodzki DM, Jakob PM, Heismann B. Ultrashort echo time imaging using pointwise encoding time reduction with radial acquisition (PETRA). Magn Reson Med 2012;67(2):510–8.

24. Kobayashi N, Goerke U, Wang L, et al. Gradient-modulated PETRA MRI. Tomography 2015;1(2): 85–90.

25. Ernst RR, Bodenhausen G, Wokaun A. Principles of nuclear magnetic resonance in one and two dimensions. Oxford: Clarendon Press; 1987. p. 610.

26. Aida N, Niwa T, Fujii Y, et al. Quiet T1-weighted pointwise encoding time reduction with radial acquisition for assessing myelination in the pediatric brain. AJNR Am J Neuroradiol 2016;37(8):1528–34.

27. Jang H, Carl M, Ma Y, et al. Inversion recovery zero echo time (IR-ZTE) imaging for direct myelin detection in human brain: a feasibility study. Quant Imaging Med Surg 2020;10(5):895–906.

28. Wood TC, Damestani NL, Lawrence AJ, et al. Silent myelin-weighted magnetic resonance imaging. Wellcome open Res 2020;5:74.

29. Marcon M, Weiger M, Keller D, et al. Magnetization transfer imaging of cortical bone in vivo using a zero echo time sequence in mice at 4.7 T: a feasibility study. MAGMA 2016;29(6):853–62.

30. Wurnig MC, Weiger M, Wu M, et al. In vivo magnetization transfer imaging of the lung using a zero echo time sequence at 4.7 Tesla in mice: initial experience. Magn Reson Med 2016;76(1):156–62.

31. Solana AB, Menini A, Sacolick LI, et al. Quiet and distortion-free, whole brain BOLD fMRI using T2-prepared RUFIS. Magn Reson Med 2016;75(4):1402–12.

32. Glover GH, Pauly JM. Projection reconstruction techniques for reduction of motion effects in MRI. Magn Reson Med 1992;28(2):275–89.

33. Brodsky EK, Holmes JH, Yu H, et al. Generalized k-space decomposition with chemical shift

correction for non-Cartesian water-fat imaging. Magn Reson Med 2008;59(5):1151–64.

34. Engstrom M, McKinnon G, Cozzini C, et al. In-phase zero TE musculoskeletal imaging. Magn Reson Med 2020;83(1):195–202.

35. Edmund JM, Andreasen D, Mahmood F, et al. Cone beam computed tomography guided treatment delivery and planning verification for magnetic resonance imaging only radiotherapy of the brain. Acta Oncol 2015;54(9):1496–500.

36. Uh J, Merchant TE, Li Y, et al. MRI-based treatment planning with pseudo CT generated through atlas registration. Med Phys 2014;41(5):051711.

37. Paradis E, Cao Y, Lawrence TS, et al. Assessing the dosimetric accuracy of magnetic resonance-generated synthetic CT images for focal brain VMAT radiation therapy. Int J Radiat Oncol Biol Phys 2015;93(5):1154–61.

38. Johansson A, Karlsson M, Yu J, et al. Voxel-wise uncertainty in CT substitute derived from MRI. Med Phys 2012;39(6):3283–90.

39. Johnstone E, Wyatt JJ, Henry AM, et al. Systematic review of synthetic computed tomography generation methodologies for use in magnetic resonance imaging-only radiation therapy. Int J Radiat Oncol Biol Phys 2018;100(1):199–217.

40. Edmund JM, Nyholm T. A review of substitute CT generation for MRI-only radiation therapy. Radiat Oncol 2017;12(1):28.

41. Wiesinger F, Bylund M, Yang J, et al. Zero TE-based pseudo-CT image conversion in the head and its application in PET/MR attenuation correction and MR-guided radiation therapy planning. Magn Reson Med 2018;80(4):1440–51.

42. Wiesinger F, Sacolick LI, Menini A, et al. Zero TE MR bone imaging in the head. Magn Reson Med 2016; 75(1):107–14.

43. Tustison NJ, Avants BB, Cook PA, et al. N4ITK: improved N3 bias correction. IEEE Trans Med Imaging 2010;29(6):1310–20.

44. Lu A, Gorny KR, Ho ML, et al. Improved delineation of air-bone interface in in-vivo high-resolution bright bone ZTE MRI at 3T. Proc 25th ISMRM 2017;P5109.

45. Leynes AP, Yang J, Wiesinger F, et al. Zero-echo-time and Dixon deep pseudo-CT (ZeDD CT): direct generation of pseudo-CT images for pelvic PET/MRI attenuation correction using deep convolutional neural networks with multiparametric MRI. J Nucl Med 2018;59(5):852–8.

46. Gong K, Yang J, Kim K, et al. Attenuation correction for brain PET imaging using deep neural network based on Dixon and ZTE MR images. Phys Med Biol 2018;63(12):125011.

47. Nie D, Cao X, Gao Y, et al. Estimating CT image from MRI data using 3D fully convolutional networks. Deep Learn Data Label Med Appl (2016) 2016; 2016:170–8.

48. Andreasen D, Van Leemput K, Hansen RH, et al. Patch-based generation of a pseudo CT from conventional MRI sequences for MRI-only radiotherapy of the brain. Med Phys 2015;42(4):1596–605.

49. Boukellouz W, Moussaoui A. Magnetic resonance-driven pseudo CT image using patch-based multimodal feature extraction and ensemble learning with stacked generalization. J King Saud Univ Computer Inf Sci 2019.

50. Bambach S, Ho ML. Bone MRI: can it replace CT? 2nd Place AI Award, Artificial Intelligence Workshop, American Society of Functional Neuroradiology, October 2020 2021. ASFNR Presents AI, American Society of Functional Neuroradiology.

51. Ronneberger O, Fischer P, Brox T. U-net: convolutional networks for biomedical image segmentation. In: Medical Image Computing and Computer-Assisted Intervention (MICCAI)9351. LNCS: Springer; 2015. p. 234–41. arXiv:1505.04597 [cs. CV].

52. Simonyan K, Zisserman A. Very deep convolutional networks for large-scale image recognition. arXiv preprint arXiv 2014;1409:1556.

53. Deng J, Dong W, Socher R, et al. ImageNet: a large-scale hierarchical image database. 2009 IEEE Conference on Computer vision and pattern recognition 2009.

54. Goodfellow I, Pouget-Abadie J, Mirza M, et al. Generative adversarial nets. Adv Neural Inf Process Syst 2014;27:2672–80.

55. Wolterink JM, Dinkla AM, Savenije MHF, et al. MR to CT synthesis using unpaired data. Simulation and Synthesis in Medical Imaging. SASHIMI. In: Lecture Notes in Computer Science, 10557. Cham: Springer; 2017. arXiv:1708.01155 [cs.CV].

56. Zhu J-Y, Park T, Isola P, et al. Unpaired image-to-image translation using cycle-consistent adversarial networks. 2017 IEEE International Conference on Computer Vision (ICCV) 2017.

57. Isola P, Zhu J-Y, Zhou T, et al. Image-to-Image translation with conditional adversarial networks. 2017 IEEE Conference on Computer vision and Pattern Recognition (CVPR) 2017.

58. Li W, Li Y, Qin W, et al. Magnetic resonance image (MRI) synthesis from brain computed tomography (CT) images based on deep learning methods for magnetic resonance (MR)-guided radiotherapy. Quant Imaging Med Surg 2020;10:1223–36.

59. Eley KA, Watt-Smith SR, Sheerin F, et al. "Black Bone" MRI: a potential alternative to CT with three-dimensional reconstruction of the craniofacial skeleton in the diagnosis of craniosynostosis. Eur Radiol 2014;24(10):2417–26.

60. Eley KA, Watt-Smith SR, Golding SJ. Three-dimensional reconstruction of the craniofacial skeleton

with gradient echo magnetic resonance imaging ("black bone"): what is currently possible? J Craniofac Surg 2017;28(2):463–7.

61. Lu A, Gorny KR, Ho ML. Zero TE MRI for craniofacial bone imaging. AJNR Am J Neuroradiol 2019;40(9): 1562–6.

62. Suchyta MA, Gibreel W, Hunt CH, et al. Using black bone magnetic resonance imaging in craniofacial virtual surgical planning: a comparative cadaver study. Plast Reconstr Surg 2018;141(6):1459–70.

63. Guo S, Zhuo J, Li G, et al. Feasibility of ultrashort echo time images using full-wave acoustic and thermal modeling for transcranial MRI-guided focused ultrasound (tcMRgFUS) planning. Phys Med Biol 2019;64(9):095008.

64. Caballero-Insaurriaga J, Rodríguez-Rojas R, Martínez-Fernández R, et al. Zero TE MRI applications to transcranial MR-guided focused ultrasound: patient screening and treatment efficiency estimation. J Magn Reson Imaging 2019;50(5):1583–92.

65. Kang Y, Hua C, Wu B, et al. Investigation of zero TE MR in preoperative planning in dentistry. Magn Reson Imaging 2018;54:77–83.

66. Weiger M, Pruessmann KP, Bracher AK, et al. High-resolution ZTE imaging of human teeth. NMR Biomed 2012;25(10):1144–51.

67. Hövener JB, Zwick S, Leupold J, et al. Dental MRI: imaging of soft and solid components without ionizing radiation. J Magn Reson Imaging 2012; 36(4):841–6.

68. Hilgenfeld T, Prager M, Heil A, et al. PETRA, MSVAT-SPACE and SEMAC sequences for metal artefact reduction in dental MR imaging. Eur Radiol 2017; 27(12):5104–12.

69. Dremmen MHG, Wagner MW, Bosemani T, et al. Does the addition of a "black bone" sequence to a fast multisequence trauma MR protocol allow MRI to replace CT after traumatic brain injury in children? AJNR Am J Neuroradiol 2017;38(11):2187–92.

70. Kralik SF, Supakul N, Wu IC, et al. Black bone MRI with 3D reconstruction for the detection of skull fractures in children with suspected abusive head trauma. Neuroradiology 2019;61(1):81–7.

71. Cho SB, Baek HJ, Ryu KH, et al. Clinical feasibility of Zero TE Skull MRI in patients with head trauma in comparison with CT: a single-center study. AJNR Am J Neuroradiol 2019;40(1):109–15.

Vessel Wall MR Imaging in the Pediatric Head and Neck

Mahmud Mossa-Basha, MD[a],*, Chengcheng Zhu, PhD[b], Lei Wu, MD[c]

KEYWORDS

- Vasculitis • MRI • Moyamoya • Vessel wall imaging • Pediatric vasculopathy

KEY POINTS

- Vessel wall MR imaging (VWI) can differentiate intracranial and extracranial vasculopathies better than conventional angiography with luminal imaging alone.
- VWI can detect inflammatory changes in large artery vasculitis earlier than luminal imaging, prompting earlier treatment and potentially preventing chronic steno-occlusive changes.
- VWI is more accurate in evaluating low-grade vascular injury than computed tomographic angiography and, as a second-line imaging tool, could reduce unnecessary therapy and additional workup.

INTRODUCTION

Vessel wall MR imaging (VWI) is an advanced MR imaging (MRI) application that has shown added clinical value in cerebrovascular disease. VWI has been applied to characterization of carotid atherosclerotic disease for more than 25 years,[1–4] but in more recent years, the application of extracranial VWI (EVWMR) has expanded to include traumatic cerebrovascular arterial injuries[5,6] and large artery vasculitis.[7] In addition, the technique can aid in differentiation,[8] characterization,[9–11] and detection[10–16] of intracranial vasculopathies. Although most studies to date have focused on adult vascular diseases, these techniques have shown promise in the evaluation of pediatric intracranial[17,18] and extracranial vasculopathies.[19] We present the existing literature on applications of VWI on pediatric intracranial and extracranial vasculopathies and technical considerations.

INTRACRANIAL VESSEL WALL MR IMAGING
Intracranial Vessel Wall Imaging Techniques

There are several technical considerations for intracranial VWI (IVWMR). First, intracranial arteries are small, tortuous structures with thin walls; the normal middle cerebral (MCA) artery wall measures 0.2 mm to 0.3 mm,[20] necessitating high resolution. Second, the vessel wall is surrounded by flowing blood and cerebrospinal fluid (CSF). Slow flow artifacts can mimic vessel wall pathology[21] and insufficient CSF suppression can mimic pathology. Blood suppression[21–23] and CSF suppression methods[24] are required to characterize the wall features reliably. Third, due to resolution requirements, scan times are long (7–10 minutes per sequence), and protocol times can be limiting. Lastly, due to the various vasculopathies to consider intracranially, multicontrast imaging (precontrast and postcontrast and T1/T2 weighting) is important. Therefore, implementation in a clinical

---

[a] Department of Radiology, University of Washington, 1959 NE Pacific Street, Seattle, WA 98195, USA;
[b] Department of Radiology, University of Washington, 325 9th Avenue, Seattle, WA 98104, USA;
[c] Department of Radiology, University of Washington, 1660 South Columbian Way, Seattle, WA 98108, USA
* Corresponding author.
E-mail address: mmossab@uw.edu

Magn Reson Imaging Clin N Am 29 (2021) 595–604
https://doi.org/10.1016/j.mric.2021.06.009
1064-9689/21/© 2021 Elsevier Inc. All rights reserved.

setting is challenging, especially for pediatric patients when anesthesia is required.

Although earlier studies used 2-dimensional (2-D) imaging methods, over the past decade 3-dimensional (3-D) IVWMR has become popular because of high isotropic resolution, large coverage, and high scan efficiency, leading to increased reliability/reproducibility, better pathology detection and characterization, and less reliance on the radiologist for image targeting. The most widely used 3-D sequence is turbo-spin-echo with variable refocusing flip angle train (VFA), termed Vista (Philips Healthcare; Best, the Netherlands), SPACE (Siemens Healthineers, Erlangen, Germany), or CUBE (GE Healthcare, Waukesha, Wisconsin). The variable flip angle train modulates the signal evaluation and allows a long echo train (up to 40–60) without significant image blurring,[25] whereas the traditional fast-spin-echo sequences often have an echo train of 10 to 20. The long echo train means acquiring more k-space lines per repetition time; therefore, the scanning efficiency is greatly improved. A 3-D IVWMR covering the whole brain with 0.5 mm to 0.6 mm isotropic resolution can be acquired within 7 to 10 minutes,[25] whereas 2-D IVWMR commonly has slice thickness of 2 mm with 0.4 to 0.5 mm in plane resolution that requires 36 to 45 seconds per slice.[8,9] The actual resolution of VFA sequences depends on the flip angle train design, which determines the point-spread function and image sharpness.[25] Due to the high resolution used in 3-D IVWMR, to achieve sufficient signal-to-noise, 3T is optimal.

A major consideration for 3-D IVWMR is blood and CSF suppression, considering volume acquisitions generate flow artifacts. The VFA train has inherent blood suppression effect due to intravoxel phase dispersion.[9] In cases of slow or turbulent flow, additional blood-suppression techniques, including motion-sensitized driven-equilibrium (MSDE)[23] and DANTE[24] can be used (Fig. 1). At 3T, anti–drive-equilibrium[26] can be applied to suppress CSF without increasing scan time, and can help limit CSF flow artifact.

Acceleration techniques, such as compressed sensing, have shown the ability to accelerate imaging without loss in image quality.[27] In IVWMR applications, compressed sensing[28] and wave-controlled aliasing in parallel imaging[29] can reduce scan times by 40% to 65% while maintaining comparable image quality with reference scans. Artificial intelligence applications, through using a reference standard, also can improve image quality from more accelerated acquisitions.[30] With further imaging acceleration, reduced anesthesia time for pediatric patients can be achieved and, with sufficient acceleration, potentially eliminate the need for anesthesia.

Intracranial Vasculopathies

In adult and pediatric inflammatory vasculopathies, IVWMR has shown promise in vasculopathy detection[8,31] and differentiation[32,33] relative to other vascular diseases. The development of new techniques for inflammatory vasculopathies are especially important considering the limitations of current angiographic techniques; digital subtraction angiography (DSA) has shown sensitivities that can be as low as 50%, and specificity in the range of 30% for inflammatory vasculopathies.[34–36] The limitations of luminal imaging, including DSA, lie in evaluation of inflammatory vasculopathies, differentiation between various vascular diseases, and detectability of small artery angiitis. IVWMR typically can depict small artery angiitis due to arterial wall inflammation spilling over and involving perivascular tissues, resulting in much more extensive inflammatory changes and enhancement, whereas luminal imaging cannot accurately depict the absence or irregularity of tiny perforator branches.[35,37]

Inflammatory vasculopathies are an important consideration in pediatric patients with strokes. Secondary central nervous system (CNS) vasculitis can develop in the setting of systemic vasculitis resulting from numerous diseases, including systemic lupus erythematosus, infectious, mitochondrial abnormalities, malignancies, radiation, and toxic/drug exposures.[38] Childhood primary angiitis of the CNS originally was considered a rare disease, representing 2% to 6% of all pediatric arteriopathies[39]; however, it has been shown to be an important cause for pediatric strokes.[40] Similar to adult primary angiitis, pediatric angiitis can affect medium or small arteries; however, the specificity of angiographic techniques for inflammatory vasculopathies for children likely is higher than for adults, due to the absence of atherosclerosis and reversible cerebral vasoconstriction syndrome in pediatric populations. Two disease entities, specifically post-varicella angiopathy and transient cerebral arteriopathy, however, do overlap in imaging appearances with vasculitis. In addition, angiographic techniques are limited in detecting small artery vasculitides, and these cases frequently require brain biopsy for diagnosis. IVWMR has the potential to limit the need for highly invasive biopsies in this subset of vasculitis.

Dlamini and colleagues[17] evaluated 26 pediatric patients with acute ischemic stroke and found that IVWMR appearances strongly correlated with

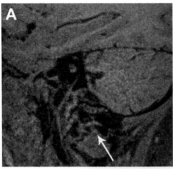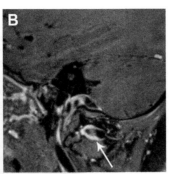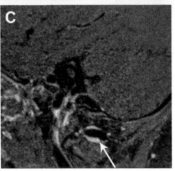

Fig. 1. (A) Accelerated sagittal T1-SPACE shows flow artifact (*arrow*) in the right V3 vertebral artifact. (B) Postcontrast T1-SPACE shows a similar flow artifact (*arrow*). (C) DANTE flow-suppressed T1-SPACE postcontrast shows suppression of the luminal flow artifact (*arrow*).

specific types of vasculopathies, including transient cerebral arteriopathy, primary angiitis, dissection, cardioembolic stroke, and dissecting aneurysm. 35% showed arterial wall enhancement, whereas 59% (10/17) of those that did not show enhancement had abnormal MR angiography (MRA) appearance including steno-occlusive (n = 8), dissection (n = 1), and pseudoaneurysm (n = 1) diagnoses.

The typical imaging appearance of an inflammatory vasculopathy, specifically primary or secondary angiitis of the CNS, is circumferential, homogeneous, intense arterial wall enhancement that may or may not be multifocal on T1-weighted postcontrast IVWMR (**Fig. 2**).[8] In pediatric patients, however, circumferential wall enhancement is not exclusive to inflammatory vasculopathies, because this also can be seen in the setting of subarachnoid hemorrhage or vasospasm.[41] Inclusion of T2-weighted imaging can help better differentiate vasculopathies; inflammatory vasculopathy typically has wall thickening that is isointense to gray matter, whereas vasospasm or subarachnoid hemorrhage-related wall changes typically show little to no wall thickening on T2-weighted imaging.[8,33,41]

Focal cerebral arteriopathy (FCA) is a vasculopathy involving 1 side of the anterior circulation or a single large intracranial anterior circulation artery and is a frequent cause of pediatric stroke.[42]

FCA can further be classified into (1) inflammatory, (2) posttraumatic dissection, and (3) subtypes not otherwise specified. In the evaluation of 16 patients with FCA, Stence and colleagues[18] found that strong arterial wall enhancement was significantly associated with progressive arteriopathy (P = .008). In the assessment of 9 inflammatory FCA patients, Perez and colleagues[42] found that there was no correlation between the presence of arterial wall enhancement and infarct size, outcomes, and arteriopathy severity. These studies are limited by small sample sizes, and further investigation is necessary.

IVWMR also has been applied to sickle cell disease (SCD).[43] In the evaluation of 69 adult and pediatric SCD patients, arterial walls were significantly thicker than normal controls (n = 38) (1.07 mm ± 0.19 mm vs 0.97 mm ± .07 mm, respectively; $P<.001$), and wall thickness was higher in SCD patients receiving chronic transfusions (P = .013). There also was a trend ($P<.1$) for wall thickness correlating with decreasing hematocrit and increasing circulating white cells.

Brain Aneurysms

There has been extensive investigation evaluating the value of IVWMR in intracranial aneurysms. Studies have shown that aneurysmal wall

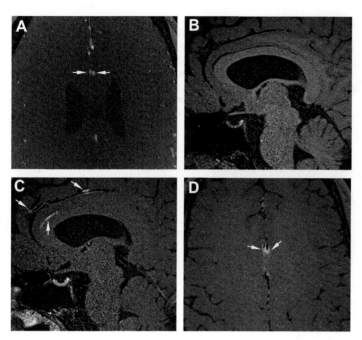

Fig. 2. An 18-year-old with history of Henoch -Schönlein purpura and cerebral vasculitis presenting with vision changes, paresthesias, and dysphasia. (*A*) Axial contrast-enhanced MRA shows mild bilateral ACA luminal narrowing with enhancing perivascular halo (*arrows*). (*B*) Sagittal precontrast, (*C*) sagittal postcontrast, and (*D*) axial postcontrast T1-SPACE show multifocal bilateral ACA wall enhancement (*arrows*), representing recurrent vasculitis.

enhancement correlates with inflammation in the aneurysm wall on histology.[44] Aneurysm wall enhancement also has shown significant association with increased scores of aneurysm vulnerability[45] and subsequent aneurysm growth.[46] Aneurysm wall enhancement and quantitative intensity of enhancement are associated with symptomatic aneurysms.[47] In an evaluation of 341 unruptured intracranial aneurysms with IVWMR, 93 of which were symptomatic, symptomatic aneurysms more frequently showed circumferential wall enhancement (66.7% vs 17.3%; $P<.001$) and quantitative wall enhancement ($P<.001$), and both were independent factors associated with symptoms. The combined wall imaging characteristics had a sensitivity of 95.7% and specificity of 73.4% for symptomatic aneurysms. Wall enhancement also is seen with pseudoaneurysms and dissecting pseudoaneurysms, likely secondary to wall inflammatory changes.[48] The wall enhancement can extend beyond the region of luminal abnormality, likely indicating further extent of wall injury.[49]

In patients with aneurysmal SAH, an increased likelihood of IVWMR wall enhancement relative to those without aneurysm rupture (29.9% vs 7.2%, respectively; odds ratio [OR] 5.5; 95% CI, 2.2–13.7) has been shown and a strong ability to predict subsequent vasospasm development when controlling for grade of hemorrhage (OR 3.9; 95% CI, 1.7–9.4).[41]

Moyamoya Vasculopathy

Moyamoya vasculopathy represents heterogeneous disease processes that lead to steno-occlusive changes involving the carotid terminus, proximal M1 middle cerebral artery (MCA), and/or proximal A1 anterior cerebral artery (ACA). Moyamoya disease (MMD) represents an idiopathic steno-occlusive process, though genetic predisposition has been indicated.[50] This is supported by the fact that the proportion of patients with afflicted first-degree relatives in Japan is 10% and in the United States 6%.[51] MMD develops bilaterally and has bimodal distribution, with peaks at 5 years and 40 years old, representing the most common cerebrovascular disease in Japanese children (3 per 100,000).[51] Moyamoya syndrome (MMS) develops secondarily in neurofibromatosis type 1, Down syndrome, SCD, radiation, and other disorders[51] and is more likely to appear unilaterally.

IVWMR has been able to better characterize MMD than luminal techniques. IVWMR improved the diagnostic accuracy of differentiating MMD from inflammatory MMS compared with luminal imaging alone, with accuracy improvement from 31.6% to 86.8% ($P<.001$).[32] MMD typically shows minimal or no wall postcontrast T1-weighted enhancement and no wall thickening. This differs from inflammatory MMS, which shows circumferential intense wall enhancement and wall thickening. This MMD does show wall enhancement,

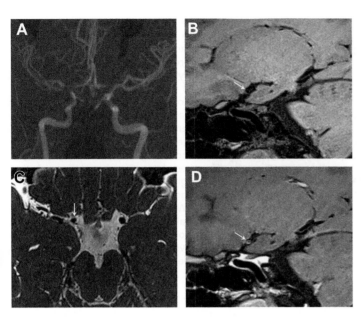

Fig. 3. A 17-year-old woman with history of polycystic kidney disease and progressive headaches. (*A*) On maximum intensity projection MRA, there is right greater than left steno-occlusive disease affecting the carotid termini, proximal ACA, and proximal MCA. (*B*) On sagittal T1-SPACE precontrast and (*D*) postcontrast images, there is mild circumferential wall enhancement of the right carotid terminus just proximal to the occlusion (*arrows on B and D*). (*C*) Axial T2-SPACE shows no wall thickening of the affected segment (*arrow*), supporting the diagnosis of MMD.

there is no wall thickening on T2-SPACE (**Fig. 3**), whereas inflammatory MMS shows wall thickening.

EXTRACRANIAL VESSEL WALL MR IMAGING
Extracranial Vessel Wall Imaging Techniques

Extracranial arteries—specifically the extracranial carotid arteries, origins of the great arteries and aorta—are large structures that generally have a straight course, making EVWMR less challenging than IVWMR. EVWMR initially relied on 2-D techniques; however, these techniques are limited for pathology characterization and detection due to thicker slices and limited coverage, especially when imaging the aorta or the length of the carotid arteries. During the past decade, clinical and research practice has moved toward 3-D EVWMR, which provides higher resolution, extended coverage, and shorter scan times.[52,53] These techniques use VFA or gradient-echo sequences for image acquisition with MSDE or DANTE preparation pulses to improve blood suppression. These techniques can achieve high spatial resolution (0.6 mm^3) in 2 to 4-minute scan times.

Acceleration techniques, such as compressed sensing[54] and motion correction methods,[55] have been implemented as well to reduce the scan time and reduce the impact of patient motion. These applications may prove useful for pediatrics, due to the need for fast, motion-resistant imaging.

Because the carotid bifurcation is close to the skin, the use of dedicated surface coils can improve image quality significantly; however, this can create barriers to wider use in clinical settings due to limited availability. A recent study demonstrated that 3-D EVWMR using standard neurovascular coils achieved good agreement with EVWMR using carotid coils for carotid plaque evaluation.[56] Further optimization of EVWMR protocols for standard neurovascular coils may improve clinical adoption.

Large Artery Inflammatory Vasculopathies

Vasculitides are a group of conditions characterized by inflammation of arterial walls, commonly classified by the size of the affected vessels. Imaging is most helpful for large vessel vasculitis, with Takayasu arteritis (TA) the most frequently encountered in children. Due to the nonspecific clinical presentation of large vessel vasculitis in early disease and the lack of specific laboratory tests for diagnosis, diagnosis can be delayed by 10 to 15.5 months in pediatric patients, which may lead to secondary organ damage before treatment can be started.[57] Imaging increasingly has been used to facilitate earlier diagnosis because of this. Traditionally, luminal imaging, such as CT angiography (CTA) and DSA, has been used predominantly for evaluation of vessel stenosis or occlusion. With the advent of VWI, however, there has been a progressive paradigm shift from luminal imaging to EVWMR for detection of vessel wall inflammation.[49,58,59] EVWMR is

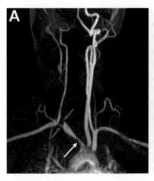
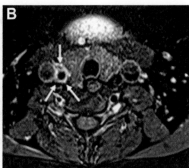

Fig. 4. An 18-year-old woman with TA who presented with elevated inflammatory markers, including C-reactive protein of 67 mg/L and erythrocyte sedimentation rate of 31 mm/h, raising concern for disease recurrence. (A) Contrast-enhanced maximum intensity projection MRA demonstrated significant stenosis of the innominate artery (*white arrow*) and the right subclavian artery origin (*red arrow*), and occlusion of the right common carotid artery at its origin (*blue arrow*). (B) On axial VWI, there is circumferential thick wall enhancement of the right common carotid artery (*arrows*), with involvement of the other proximal great arteries (not shown).

advantageous particularly in the pediatric population, due to avoidance of ionizing radiation. Furthermore, EVWMR may be more sensitive in early disease before any significant luminal narrowing develops,[58] when wall changes may still be reversible. Once stenosis or occlusion is detected on luminal imaging, vascular changes are irreversible due to fibrosis and scarring in the arterial wall. Large artery vasculitis frequently shows circumferential artery wall enhancement, wall thickening (**Fig. 4**), and T2-signal abnormality on EVWMR. In addition to earlier diagnosis, EVWMR also can be used for disease activity monitoring when the acute-phase markers are normal because luminal imaging does not track disease activity well, whether or not fixed stenoses have developed[60] (**Fig. 5**).

TA is the third most common vasculitis and the most common large vessel vasculitis in pediatric populations, although it is rare in children younger than 16 years.[61] TA is more common in female patients and Asian populations. The disease classically involves the aorta and its major branches (see **Fig. 4**). Chronic inflammation of the vessel wall may lead to stenosis and rarely thrombosis and aneurysm if left untreated.

As the availability and familiarity with VWI continue to increase, its impact on diagnosis and management of large vessel vasculitis also likely will increase. Specifically, EVWMR may facilitate earlier diagnosis, which could help prevent end organ damage and provide more accurate assessment of disease activity, which could allow for better titration of medications or even discontinuation of medication in quiescent disease. Finally, lack of ionizing radiation makes VWI particularly advantageous in the pediatric population.

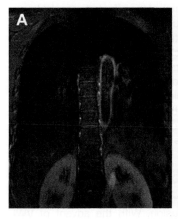
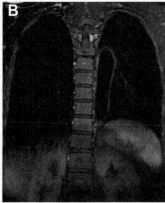

Fig. 5. A 19-year-old woman 1 year after onset of generalized fatigue and extremity pain. She initially was diagnosed with late onset Still disease. (A) On coronal postcontrast VWI, there was circumferential enhancement and wall thickening of the aortic arch and descending thoracic aorta, more than expected for age and presumed to represent large artery vasculitis. Immunomodulation therapy was initiated, which led to improvement in some symptoms. (B) On follow-up VWI 2 years later, enhancement and wall thickening decreased, coinciding with improved symptoms and laboratory values.

Craniocervical Dissections

Craniocervical artery dissection (CAD) can occur either spontaneously or as a result of nonpenetrating trauma, known as blunt cerebrovascular injury (BCVI). Both etiologies are relatively rare, with 2.6 per 100,000 incidence of spontaneous CAD and 0.33% incidence of BCVI in pediatric patients after blunt trauma.[5,62] Nevertheless, these are clinically significant due to the risk of stroke if untreated.[63,64] Spontaneous CAD is increasingly recognized as a leading cause of stroke, particularly in young patients, accounting for up to 20% of cases.[5] The risk of BCVI-related stroke in children is 37.4%, with a mortality risk of 12.7%.[62]

On VWI, intramural hematoma is seen in 87% to 100% and eccentric wall enhancement in 67% of dissection cases.[49] Intramural hematoma signal intensity depends on the age of injury, with most showing bright T1-weighted signal, typically in the subacute phase. Enhancement likely is secondary to inflammation, nonflowing blood, and/or vasa vasorum injury.

Although CTA largely has supplanted DSA for diagnosis due to availability, cost, and noninvasiveness, detection of low-grade injuries can be challenging on CTA. In 1 series, 10% of carotid and 20% of vertebral artery injuries were overlooked on CTA, all of which were low grade.[65] EVWMR may be more accurate compared with CTA because of its ability to demonstrate not only luminal irregularity but also associated intramural hematomas (**Fig. 6**). Interobserver agreement in low-grade injuries on CTA can be suboptimal, with kappa values ranging from 0.35 to 0.52.[66] In contrast, EVWMR has been shown to be more accurate in identifying and grading BCVI compared with CTA, particularly in low-grade injuries.[6] Furthermore, the false-positive rate of EVWMR is lower compared with CTA (0.03 vs 0.35) because subtle vessel contour irregularity representing artifact or vasospasm is less likely to be misclassified as BCVI (**Fig. 7**). Given the risk of hemorrhagic events associated with antithrombotic therapy — the mainstay of treatment of CAD — EVWMR can be helpful in confirming arterial dissection before initiating such therapy in equivocal cases, particularly in patients at higher risk for intracranial or systemic hemorrhage. This approach can reduce the number of costly hospital admissions, follow-up patient visits, and serial imaging studies. Finally, intraluminal contrast enhancement on EVWMR is associated with acute ischemic strokes in patients with CAD. Therefore, EVWMR may be useful in identifying and stratifying patients at higher risk of stroke during the latent period.

CONCLUSION

VWI has the potential to improve diagnostic accuracy for pediatric vasculopathies, in both intracranial and extracranial vascular beds, specifically as it relates to detection of arterial wall inflammation and differentiation of arterial diseases. Ongoing work determining the impact of VWI and its ability to predict outcomes and stroke events is needed to better establish the role of VWI in clinical diagnostic algorithms.

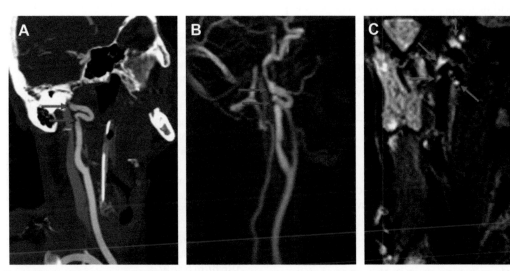

Fig. 6. Right cervical internal carotid artery (ICA) BCVI after motor vehicle accident. Right cervical ICA pseudoaneurysm and dissection (*arrows*) on (*A*) maximum intensity projection CTA and (*B*) maximum intensity projection MRA. (*C*) T1-SPACE demonstrates associated intramural hematomas (*arrows*).

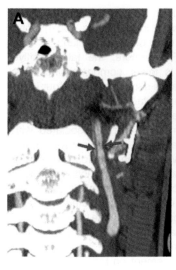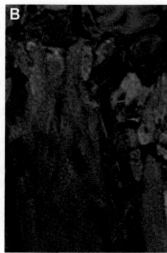

Fig. 7. Status post 25-m fall. (*A*) Coronal CTA was interpreted as a Denver grade 1 injury of the left cervical internal carotid artery due to subtle luminal irregularity (*arrows*). (*B*) Subsequent T1-SPACE demonstrates no abnormality (*arrows*) in the questioned segment, ruling out injury. In retrospect, the luminal irregularity was due to streak artifact from adjacent mandibular metallic hardware.

CLINICS CARE POINTS

- Inflammatory vasculopathy typically shows circumferential, intense, homogeneous arterial wall lesion enhancement on T1 postcontrast, and iso-intense wall thickening relative to grey matter on T2-weighted imaging.

- Moyamoya disease shows minimal to no enhancement and no appreciable wall thickening.

- Vasospastic processes typically show no wall thickening or enhancement.

- Use of flow suppression techniques can be advantageous to avoid flow artifacts that can mimic wall pathology.

- Depending on the stage of hemorrhage evolution, there can be variable appearances of arterial dissections. In the subacute phase, there is typically T1-weighted hyperintensity that may or may not enhance.

DISCLOSURES

Dr Mossa-Basha has received funding from NIH R01NS092207. Drs Zhu and Wu have no financial disclosures related to this work.

REFERENCES

1. de Havenon A, Tirschwell D, Majersik JJ, et al. Carotid intraplaque hemorrhage on vessel wall MRI does not correlate with TCD emboli monitoring in patients with recently symptomatic carotid atherosclerosis. Neuroradiol J 2017;30(5):486–9.

2. Mossa-Basha M, Wasserman BA. Low-grade carotid stenosis: implications of MR imaging. Neuroimaging Clin N Am 2016;26(1):129–45.

3. Saba L, Mossa-Basha M, Abbott A, et al. Multinational survey of current practice from imaging to treatment of atherosclerotic carotid stenosis. Cerebrovasc Dis 2021;1–13.

4. Saba L, Yuan C, Hatsukami TS, et al. Carotid artery wall imaging: perspective and guidelines from the ASNR vessel wall imaging study group and expert consensus recommendations of the American Society of Neuroradiology. AJNR Am J Neuroradiol 2018; 39(2):E9–31.

5. Rutman AM, Vranic JE, Mossa-Basha M. Imaging and management of blunt cerebrovascular injury. Radiographics 2018;38(2):542–63.

6. Vranic JE, Huynh TJ, Fata P, et al. The ability of magnetic resonance black blood vessel wall imaging to evaluate blunt cerebrovascular injury following acute trauma. J Neuroradiol 2020;47(3):210–5.

7. Bley TA, Uhl M, Carew J, et al. Diagnostic value of high-resolution MR imaging in giant cell arteritis. AJNR Am J Neuroradiol 2007;28(9):1722–7.

8. Mossa-Basha M, Hwang WD, De Havenon A, et al. Multicontrast high-resolution vessel wall magnetic resonance imaging and its value in differentiating intracranial vasculopathic processes. Stroke 2015; 46(6):1567–73.

9. Alexander MD, Yuan C, Rutman A, et al. High-resolution intracranial vessel wall imaging: imaging beyond the lumen. J Neurol Neurosurg Psychiatry 2016;87(6):589–97.

10. de Havenon A, Mossa-Basha M, Shah L, et al. High-resolution vessel wall MRI for the evaluation of

intracranial atherosclerotic disease. Neuroradiology 2017;59(12):1193–202.

11. Mossa-Basha M, Alexander M, Gaddikeri S, et al. Vessel wall imaging for intracranial vascular disease evaluation. J Neurointerv Surg 2016;8(11):1154–9.

12. Brinjikji W, Mossa-Basha M, Huston J, et al. Intracranial vessel wall imaging for evaluation of steno-occlusive diseases and intracranial aneurysms. J Neuroradiol 2017;44(2):123–34.

13. de Havenon A, Yuan C, Tirschwell D, et al. Nonstenotic culprit plaque: the utility of high-resolution vessel wall MRI of intracranial vessels after ischemic stroke. Case Rep Radiol 2015;2015:356582.

14. Mossa-Basha M, Watase H, Sun J, et al. Inter-rater and scan-rescan reproducibility of the detection of intracranial atherosclerosis on contrast-enhanced 3D vessel wall MRI. Br J Radiol 2019;92(1097):20180973.

15. Sarikaya B, Colip C, Hwang WD, et al. Comparison of time-of-flight MR angiography and intracranial vessel wall MRI for luminal measurements relative to CT angiography. Br J Radiol 2021;94(1118):20200743.

16. Tian X, Tian B, Shi Z, et al. Assessment of intracranial atherosclerotic plaques using 3D black-blood MRI: Comparison with 3D time-of-flight MRA and DSA. J Magn Reson Imaging 2021;53(2):469–78.

17. Dlamini N, Yau I, Muthusami P, et al. Arterial wall imaging in pediatric stroke. Stroke 2018;49(4):891–8.

18. Stence NV, Pabst LL, Hollatz AL, et al. Predicting progression of intracranial arteriopathies in childhood stroke with vessel wall imaging. Stroke 2017;48(8):2274–7.

19. Mossa-Basha M, Alexander M, Maki J, et al. Exploring Other Vascular Dimensions: Comparison of 3-Dimensional and 2-Dimensional Vessel Wall Imaging Techniques for the Assessment of Large Artery Vasculopathies. In: Paper presented at: 24th Annual International Society of Magnetic Resonance in Medicine Meeting; May 7-13, 2016. 2016. Singapore.

20. Jain KK. Some observations on the anatomy of the middle cerebral artery. Can J Surg 1964;7:134–9.

21. Kalsoum E, Chabernaud Negrier A, Tuilier T, et al. Blood flow mimicking aneurysmal wall enhancement: A diagnostic pitfall of vessel wall MRI using the postcontrast 3D turbo spin-echo MR imaging sequence. AJNR Am J Neuroradiol 2018;39(6):1065–7.

22. Balu N, Zhou Z, Hippe DS, et al. Accelerated multi-contrast high isotropic resolution 3D intracranial vessel wall MRI using a tailored k-space undersampling and partially parallel reconstruction strategy. Magma 2019;32(3):343–57.

23. Zhu C, Graves MJ, Yuan J, et al. Optimization of improved motion-sensitized driven-equilibrium (iMSDE) blood suppression for carotid artery wall imaging. J Cardiovasc Magn Reson 2014;16(1):61.

24. Wang J, Helle M, Zhou Z, et al. Joint blood and cerebrospinal fluid suppression for intracranial vessel wall MRI. Magn Reson Med 2016;75(2):831–8.

25. Zhu C, Haraldsson H, Tian B, et al. High resolution imaging of the intracranial vessel wall at 3 and 7 T using 3D fast spin echo MRI. Magma 2016;29(3):559–70.

26. Yang H, Zhang X, Qin Q, et al. Improved cerebrospinal fluid suppression for intracranial vessel wall MRI. J Magn Reson Imaging 2016;44(3):665–72.

27. Vranic JE, Cross NM, Wang Y, et al. Compressed sensing-sensitivity encoding (CS-SENSE) accelerated brain imaging: Reduced scan time without reduced image quality. AJNR Am J Neuroradiol 2019;40(1):92–8.

28. Zhu C, Tian B, Chen L, et al. Accelerated whole brain intracranial vessel wall imaging using black blood fast spin echo with compressed sensing (CS-SPACE). Magma 2018;31(3):457–67.

29. Conklin J, Longo MGF, Cauley SF, et al. Validation of highly accelerated wave-CAIPI SWI compared with conventional SWI and T2*-weighted gradient recalled-echo for routine clinical brain MRI at 3T. AJNR Am J Neuroradiol 2019;40(12):2073–80.

30. Mardani M, Gong E, Cheng JY, et al. Deep generative adversarial neural networks for compressive sensing MRI. IEEE Trans Med Imaging 2019;38(1):167–79.

31. de Havenon ACL, Park M, Mossa-Basha M. Intracranial vessel wall MRI: a review of current indications and future applications. Neurovascular Imaging 2016;2(10).

32. Mossa-Basha M, de Havenon A, Becker KJ, et al. Added value of vessel wall magnetic resonance imaging in the differentiation of moyamoya vasculopathies in a non-asian cohort. Stroke 2016;47(7):1782–8.

33. Mossa-Basha M, Shibata DK, Hallam DK, et al. Added value of vessel wall magnetic resonance imaging for differentiation of nonocclusive intracranial vasculopathies. Stroke 2017;48(11):3026–33.

34. Birnbaum J, Hellmann DB. Primary angiitis of the central nervous system. Arch Neurol 2009;66(6):704–9.

35. Hajj-Ali RA, Singhal AB, Benseler S, et al. Primary angiitis of the CNS. Lancet Neurol 2011;10(6):561–72.

36. MacLaren K, Gillespie J, Shrestha S, et al. Primary angiitis of the central nervous system: emerging variants. QJM 2005;98(9):643–54.

37. Campi A, Benndorf G, Filippi M, et al. Primary angiitis of the central nervous system: serial MRI of brain and spinal cord. Neuroradiology 2001;43(8):599–607.

38. Elbers J, Benseler SM. Central nervous system vasculitis in children. Curr Opin Rheumatol 2008; 20(1):47–54.

39. Friedman NR. Small vessel childhood primary angiitis of the CNS: first steps toward a standardised treatment regimen. Lancet Neurol 2010;9(11): 1042–4.

40. Benseler S, Schneider R. Central nervous system vasculitis in children. Curr Opin Rheumatol 2004; 16(1):43–50.

41. Mossa-Basha M, Huynh TJ, Hippe DS, et al. Vessel wall MRI characteristics of endovascularly treated aneurysms: association with angiographic vasospasm. J Neurosurg 2018;131(3):859–67.

42. Perez FA, Oesch G, Amlie-Lefond CM. MRI vessel wall enhancement and other imaging biomarkers in pediatric focal cerebral arteriopathy-inflammatory subtype. Stroke 2020;51(3):853–9.

43. Yuan S, Jordan LC, Davis LT, et al. A cross-sectional, case-control study of intracranial arterial wall thickness and complete blood count measures in sickle cell disease. Br J Haematol 2021;192(4):769–77.

44. Shimonaga K, Matsushige T, Ishii D, et al. Clinicopathological insights from vessel wall imaging of unruptured intracranial aneurysms. Stroke 2018; 49(10):2516–9.

45. Hartman JB, Watase H, Sun J, et al. Intracranial aneurysms at higher clinical risk for rupture demonstrate increased wall enhancement and thinning on multicontrast 3D vessel wall MRI. Br J Radiol 2019; 92(1096):20180950.

46. Gariel F, Ben Hassen W, Boulouis G, et al. Increased wall enhancement during follow-up as a predictor of subsequent aneurysmal growth. Stroke 2020;51(6): 1868–72.

47. Fu Q, Wang Y, Zhang Y, et al. Qualitative and quantitative wall enhancement on magnetic resonance imaging is associated with symptoms of unruptured intracranial aneurysms. Stroke 2021;52(1):213–22.

48. Lehman VT, Brinjikji W, Mossa-Basha M, et al. Conventional and high-resolution vessel wall MRI of intracranial aneurysms: current concepts and new horizons. J Neurosurg 2018;128(4):969–81.

49. Young CC, Bonow RH, Barros G, et al. Magnetic resonance vessel wall imaging in cerebrovascular diseases. Neurosurg Focus 2019;47(6):E4.

50. Akagawa H, Mukawa M, Nariai T, et al. Novel and recurrent RNF213 variants in Japanese pediatric patients with moyamoya disease. Hum Genome Var 2018;5:17060.

51. Scott RM, Smith ER. Moyamoya disease and moyamoya syndrome. N Engl J Med 2009;360(12): 1226–37.

52. Balu N, Yarnykh VL, Chu B, et al. Carotid plaque assessment using fast 3D isotropic resolution black-blood MRI. Magn Reson Med 2011;65(3): 627–37.

53. Zhu C, Sadat U, Patterson AJ, et al. 3D high-resolution contrast enhanced MRI of carotid atheroma–a technical update. Magn Reson Imaging 2014;32(5):594–7.

54. Jia S, Zhang L, Ren L, et al. Joint intracranial and carotid vessel wall imaging in 5 minutes using compressed sensing accelerated DANTE-SPACE. Eur Radiol 2020;30(1):119–27.

55. Dyverfeldt P, Deshpande VS, Kober T, et al. Reduction of motion artifacts in carotid MRI using free-induction decay navigators. J Magn Reson Imaging 2014;40(1):214–20.

56. Brinjikji W, DeMarco JK, Shih R, et al. Diagnostic accuracy of a clinical carotid plaque MR protocol using a neurovascular coil compared to a surface coil protocol. J Magn Reson Imaging 2018;48(5):1264–72.

57. Abularrage CJ, Slidell MB, Sidawy AN, et al. Quality of life of patients with Takayasu's arteritis. J Vasc Surg 2008;47(1):131–6. discussion 136-137.

58. Choe YH, Han BK, Koh EM, et al. Takayasu's arteritis: assessment of disease activity with contrast-enhanced MR imaging. AJR Am J Roentgenol 2000;175(2):505–11.

59. Mandell DM, Mossa-Basha M, Qiao Y, et al. Intracranial vessel wall MRI: Principles and expert consensus recommendations of the American Society of Neuroradiology. AJNR Am J Neuroradiol 2017; 38(2):218–29.

60. Sun Y, Ma L, Ji Z, et al. Value of whole-body contrast-enhanced magnetic resonance angiography with vessel wall imaging in quantitative assessment of disease activity and follow-up examination in Takayasu's arteritis. Clin Rheumatol 2016; 35(3):685–93.

61. Soliman M, Laxer R, Manson D, et al. Imaging of systemic vasculitis in childhood. Pediatr Radiol 2015;45(8):1110–25.

62. Harris DA, Sorte DE, Lam SK, et al. Blunt cerebrovascular injury in pediatric trauma: a national database study. J Neurosurg Pediatr 2019;1–10.

63. Bonow RH, Witt CE, Mosher BP, et al. Transcranial doppler microemboli monitoring for stroke risk stratification in blunt cerebrovascular injury. Crit Care Med 2017;45(10):e1011–7.

64. Wu L, Christensen D, Call L, et al. Natural history of blunt cerebrovascular injury: experience over a 10-year period at a level I trauma center. Radiology 2020;297(2):428–35.

65. Bub LD, Hollingworth W, Jarvik JG, et al. Screening for blunt cerebrovascular injury: evaluating the accuracy of multidetector computed tomographic angiography. J Trauma 2005;59(3):691–7.

66. Roberts DJ, Chaubey VP, Zygun DA, et al. Diagnostic accuracy of computed tomographic angiography for blunt cerebrovascular injury detection in trauma patients: a systematic review and meta-analysis. Ann Surg 2013;257(4):621–32.

Magnetic Resonance Fingerprinting of the Pediatric Brain

Sheng-Che Hung, MD, PhD[a,b], Yong Chen, PhD[c], Pew-Thian Yap, PhD[a,b], Weili Lin, PhD[a,b],*

KEYWORDS

- Quantitative MR imaging • Adolescent • Pediatric • MR imaging • Brain
- Magnetic resonance fingerprinting (MRF)

KEY POINTS

- Magnetic resonance fingerprinting (MRF) is a new quantitative MR imaging technique for rapid and simultaneous quantification of multiple tissue properties.
- MRF can reliably and accurately characterize intrinsic tissue properties, such as T1 and T2 relaxation times.
- MRF has many potential applications in children, including evaluation of brain development and differentiation of normal from pathologic tissues.

INTRODUCTION

With continuing advancements of MR imaging technologies, quantitative imaging approaches have gained substantial traction in both clinical and research applications. For example, diffusion-weighted imaging, perfusion-weighted imaging, functional MR imaging, and MR have already been widely used to provide great insights into normal brain development and various neurologic disorders in children.[1–4] Quantitative imaging approaches yield findings that are objective and potentially more reproducible when system-related biases are controlled. Despite these potential advantages, qualitative T1-weighted and T2-weighted images remain the most widely used MR images in clinical practice, and clinical interpretations/diagnoses largely rely on qualitative or semiquantitative visual assessments. T1 and T2 relaxation times are fundamental MR imaging–specific properties that are governed by intrinsic tissue composition, microenvironment, temperature, and magnetic field strength. Compared with conventional MR imaging, directly measuring T1 and T2 relaxation times can potentially provide more quantitative and objective assessments of tissue characteristics and pathologic processes.[5,6] However, technical limitations—particularly long acquisition time—make these approaches more vulnerable to motion and prone to system-related instabilities, hampering their wide clinical adoption.

MR fingerprinting (MRF) is a novel imaging framework using fundamentally different data acquisition and postprocessing schemes from those of conventional MR imaging relaxometry approaches. In brief, traditional relaxometry methods acquire multiple datasets where one imaging parameter, such as flip angle (FA), repetition time (TR), and echo time (TE) is varied for each dataset depending on the MR intrinsic parameter of interest.

Sheng-Che Hung and Yong Chen contributed equally.

[a] Department of Radiology, School of Medicine, University of North Carolina at Chapel Hill, 2006 Old Clinic, CB#7510, 101 Manning Dr, Chapel Hill, NC 27599, USA; [b] Biomedical Research Imaging Center, School of Medicine, University of North Carolina at Chapel Hill, 125 Mason Farm Road, Marsico Hall, suite 1200, Chapel Hill, NC 27599, USA; [c] Department of Radiology, Case Western Reserve University, 10900 Euclid Avenue, Cleveland, OH 44106, USA

* Corresponding author. Department of Radiology and Biomedical Research Imaging Center, University of North Carolina at Chapel Hill, CB#7513, Chapel Hill, NC 27599.
E-mail address: weili_lin@med.unc.edu

Magn Reson Imaging Clin N Am 29 (2021) 605–616
https://doi.org/10.1016/j.mric.2021.06.010
1064-9689/21/© 2021 Elsevier Inc. All rights reserved.

Subsequently, all datasets are combined to derive either proton density, T1 or T2, respectively. There are several limitations associated with these conventional approaches. First, the total data acquisition time can be long because multiple datasets are needed. Second, because all of the acquired datasets are used to compute tissue parameters, subject motion between scans could lead to inaccurate results. Finally, system-related biases such as field inhomogeneities, could further affect the accuracy of the estimated tissue properties. In contrast, MRF uses a set of pseudo-randomized acquisition parameters including FA, TR, and TE, in a single scan, to generate unique signal evolutions depending on specific tissue parameters. Subsequently, tissue properties can be estimated using a template-matching method by comparing the experimentally acquired signal evolutions with a preestablished dictionary voxel-by-voxel.[7] This approach allows for reliable and accelerated parallel quantitative measurements of multiple tissue properties using highly undersampled data.[7–9] In the following sections, we introduce the technical background and the novel applications of machine learning (ML) to accelerate MRF and review the clinical applications of MRF in pediatric neuroimaging.

TECHNICAL BACKGROUND
Overview of Basic Concepts

In this section, we first provide an overview of data acquisition and postprocessing methods of the MRF technique.

Data acquisition

MRF has been implemented based on several types of MR pulse sequences.[10–14] In this section, we review different MRF sequences, imaging parameters, and 2-dimensional (2D) versus 3D acquisition.

The first MRF acquisition approach pioneered by Case Western Reserve University was based on an inversion-recovery balanced steady-state free precession (IR-bSSFP) sequence.[7] The main reasons that IR-bSSFP was originally chosen include its high signal-to-noise efficiency and sensitivity to multiple important tissue parameters, including T1, T2, proton density (M0), and off-resonance frequency. However, the presence of magnetic field inhomogeneities represents a major concern for bSSFP sequences, which could potentially introduce banding artifacts in the acquired tissue property maps. The fast imaging with steady-state free precession (FISP) sequence is also a part of the SSFP family and has been previously used for rapid quantification of water diffusion and magnetic transfer.[15,16] Compared with the bSSFP sequences, FISP is less sensitive to magnetic field

inhomogeneities and immune to banding artifacts at a cost of reduced signal-to-noise ratio. Recently, significant effort has been made to develop FISP-based MRF techniques with great success of applying them in brain, abdomen, cardiac, and pediatric applications.[10,17–21] Finally, the MRF framework enables the combination of different types of pulse sequences in a single acquisition to extract multiple tissue properties of interest.[12,22]

Because hundreds to thousands of MRF signals are needed in order to achieve accurate estimates of tissue properties, it is imperative to use acquisition approaches capable of acquiring images in a clinically acceptable time. To this end, the highly undersampled spiral approach has been used where one spiral interleaf is acquired for one MRF time frame, yielding highly aliased images (**Fig. 1**).[7] Although other k-space sampling schemes such as Cartesian, radial, echo planar imaging, and rosette trajectories have also been implemented in the MRF framework,[21,23–26] we focus on spiral trajectory approaches because they provide high scan efficiency and are widely used.

Significant progress has also been made to translate the 2D MRF originally proposed by Ma and colleagues[7] to 3D techniques capable of providing volumetric quantitative imaging.[13,17,27,28] With the addition of a linear slice-encoding gradient, 3D MRF data are typically acquired sequentially through the partition encoding direction. The same acquisition parameters, such as FA pattern and in-plane spiral readouts, are repeated for each partition, and a constant waiting time is applied between partitions for longitudinal magnetization recovery. With the extra encoding dimension, fast imaging approaches have been explored to further accelerate along the partition encoding direction. For example, Ma and colleagues[13] proposed an interleaved sampling pattern to uniformly undersample data along the slice-encoding direction (**Fig. 2**). Although this approach creates incoherent artifacts, these artifacts can be mitigated using a pattern matching algorithm. Whole-brain coverage (~ 14 cm volume) with a spatial resolution of $1.2 \times 1.2 \times 3$ mm^3 in less than 5 minutes can be achieved. Nevertheless, the achieved spatial resolution may not be sufficient for clinical applications, particularly for pediatric subjects.

Tissue quantification using pattern matching

One major feature of the MRF technique is the use of pattern matching to extract tissue properties (see **Fig. 1**). Conventional MR acquisition approaches, where a fixed and identical set of imaging parameters is used for each k-space line, yield identical magnetization evolution time courses for the entirety of k-space. In contrast, MRF uses a

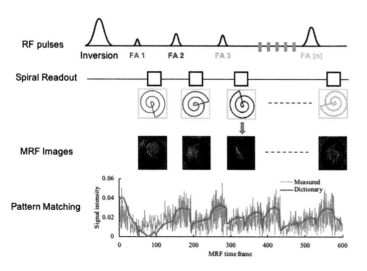

Fig. 1. MRF data acquisition and pattern matching. Pseudorandomized acquisition parameters, including flip angles and TRs, are used in the acquisition, and each MRF image is highly undersampled and aliased. The tissue properties for each pixel are then extracted by matching the corresponding MRF signal evolution to a predefined dictionary.

pseudorandomized acquisition approach to generate incoherent magnetization time courses, such that magnetization evolution time courses oscillate in a manner defined by variable acquisition parameters and unique tissue properties. An MRF dictionary consists of all possible signal evolutions either using the Bloch equation simulations or then creating an extended phase graph. Subsequently, the MRF-acquired magnetization evolution time courses are then matched, voxel-by-voxel, to an entry of this dictionary using an appropriate pattern recognition algorithm and from which unique tissue properties such as T1, T2, and spin density can be calculated.

Partial volume analysis using magnetic resonance fingerprinting

It is likely that multiple tissue types are contained in most imaging voxels. To this end, partial volume analysis approaches can be applied to model signal evolution and potentially extract additional information.[29] Assuming "n" types of tissues in a voxel, this partial volume problem can be described as follows:

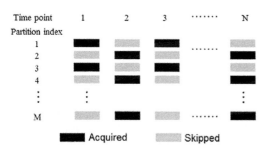

Fig. 2. Interleaved undersampling scheme in slice-encoding direction for 3D MRF (Undersampling factor, 2).

$$S_v = \sum_{i=1}^{n} w_i D_i,$$

where S_v represents the MRF signal evolution from one voxel, D_i represents signal evolution for a given tissue with known tissue properties, and w_i is the fraction for each individual tissue within this voxel. This partial volume analysis was applied to calculate tissue fraction maps for gray matter, white matter (WM), and cerebrospinal fluid in brain imaging.[7] More recently, a 3-component model was proposed to model 3 water pools including myelin water, intracellular/extracellular water, and free water. Subsequently, the myelin water fraction (MWF) defined as the percentage of myelin water to the total water can be calculated. MWF has been shown to provide better detection of myelin content during early brain development.[18]

Technical Considerations for Pediatric Neuroimaging

As a new quantitative imaging method, the performance and robustness of MRF has been extensively validated in multiple studies across different human organs. Here we provide a brief review of a few studies that could affect pediatric neuroimaging.

Repeatability and reproducibility

Compared with conventional qualitative contrast-weighted imaging, quantitative MR measurements should yield more consistent results independent of scanners, vendors, and imaging sites. However, experimental results along this direction are often lacking, which has been one of the major barriers for MRF clinical adoption. To demonstrate the robustness of MRF for future clinical applications, multiple studies have been conducted to examine the repeatability and reproducibility of techniques across MR scanners, field strengths, and vendor platforms.[30–32] With 10 healthy volunteers who were imaged across 10 3.0 T Siemens scanners at 4 image sites, the 2D FISP-based MRF yielded 3.4% and 8.0% variabilities for T1 and T2 in solid brain tissues, respectively.[30] The intrascanner repeatability was 2.0% to 3.1% for T1 and 3.1% to 7.9% for T2. In another study performed on 9 healthy volunteers at 2 imaging centers, Buonincontri and colleagues demonstrated an excellent repeatability (coefficients of variation: 2%–3% for T1, 5%–8% for T2, 3% for M0) and a good reproducibility (coefficients of variation: 3%–8% for T1, 8%–14% for T2, 5% for M0) for 2D MRF across 5 GE scanners (2 at 3.0 T and 3 at 1.5 T).[31] Using a 3D MRF method, our group has also demonstrated that the quantitative measures derived from MRF showed improved intrascanner and interscanner variability as compared with that of conventional contrast-weighted MR imaging.[32] All of these results suggest that quantitative tissue measurements obtained using MRF can serve as good candidates for longitudinal assessments of pathologies and monitoring treatment responses.

Field inhomogeneities

One of the major confounding factors for accurate tissue property mapping is system-dependent B1 inhomogeneities; this could lead to spatially varying signal behaviors and inconsistent image quality between studies. Multiple approaches have thus been developed to improve the performance of MRF quantification in the presence of B1 field inhomogeneities. In combination with a rapid Bloch-Siegert B1 mapping, Chen and colleagues[19] have shown that accurate T1 and T2 mapping can be achieved by using a 2D FISP-based MRF in abdominal imaging. A similar approach has been adopted in 3D MRF to improve performance of volumetric brain imaging.[13] Alternatively, MRF with simultaneous B1 mapping has also been developed where sensitivity to B1 was increased by adding abrupt changes in the FA pattern during acquisition.[33] In a recent pediatric study, we incorporated multiple B1-insensitive preparation modules and low-power excitation pulses in MRF. The results showed that transmit B1 inhomogeneities can be mitigated in pediatric neuroimaging.[18] **Fig. 3** shows the T1 and T2 maps obtained using 2D MRF, and the results are consistent with the reference maps where B1 field correction was performed. Finally, using different setups for receive coils, we have also demonstrated consistent quantitative measurements independent of receiver B1 field inhomogeneities.[32]

Motion robustness

It is well known that subject motion during data acquisition can lead to substantial image quality degradation. This is particularly challenging for pediatric MR imaging because young children have difficulty keeping still without sedation. Compared with conventional Cartesian MR imaging, most MRF approaches use a non-Cartesian spiral trajectory for in-plane encoding, which has been shown to be less sensitive to motion when compared with Cartesian encoding.[7] In addition, using the pattern matching algorithm, 2D MRF also exhibits a certain degree of motion tolerance. As shown by Ma and colleagues,[7] the motion-corrupted time frames behaved like noise during the pattern matching process, and accurate quantification was obtained in spite of severe subject motion. However, further investigation demonstrated that motion tolerance of 2D MRF approaches depended greatly on the magnitude and timing of subject motion. Alternatively, several studies propose using iterative reconstruction methods to retrospectively correct motions in MRF.[34,35] However, iterative approaches are time consuming and difficult to extend to 3D MRF acquisitions. Another major limitation of the 2D MRF-based approach is its inability to correct through-slice motion because proton signals would move in and out of the image slices. Extending 2D to 3D MRF provides an opportunity to correct motion in all directions. By using a 3D spiral projection acquisition scheme, Kurzawski and colleagues[36] demonstrated improved motion robustness of 3D MRF for brain imaging. Our group has developed a new approach combining 3D MRF with fat navigators for motion correction.[37] A rapid fat navigator sampling with a spatial resolution of $2 \times 2 \times 3$ mm^3 and whole brain coverage can be achieved using non-Cartesian spiral GRAPPA in 0.5 sec. Representative T1 and T2 maps obtained with and without motion correction are shown in **Fig. 4.** Note that this approach does not increase scan time for MRF. To date, most of the studies focusing on improving MRF motion robustness have been performed in adults, and future studies of children are needed to further evaluate pediatric applicability.

Integration with Machine Learning

ML has received increasing interest in the MR imaging community. Specifically, ML has been integrated into almost every step of MRF including data acquisition, dictionary generation, and tissue characterization. In this section, we review some ML approaches that could potentially enhance the applications of MRF in pediatric neuroimaging.

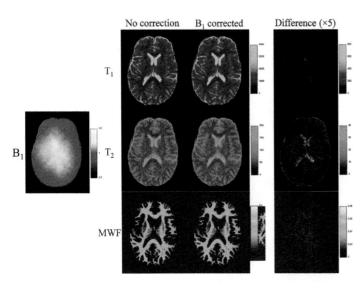

Fig. 3. Effect of B1 field inhomogeneity. The B1 map was acquired using the Bloch-Siegert method. Corresponding T1, T2, and MWF maps obtained with and without B1 correction are shown. The difference maps were calculated using the B1-corrected maps as the reference. (Reprint from Chen et al., Neuroimage 2019)

Improving postprocessing speed

One important feature of MRF compared with most other quantitative MR imaging methods is the use of pattern matching to extract tissue properties, which can operate robustly in the presence of substantial noise and motion artifacts. However, this approach is relatively slow and requires large memory capacity to store both image datasets and an MRF dictionary. Therefore, one logical area for application of ML in MRF is to accelerate tissue parameter estimations by replacing pattern matching with ML. Cohen and colleagues[38] proposed a fully connected convolutional neural network (CNN) capable of accurate tissue quantification that was 300 to 5000 times faster than that of using pattern matching. This method should potentially improve the workflow of MRF in a clinical setting.

Acceleration of image acquisition

Another limitation of pattern matching is that it treats each voxel independently, and hence does not take full advantage of information acquired in MRF. Because of this limitation, hundreds to thousands of MRF time courses are typically required for accurate tissue characterization using pattern matching, which prolongs the overall acquisition. However, valuable information exists in local regions of each signal evolution, and measures from neighboring pixels could enable better tissue characterization. Advanced postprocessing methods extracting additional features embedded in both spatial and temporal domains can potentially improve performance, and therefore reduce acquisition time by decreasing the required number of time courses for tissue parameter estimations. Deep learning is an ideal solution for information retrieval from MRF measurements. In a proof-of-concept study, we developed an advanced CNN model with 2 major modules, a feature extraction module and a UNet module, to accelerate MRF acquisition with improved tissue property mapping (**Fig. 5**).[39] The feature extraction module consists of a few fully connected layers, which is designed to mimic singular value decomposition (SVD) to reduce the dimension of signal evolutions.[40] Although SVD functions as a single-layer linear mapping, the proposed feature extraction module provides a multilayer nonlinear mapping from the signal to the extracted features, which can be used to improve the robustness and accuracy of tissue quantification. The second UNet module is used to capture spatial information of the feature map and finally generate the estimated tissue property.[41] Our results on quantitative brain imaging demonstrate that accurate T1 and T2 relaxation time mapping can be achieved with 4 times acceleration in MRF acquisition.[39] A similar approach has been applied to enable rapid submillimeter 2D MRF (0.8 mm in-plane resolution) in ~7.5 sec per slice.[42] An example using the aforementioned approach in a 10-year-old subject is shown in **Fig. 6**.

Rapid whole-brain tissue property mapping

Compared with traditional relaxometry MR imaging approaches, MRF has significantly improved overall acquisition speed. Nevertheless, the scan time is still relatively long for volumetric imaging, especially for a whole brain coverage as is often preferred in pediatric neuroimaging. In addition, high spatial resolution (1 mm isotropic or less) is

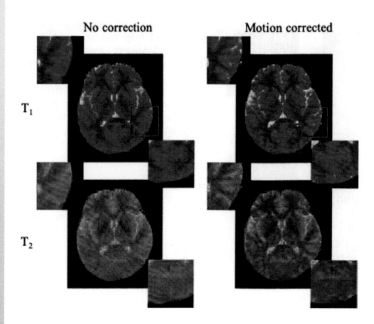

Fig. 4. Representative T1 and T2 maps obtained before and after k-space correction using fat navigator signal. The subject was instructed to move intentionally during the 3D MRF scan.

often desired for imaging children, which poses grea technical challenges in efficient data sampling. Combining parallel imaging and deep learning, we have developed a novel 3D MRF capable of achieving high-resolution (1 mm^3) and whole-brain coverage (18-cm volume) MRF in 7 minutes.[27] Preliminary evaluation of this new approach on 6 pediatric subjects has been conducted. Example images from a 5-year-old subject are shown in **Fig. 7**. The extracted quantitative measures agree well with the results obtained using pattern matching as well as our previous findings from a similar age.[18]

CLINICAL APPLICATIONS

In summary, MRF offers several major advantages in pediatric imaging when compared with traditional MR relaxometry approaches. First, the acquisition time is shorter. Second, MRF is intrinsically less sensitive to motion because of the use of a spiral trajectory acquisition scheme. This advantage is particularly critical for pediatric applications because it can potentially reduce the need for anesthesia.[43] Third, simultaneous acquisition of multiple parameters mitigates errors of misregistration among different scans. Fourth, there are excellent reliability and reproducibility of MRF-derived measurements across scanners/platforms/vendors, making MRF a suitable tool for longitudinal assessment of pediatric developmental trajectories or treatment responses. Finally, the new 3D MRF sequence enables whole-brain coverage with isotropic high resolution.[27] Therefore, MRF has gained increasing popularity since its inception in 2013. The latest applications of MRF in several fields of pediatric neuroimaging, including early brain development, brain tumors and epilepsy, are reviewed.[18,44–46]

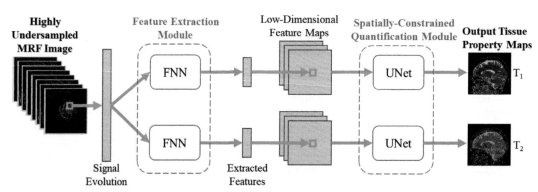

Fig. 5. Schematic drawing of the CNN model with 2 modules for tissue property mapping.

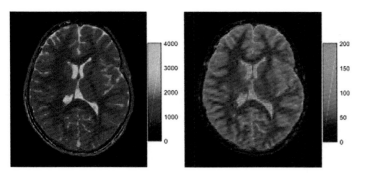

Fig. 6. T1 and T2 maps obtained from a 10-year-old female pediatric subject using submillimeter 2D MRF with residual channel attention UNet.

Assessment of Brain Myelination

Understanding healthy brain development should facilitate earlier identification of neuropsychiatric disorders, so that appropriate treatments or interventions can be implemented promptly.[47] Recently, there has been renewed interest in linking dysregulated myelination to the pathophysiologic mechanisms of neurodevelopmental disorders, such as attention deficit hyperactivity disorder (ADHD) and autism spectrum disorder (ASD). It is well known that ADHD and ASD are associated with widespread altered WM integrity.[48,49] A recent genome-wide association meta-analysis of 20,183 ADHD patients and 35,191 controls has identified 12 independent foci; several of these foci are associated with myelination and oligodendrocyte function and suggest a potential role of dysregulated myelination in the underlying pathogenesis of ADHD.[50,51] Likewise, precocious maturation of myelination has been observed in both patients and a mouse model of autism.[52,53] In patients with ASD, altered WM has

been shown in young ASD children but may disappear or reverse later in life.[52] In addition, an accelerated myelination trajectory of the WM has been observed in the frontal brain of neonatal mice but not seen in adult mice with autism.[53] Thus, developing a noninvasive, accurate, and robust technique enabling longitudinal quantitative measurements of myelin can help shed light on the pathogenetic mechanisms of these neurodevelopmental disorders.

In a pilot study, we successfully demonstrated the feasibility of using MRF to quantify brain MWF in 28 typically developing children younger than 5 years without sedation.[18] We measured the MWF in multiple WM regions and demonstrated that MWF is almost undetectable at 0 to 6 months old and gradually increases after about 6 months of age (**Fig. 8**). Depending on the brain regions, there is also a phase of rapid increase in MWF between 6 to 12 months and 6 to 18 months old. These age-dependent and spatially dependent myelin maturation trajectories are consistent

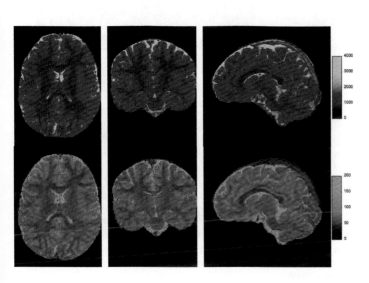

Fig. 7. 3D MRF (1 mm³) acquired from a 5-year-old subject in axial, coronal, and sagittal views. About 140 slices were acquired in 6 minutes, and the quantitative maps were obtained using an adult-trained CNN model.

with findings reported in the literature using post-mortem brain tissues[54,55]; this implies that MRF can be a promising quantitative tool for in vivo evaluation of myelination development in pediatric neurodevelopmental disorders.

Brain Tumors

Pediatric central nervous system tumors are the second most common childhood malignancy and account for the most common cause of cancer-related death in children. A variety of multimodality imaging techniques have been used to image brain tumors, but the results are variable.[56–63] Because of the advantages of multiparametric capabilities and repeatability, the potential clinical efficacy of MRF in characterizing brain tumors has also been studied in pediatric patients.

In a preliminary study of 23 pediatric brain tumors (19 low-grade glioma, 4 high-grade glioma), De Blank and colleagues[44] used MRF-derived T1 and T2 values to characterize regions of solid tumor, peritumoral WM, and contralateral WM. They demonstrated that T1 and T2 values can differentiate the solid tumor portions from the contralateral normal-appearing WM, as well as high-grade gliomas from low-grade gliomas.

Epilepsy

Epilepsy is one of the most prevalent chronic neurologic disorders, affecting an estimated half million children in the United States.[64] The direct annual health care cost with epilepsy ranged from approximately 10,000 to 47,000 dollars per patient and were higher in patients with uncontrolled seizures.[65] Approximately 30% of epilepsy patients are resistant to medications but are potentially curable by surgery.[66] Accurate detection and delineation of epileptogenic lesions is important during presurgical evaluation of medically intractable epilepsies.

At the time of writing this review, there have been no dedicated studies of MRF in pediatric patients with epilepsy. In a study of 15 patients with medically intractable epilepsy (2 adolescents and 13 adults), Ma and colleagues reported that additional findings, including additional lesions or subtle signal differences between epileptogenic and epileptogenic lesions, were observed in 4 of the 15 patients when 3D high-resolution MRF images were made available to radiologists.[46] The additional lesions identified by MRF included 1 mild malformation of cortical development, 2 heterotopias, and 1 tuber. Of note, these were adult patients, and studies focusing on pediatric epileptic patients are still lacking.

Mesial temporal lobe epilepsy (MTLE) is the most common form of focal epilepsy in adolescents and young adults, with hippocampal sclerosis (HS) as the top cause of MTLE. The clinical diagnosis of HS is traditionally made by visual comparisons of abnormally elevated T2/FLAIR signal between the

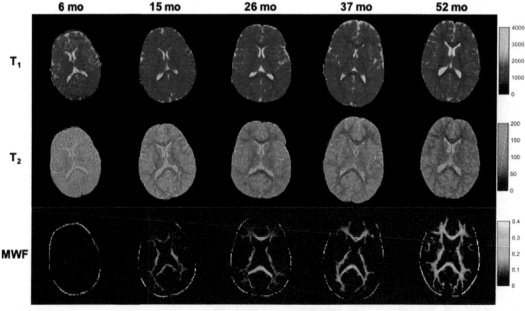

Fig. 8. Representative T1, T2, and MWF maps from 5 subjects at different ages. A similar slice location covering the genu and splenium of the corpus callosum was selected. Both T1 and T2 decrease, whereas MWF increases with age. (Reprint from Chen et al., Neuroimage 2019)

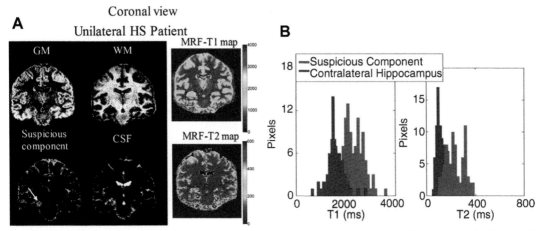

Fig. 9. Representative tissue fraction segmentation maps in a patient with unilateral hippocampal sclerosis. The histogram shows the different T1 and T2 distributions between healthy and suspicious hippocampi. (Reprint from Liao et al., Radiology 2018)

hippocampi, assuming that the contralateral hippocampus is healthy. The false-negative rate of this qualitative approach is approximately 15%, including patients with bilateral hippocampal involvement or early HS with minimal T2 signal changes. It is well known that T2 relaxometry can improve detection of early hippocampal damage and lateralization of HS in patients with MTLE.[67] In a recent study of 2D MRF comparing 33 MTLE patients with HS (32 adults) and 30 healthy controls, Liao and colleagues[45] demonstrated that MRF-derived T1 and T2 values can distinguish HS from healthy hippocampus and can improve the accuracy of MTLE diagnosis when compared with traditional visual assessment (96.9% vs 69.7%) **(Fig. 9)**.

These 2 studies suggest that MRF is a promising imaging technique to improve sensitivity and accuracy of identifying epileptic lesions, which might optimize management and guide surgical strategy in patients with epilepsy.

FUTURE DIRECTIONS AND CONCLUSION

MRF is a promising quantitative MR imaging technique that can calculate unbiased and accurate tissue properties. These tissue values can then be used as biomarkers to differentiate normal and abnormal tissues or for longitudinal monitoring. The advantages of a short acquisition time and motion robustness offer potential clinical pediatric applications. However, most current evidence involves relatively small sample sizes and heterogeneous populations, and further investigations are warranted.

CLINICS CARE POINTS

- MRF can measure multiple quantitative MR parameters in a single acquisition.
- Compared to conventional quantitative MRI methods, MRF is advantageous for pediatric patients due to the shorter acquisition time and better motion tolerance.
- 3D MRF can provide whole brain coverage and high-resolution images.
- MRF is a promising tool for measuring myelination development, differentiating low-grade and high-grade brain tumors, and identifying epileptogenic lesions.

ACKNOWLEDGMENTS

This work was supported in part by United States National Institutes of Health (NIH) grants EB006733 and U01MH110274.

REFERENCES

1. Feldman HM, Yeatman JD, Lee ES, et al. Diffusion tensor imaging: a review for pediatric researchers and clinicians. J Dev Behav Pediatr 2010;31(4): 346–56.

2. Huisman TA, Sorensen AG. Perfusion-weighted magnetic resonance imaging of the brain: techniques and application in children. Eur Radiol 2004;14(1):59–72.

3. Zhang H, Shen D, Lin W. Resting-state functional MRI studies on infant brains: a decade of gap-filling efforts. Neuroimage 2019;185:664–84.

4. Soares DP, Law M. Magnetic resonance spectroscopy of the brain: review of metabolites and clinical applications. Clin Radiol 2009;64(1):12–21.

5. Jackson GD, Connelly A, Duncan JS, et al. Detection of hippocampal pathology in intractable partial epilepsy: increased sensitivity with quantitative magnetic resonance T2 relaxometry. Neurology 1993;43(9):1793–9.

6. Leppert IR, Almli CR, McKinstry RC, et al. T(2) relaxometry of normal pediatric brain development. J Magn Reson Imaging 2009;29(2):258–67.

7. Ma D, Gulani V, Seiberlich N, et al. Magnetic resonance fingerprinting. Nature 2013;495(7440):187–92.

8. Jiang Y, Ma D, Keenan KE, et al. Repeatability of magnetic resonance fingerprinting T1 and T2 estimates assessed using the ISMRM/NIST MRI system phantom. Magn Reson Med 2017;78(4):1452–7.

9. Badve C, Yu A, Rogers M, et al. Simultaneous T1 and T2 brain relaxometry in asymptomatic volunteers using magnetic resonance fingerprinting. Tomography 2015;1(2):136–44.

10. Jiang Y, Ma D, Seiberlich N, et al. MR fingerprinting using fast imaging with steady state precession (FISP) with spiral readout. Magn Reson Med 2015;74(6):1621–31.

11. Jiang Y, Ma D, Jerecic R, et al. MR fingerprinting using the quick echo splitting NMR imaging technique. Magn Reson Med 2017;77(3):979–88.

12. Korzdorfer G, Jiang Y, Speier P, et al. Magnetic resonance field fingerprinting. Magn Reson Med 2019;81(4):2347–59.

13. Ma D, Jiang Y, Chen Y, et al. Fast 3D magnetic resonance fingerprinting for a whole-brain coverage. Magn Reson Med 2018;79(4):2190–7.

14. Wang CY, Coppo S, Mehta BB, et al. Magnetic resonance fingerprinting with quadratic RF phase for measurement of T2 (*) simultaneously with deltaf , T1 , and T2. Magn Reson Med 2019;81(3):1849–62.

15. Lu L, Erokwu B, Lee G, et al. Diffusion-prepared fast imaging with steady-state free precession (DP-FISP): a rapid diffusion MRI technique at 7 T. Magn Reson Med 2012;68(3):868–73.

16. Shah T, Lu L, Dell KM, et al. CEST-FISP: a novel technique for rapid chemical exchange saturation transfer MRI at 7 T. Magn Reson Med 2011;65(2):432–7.

17. Chen Y, Panda A, Pahwa S, et al. Three-dimensional MR fingerprinting for quantitative breast imaging. Radiology 2019;290(1):33–40.

18. Chen Y, Chen MH, Baluyot KR, et al. MR fingerprinting enables quantitative measures of brain tissue relaxation times and myelin water fraction in the first five years of life. Neuroimage 2019;186:782–93.

19. Chen Y, Jiang Y, Pahwa S, et al. MR fingerprinting for rapid quantitative abdominal imaging. Radiology 2016;279(1):278–86.

20. Hamilton JI, Jiang Y, Chen Y, et al. MR fingerprinting for rapid quantification of myocardial T1 , T2 , and proton spin density. Magn Reson Med 2017;77(4):1446–58.

21. Yu AC, Badve C, Ponsky LE, et al. Development of a combined MR fingerprinting and diffusion examination for prostate cancer. Radiology 2017;283(3):729–38.

22. Sharafi A, Medina K, Zibetti MWV, et al. Simultaneous T1 , T2 , and T1rho relaxation mapping of the lower leg muscle with MR fingerprinting. Magn Reson Med 2021;86(1):372–81.

23. Jaubert O, Cruz G, Bustin A, et al. Water-fat Dixon cardiac magnetic resonance fingerprinting. Magn Reson Med 2020;83(6):2107–23.

24. Jaubert O, Arrieta C, Cruz G, et al. Multi-parametric liver tissue characterization using MR fingerprinting: simultaneous T1 , T2 , T2 *, and fat fraction mapping. Magn Reson Med 2020;84(5):2625–35.

25. Koolstra K, Beenakker JM, Koken P, et al. Cartesian MR fingerprinting in the eye at 7T using compressed sensing and matrix completion-based reconstructions. Magn Reson Med 2019;81(4):2551–65.

26. Liu Y, Hamilton J, Eck B, et al. Myocardial T1 and T2 quantification and water-fat separation using cardiac MR fingerprinting with rosette trajectories at 3T and 1.5T. Magn Reson Med 2021;85(1):103–19.

27. Chen Y, Fang Z, Hung SC, et al. High-resolution 3D MR Fingerprinting using parallel imaging and deep learning. Neuroimage 2020;206:116329.

28. Liao C, Bilgic B, Manhard MK, et al. 3D MR fingerprinting with accelerated stack-of-spirals and hybrid sliding-window and GRAPPA reconstruction. Neuroimage 2017;162:13–22.

29. Deshmane A, McGivney DF, Ma D, et al. Partial volume mapping using magnetic resonance fingerprinting. NMR Biomed 2019;32(5):e4082.

30. Korzdorfer G, Kirsch R, Liu K, et al. Reproducibility and repeatability of MR fingerprinting relaxometry in the human brain. Radiology 2019;292(2):429–37.

31. Buonincontri G, Biagi L, Retico A, et al. Multi-site repeatability and reproducibility of MR fingerprinting of the healthy brain at 1.5 and 3.0T. Neuroimage 2019;195:362–72.

32. Lu L, Chen Y, Shen C, et al. Initial assessment of 3D magnetic resonance fingerprinting (MRF) towards quantitative brain imaging for radiation therapy. Med Phys 2020;47(3):1199–214.

33. Buonincontri G, Sawiak SJ. MR fingerprinting with simultaneous B1 estimation. Magn Reson Med 2016;76(4):1127–35.

34. Cruz G, Jaubert O, Schneider T, et al. Rigid motion-corrected magnetic resonance fingerprinting. Magn Reson Med 2019;81(2):947–61.

35. Mehta BB, Ma D, Pierre EY, et al. Image reconstruction algorithm for motion insensitive MR Fingerprinting (MRF): MORF. Magn Reson Med 2018; 80(6):2485–500.

36. Kurzawski JW, Cencini M, Peretti L, et al. Retrospective rigid motion correction of three-dimensional magnetic resonance fingerprinting of the human brain. Magn Reson Med 2020;84(5):2606–15.

37. Chen Y, Zong X, Ma D, et al. Improving motion robustness of 3D MR Fingerprinting using fat navigator. Proceedings of the 29th Meeting of the International Society for Magnetic Resonance in Medicine. 2020. p. 871.

38. Cohen O, Zhu B, Rosen MS. MR fingerprinting Deep RecOnstruction NEtwork (DRONE). Magn Reson Med 2018;80(3):885–94.

39. Fang Z, Chen Y, Liu M, et al. Deep learning for fast and spatially constrained tissue quantification from highly accelerated data in magnetic resonance fingerprinting. IEEE Trans Med Imaging 2019; 38(10):2364–74.

40. McGivney DF, Pierre E, Ma D, et al. SVD compression for magnetic resonance fingerprinting in the time domain. IEEE Trans Med Imaging 2014; 33(12):2311–22.

41. Ronneberger O, Fischer P, Brox T. U-Net: convolutional networks for biomedical image segmentation. In: Navab N, Hornegger J, Wells W, et al, editors. Medical Image Computing and Computer-Assisted Intervention – MICCAI 2015. MICCAI 2015. Lecture Notes in Computer Science, vol 9351. Cham: Springer; 2015. p. 234–41. https://doi.org/10.1007/978-3-319-24574-4_28.

42. Fang Z, Chen Y, Hung SC, et al. Submillimeter MR fingerprinting using deep learning-based tissue quantification. Magn Reson Med 2020;84(2): 579–91.

43. Andropoulos DB, Greene MF. Anesthesia and developing brains - implications of the FDA warning. N Engl J Med 2017;376(10):905–7.

44. de Blank P, Badve C, Gold DR, et al. Magnetic resonance fingerprinting to characterize childhood and young adult brain tumors. Pediatr Neurosurg 2019; 54(5):310–8.

45. Liao C, Wang K, Cao X, et al. Detection of lesions in mesial temporal lobe epilepsy by using MR fingerprinting. Radiology 2018;288(3):804–12.

46. Ma D, Jones SE, Deshmane A, et al. Development of high-resolution 3D MR fingerprinting for detection and characterization of epileptic lesions. J Magn Reson Imaging 2019;49(5):1333–46.

47. Lenroot RK, Giedd JN. Brain development in children and adolescents: insights from anatomical magnetic resonance imaging. Neurosci Biobehav Rev 2006;30(6):718–29.

48. van Ewijk H, Heslenfeld DJ, Zwiers MP, et al. Diffusion tensor imaging in attention deficit/hyperactivity disorder: a systematic review and meta-analysis. Neurosci Biobehav Rev 2012;36(4):1093–106.

49. Travers BG, Adluru N, Ennis C, et al. Diffusion tensor imaging in autism spectrum disorder: a review. Autism Res 2012;5(5):289–313.

50. Demontis D, Walters RK, Martin J, et al. Discovery of the first genome-wide significant risk loci for attention deficit/hyperactivity disorder. Nat Genet 2019; 51(1):63–75.

51. Lesch KP. Editorial: can dysregulated myelination be linked to ADHD pathogenesis and persistence? J Child Psychol Psychiatry 2019;60(3):229–31.

52. Uddin LQ, Supekar K, Menon V. Reconceptualizing functional brain connectivity in autism from a developmental perspective. Front Hum Neurosci 2013;7: 458.

53. Khanbabaei M, Hughes E, Ellegood J, et al. Precocious myelination in a mouse model of autism. Transl Psychiatry 2019;9(1):251.

54. Dubois J, Dehaene-Lambertz G, Kulikova S, et al. The early development of brain white matter: a review of imaging studies in fetuses, newborns and infants. Neuroscience 2014;276:48–71.

55. Paus T, Collins DL, Evans AC, et al. Maturation of white matter in the human brain: a review of magnetic resonance studies. Brain Res Bull 2001;54(3): 255–66.

56. Bulakbasi N, Kocaoglu M, Ors F, et al. Combination of single-voxel proton MR spectroscopy and apparent diffusion coefficient calculation in the evaluation of common brain tumors. AJNR Am J Neuroradiol 2003;24(2):225–33.

57. Cha S, Lupo JM, Chen MH, et al. Differentiation of glioblastoma multiforme and single brain metastasis by peak height and percentage of signal intensity recovery derived from dynamic susceptibility-weighted contrast-enhanced perfusion MR imaging. AJNR Am J Neuroradiol 2007;28(6):1078–84.

58. Crisi G, Orsingher L, Filice S. Lipid and macromolecules quantitation in differentiating glioblastoma from solitary metastasis: a short-echo time single-voxel magnetic resonance spectroscopy study at 3 T. J Comput Assist Tomogr 2013;37(2):265–71.

59. Fan G, Sun B, Wu Z, et al. In vivo single-voxel proton MR spectroscopy in the differentiation of high-grade gliomas and solitary metastases. Clin Radiol 2004; 59(1):77–85.

60. Halshtok Neiman O, Sadetzki S, Chetrit A, et al. Perfusion-weighted imaging of peritumoral edema can aid in the differential diagnosis of glioblastoma mulltiforme versus brain metastasis. Isr Med Assoc J 2013;15(2):103–5.

61. Kinoshita M, Goto T, Okita Y, et al. Diffusion tensor-based tumor infiltration index cannot discriminate vasogenic edema from tumor-infiltrated edema. J Neurooncol 2010;96(3):409–15.

62. Min ZG, Niu C, Rana N, et al. Differentiation of pure vasogenic edema and tumor-infiltrated edema in patients with peritumoral edema by analyzing the relationship of axial and radial diffusivities on 3.0T MRI. Clin Neurol Neurosurg 2013;115(8):1366–70.

63. Price SJ, Jena R, Burnet NG, et al. Improved delineation of glioma margins and regions of infiltration with the use of diffusion tensor imaging: an image-guided biopsy study. AJNR Am J Neuroradiol 2006;27(9):1969–74.

64. Zack MM, Kobau R. National and state estimates of the numbers of adults and children with active epilepsy - United States, 2015. MMWR Morb Mortal Wkly Rep 2017;66(31):821–5.

65. Begley CE, Durgin TL. The direct cost of epilepsy in the United States: a systematic review of estimates. Epilepsia 2015;56(9):1376–87.

66. Kalilani L, Sun X, Pelgrims B, et al. The epidemiology of drug-resistant epilepsy: a systematic review and meta-analysis. Epilepsia 2018;59(12):2179–93.

67. Bernasconi A, Bernasconi N, Caramanos Z, et al. T2 relaxometry can lateralize mesial temporal lobe epilepsy in patients with normal MRI. Neuroimage 2000;12(6):739–46.

Magnetic Resonance Elastography of the Brain

Manjunathan Nanjappa, PhD[a], Arunark Kolipaka, PhD, FAHA, FSCMR[b],*

KEYWORDS

• MRE • MR imaging • Stiffness • Elasticity • Palpation • Pediatric • Brain tumor • Elastography

KEY POINTS

• Magnetic resonance elastography (MRE) provides noninvasive quantitative assessment of tissue stiffness and biomechanical properties.
• MRE is a preferred method for diagnosing chronic liver diseases and hepatic fibrosis.
• Early MRE studies in the pediatric and adult brain show promise for clinical implementation.

INTRODUCTION

In clinical medicine, assessment of mechanical properties of biological tissues helps to diagnose various diseases. It is well-known that the biomechanical properties of various tissues vary with different physiologic stages and pathologic conditions. For instance, a malignant tumor in the breast is stiffer than a benign tumor or normal tissue.[1] Manual palpation is a useful diagnostic tool to distinguish normal and abnormal tissues. However, noninvasive palpation can only be performed on superficial tissues and cannot be applied to internal organs without surgery. In particular, palpation is impossible to apply to the brain due to the surrounding cranial vault. Another limitation of palpation is that it is qualitative, which may potentially bias diagnosis. Diagnostic imaging has technologically advanced, making it possible to noninvasively interrogate the pediatric brain using various cross-sectional modalities such as computed tomography (CT), magnetic resonance imaging (MR), and ultrasound (US). However, conventional techniques do not provide information about tissue biomechanical properties, useful when planning for surgery.

Decades of MR research on brain development in the pediatric and adolescent population using MR imaging have provided rich information regarding structural changes in gray matter and white matter volume,[2] cerebrospinal fluid (CSF) content,[3] and myelination.[4] MRI can also calculate functional parameters such as cerebral blood flow, and cerebral blood volume, during different activities and at rest. During normal aging and development, neural and behavioral changes occur rapidly.[5–7] The correlation between structural and functional changes with biomechanical properties has not been fully elucidated. Greater knowledge of tissue biomechanics could potentially lead to new biomarkers for of disease. For example, neurodevelopmental disorders such as cerebral palsy do not always show characteristic structural brain MRI lesions.[8–10] In such instances, added biomechanical information may help to diagnose and understand the underlying pathophysiology.

Increased understanding of biomechanical properties, such as stiffness of the developing pediatric brain, has potential importance in clinical and diagnostic medicine. However, the availability

a Department of Radiology, The Ohio State University Wexner Medical Center, 460 West 12th Avenue, Room No 333 3rd Floor, Columbus, OH 43210, USA; b Department of Radiology, The Ohio State Wexner Medical Center, 395 West 12th Avenue, 4th Floor, Columbus, OH 43210, USA
* Corresponding author.
E-mail address: Arunark.Kolipaka@osumc.edu

Magn Reson Imaging Clin N Am 29 (2021) 617–630
https://doi.org/10.1016/j.mric.2021.06.011
1064-9689/21/© 2021 Elsevier Inc. All rights reserved.

of such data in the literature is very limited, and only a few studies have been conducted with limited age groups and numbers of subjects.[10–12] The most established way to assess stiffness of soft tissues noninvasively is by using elastographic techniques with the help of MR and/or US systems. These methods rely on the propagation of mechanical waves in tissues. In particular, MR elastography (MRE) offers the ability to obtain quantitative measurements of tissue elasticity noninvasively and three-dimensionally.

ELASTICITY OF SOFT TISSUE

In materials science, elasticity is defined as an object's ability to resist deformation when subjected to a mechanical force, and return to its original shape and size when the force is removed. The force applied to the object is called stress, and the displacement of an object in response is called strain. The slope of the stress-strain curve is the elastic modulus, a physical parameter that reflects the stiffness of a material. According to Hooke's law, pure elastic material has a linear stress and strain relation that behaves like a spring. Soft tissues in the human body usually have an inhomogeneous structure that is viscoelastic, showing both elastic and viscous properties. Therefore, the elastic modulus of these tissues comprises a storage modulus representing the elasticity component, and a loss modulus representing the viscosity component. The human brain is a soft tissue composed of neurons, neural stem cells, glial cells, and blood vessels; its mechanical properties arise from the geometric organization of these tissue components and their network complexity.

MAGNETIC RESONANCE ELASTOGRAPHY

Many static, quasistatic, and dynamic MR elastography (MRE) techniques have been developed over the years.[13–17] Dynamic MRE is the most commonly used technique because of its efficiency and simplicity. This is a noninvasive and in vivo diagnostic technique to assess biological tissues' stiffness using either a 1.5-T or 3-T MR scanner with additional hardware and software.[17–21] MRE measures oscillating shear wave displacement fields in soft tissues, induced by an externally applied harmonic motion.

Measurement of shear wave displacements is obtained by modulating the MR gradients at the frequency of applied harmonic motion. Repeated measurements are performed with a linear phase difference between the externally applied motion and the MR gradient fields. This phase difference results in varying phase contrast across the MR images.

In MRE, there are 3 steps involved:

1. Inducing mechanical motion in soft tissues
2. Encoding waves in the phase of MR images
3. Generating an elastogram using an inversion algorithm

This article provides an overview of MRE to provide high-level understanding of the technique. A detailed review of brain MRE methods can be found in Hiscox and colleagues, 2016.[22]

EXTERNAL MECHANICAL OSCILLATOR

To estimate the elasticity of an object, one must apply an external load/force before deformation measurements can be obtained. In MRE, a continuous, single-frequency, stable mechanical shear wave motion is induced in soft tissues using a special hardware setup synchronous with the MR acquisition pulse sequence. A schematic of the MRE setup is shown in **Fig. 1**. The motion inducer consists of two components, namely an active driver and passive driver. The active driver is an electromechanical device (such as a subwoofer), able to generate mechanical vibrations at controllable frequencies and amplitudes. This active driver is placed outside the scanner room, so that its electromagnets will not interfere with the scanner magnetic field, and is controlled through the signal generator.

Mechanical waves are transmitted via an MR-compatible plastic tube and delivered to the tissue of interest using a passive driver. The passive driver is a soft, pillowlike structure placed inside the receiver coil. It is important to position the passive driver in contact with the body surface, and as close as possible to the region of interest. The frequencies generated from this driver are in the audible range (40–200 Hz),[23] which is safer for the patient and does not interfere with the MR scanner. One size of passive driver may not fit all patients and regions of interest; therefore, passive drivers of various sizes and shapes have been developed to optimize shear wave delivery and increase patient comfort. For pediatric and smaller patients, small soft drivers are available, similar to the one shown in **Fig. 2**.

IMAGING SHEAR WAVES

The fundamental concept of MRE, measuring propagating (harmonic) waves in soft tissue, stemmed from conventional phase-contrast MR

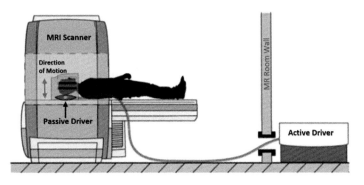

Fig. 1. The MRE technique: the patient's head is vibrated in the MR imaging scanner with a pneumatic actuator, displacement wavefields are acquired, and the inversion algorithm calculates viscoelastic shear stiffness. (Reproduced from G. McIlvain et al., "Brain Stiffness Relates to Dynamic Balance Reactions in Children With Cerebral Palsy," J. Child Neurol., vol. 35, no. 7, pp. 463–471, 2020, https://doi.org/10.1177/0883073820909274.)

imaging. Steady-state motion of nuclear spins in the presence of magnetic field gradients causes a phase shift in the image. In phase-contrast imaging, flow-encoding gradients are deployed to track moving spins. During image readout, moving spins of blood and surrounding static tissues accumulate different phase shifts in MR phase images. Similarly, propagation of shear waves in the target tissue can be captured and visualized using modified phase-contrast MR sequences where the motion-encoding gradients (MEGs) are synchronized to vibrational input. Imaging of the shear waves can be performed using a wide range of sequences, such as gradient echo (GRE), spin-echo (SE), echo-planar imaging (EPI) (**Fig. 3**), or balanced steady-state free precession imaging.

The MEGs are applied in all 3 orthogonal planes of motion to measure the three-dimensional (3D) wave vector. The frequency of MEGs applied is typically the same as the mechanical frequency and is synchronized using trigger pulses. Several wave images are acquired at different time points by varying the phase offset between the MEGs and mechanical motion. Each MR image produces a vector component of the tissue motion in the direction of MEGs. Therefore, the adjusted relative phase offsets between driver and MEGs in multiple acquisitions provide the full vector of motion within the tissue.

ELASTOGRAM

The proportionality relationship between the transverse stress (shear stress) and shear strain (deformation) in an isotropic linear elastic material can be described by the mechanical property called shear modulus (μ). According to Hooke's law, the shear modulus is directly proportional to the speed

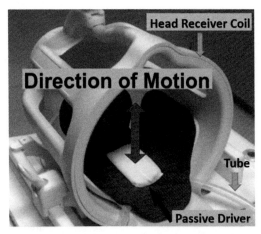

Fig. 2. Soft pillow-like passive driver used with head-coil for brain MRE applications. During image acquisition, the passive driver is positioned beneath the head to induce shear waves in the brain. An active driver connects to the passive driver via a plastic tube to induce vibrations. (Reproduced from K.M. Pepin et al., "MR Elastography Analysis of Glioma Stiffness and IDH1-Mutation Status" AJNR Am J Neuroradiol 10.3174/ajnr.A5415, http://dx.doi.org/10.3174/ajnr.A5415.)

of propagation of planar shear waves in a medium and the density of the medium[24]:

$$\mu = v^2 \rho \qquad (1)$$

Shear wave propagation speed can be calculated from the externally applied mechanical frequency (f) and wavelength (λ) of the propagating wave:

$$v = f \lambda \qquad (2)$$

Therefore, complex-valued displacement filed maps (wave images) obtained are inverted using different algorithms to calculate complex modulus, where the real part represents storage modulus and the imaginary part represents loss modulus. In MRE stiffness calculations, most of the soft tissue density is assumed to be equivalent to that of water ($\rho = 1$ g cm^{-3}).[25] Furthermore, the propagating wave field is a complex phenomenon comprising geometric complexities such as reflections, refractions, and interferences, which are minimized using band-pass and directional filters. Different inversion algorithms are currently being used to estimate the stiffness of soft tissue.[26] The most common of these is a direct inversion to estimate brain stiffness. Direct inversion assumes that the waves are propagating in a uniform, infinite, isotropic, and homogeneous medium. Modeling of fiber orientation would enable anisotropic brain stiffness estimation[27–29], but this is computationally complex. For simplicity, most current brain applications use isotropic stiffness estimations.

MAGNETIC RESONANCE ELASTOGRAPHY OF THE BRAIN

As an emerging diagnostic tool, the use of MRE in routine clinical care is still limited. Although MRE is considered the most accurate noninvasive tool for quantifying liver fibrosis,[30,31] its usage in other organs is still under investigation. Over the last 2 decades, several studies have established that MRE is capable of measuring 2D and 3D[32–34] shear wave fields in the human brain. The stiffness estimation in the brain is sensitive to experimental choices such as vibrational frequency, acquisition strategy, and postprocessing pipelines, which makes it challenging to quantitatively assess reproducibility across sites. Therefore, keeping all MRE acquisition parameters consistent is essential for biomarker qualification.[35]

Many studies have quantified the shear modulus of the brain in healthy and disease populations, with values ranging from 2.8 to 12.9 kPa for gray matter and 2.5 to 15.2 kPa for white matter.[33,34,36,37] Although most studies are consistent with white matter being significantly stiffer than gray matter, a few studies have reported otherwise.[38] This variability points to there being no gold standard method to measure brain tissue elasticity in vivo.[36,39] **(Fig. 4)**.

Several MRE studies of the healthy aging population indicate that the stiffness of brain tissue decreases with age **(Fig. 5)**.[29,40–42] Regarding the effect of sex, early studies suggested that the females demonstrated significantly higher global stiffness[41] than their male counterparts, whereas recent studies indicate that the effect of sex is significant only in the temporal and occipital lobes.[40]

The first MRE study to establish sensitivity of brain stiffness to a disease state was performed in 2010 by Wuerfel and colleagues[43] in patients with multiple sclerosis (MS), showing that brain stiffness is decreased in patients with MS compared with age-matched controls. A subsequent study of MS disease course also concluded that the chronic form of this disease leads to altered cerebral geometry and stiffness.[44]

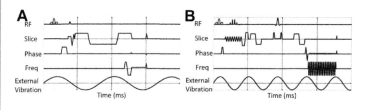

Fig. 3. MRE pulse sequence diagrams depicting the radiofrequency (RF) pulses, gradients in the frequency encoding, phase encoding, and slice select directions, with applied external motion. On the left is a GRE MRE sequence for imaging 60-Hz mechanical motion using 16-millisecond gradient-moment-nulled (GMN) MEG applied along slice encoding direction. On the right is an SE-EPI MRE sequence for imaging 60-Hz motion using 2 bipolar 6.5-m MEGs, 1 on each side of the refocusing pulse and synchronized to motion. Both sequences are shown with GMN imaging gradients and spatial presaturation pulses. (Adapted from R. L. E. Matthew, C. Murphy et al., "Phase Correction for Interslice Discontinuities in Multislice EPI MR Elastography," vol. 269, no. 5232, p. 5232, 2012.)

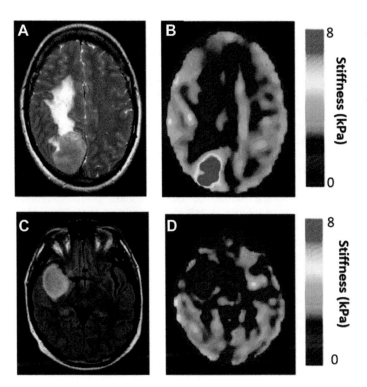

Fig. 4. *(A)* Axial T2-weighted MR of a woman with right parietal meningioma and surrounding edema and *(B)* MRE map showing stiff tumor with soft surrounding edema. *(C)* T2-weighted MR of a man with right temporal glioma and *(D)* MRE showing tumor to be softer than normal brain tissue. (Adapted from L. V. Hiscox et al., "Magnetic resonance elastography (MRE) of the human brain: Technique, findings and clinical applications," Phys. Med. Biol., vol. 61, no. 24, pp. R401–R437, 2016, https://doi.org/10.1088/0031-9155/61/24/R401.)

Some MRE studies indicate conflicting results for global and regional brain stiffness in disease pathologies. For example, one study reported that stiffness increased in the parietal and occipital lobes in patients with normal hydrocephalus (NPH),[45] whereas another study reported increased global stiffness in NPH.[44] Multicenter studies with standardized experimental setups are essential to establish uniform stiffness measurements for clinical care.

MRE studies focused on neurodegenerative disease reported that global brain stiffness

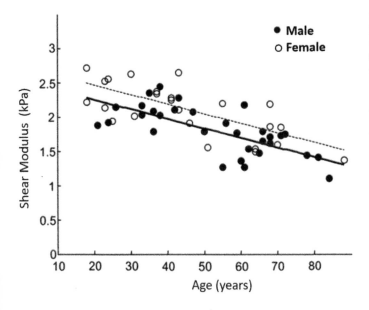

Fig. 5. Summary of the relationship between global brain (shear modulus) viscoelasticity and age. The shear modulus from this model decreases significantly with age and is larger in women compared with men. (Reproduced From I. Sack et al., "The impact of aging and gender on brain viscoelasticity," Neuroimage, vol. 46, no. 3, pp. 652–657, 2009, https://doi.org/10.1016/j.neuroimage.2009.02.040.)

decreased in subjects with Alzheimer disease (AD).[46] The variation of brain stiffness in AD was not only caused by amyloid deposition but also by degradation of extracellular matrix, loss of cytoskeletal structure, and altered synaptic connectivity (Fig. 6). This study also showed the specificity of stiffness changes (ie, decrease in stiffness) in the heteromodal association cortices that are hardest hit by the disease. The brain stiffness changes in 4 classes of dementia were compared in a recent study: patients with AD and frontotemporal dementia showed decreased cerebral stiffness in frontal and temporal regions, and patients with AD additionally showed softening of the parietal lobe and sensorimotor region. Patients with normal pressure hydrocephalus showed decreased stiffness of parietal, occipital, and sensorimotor regions, whereas dementia with Lewy bodies did not show stiffness changes in any regions. These findings further support the regional brain stiffness specificity[47] of previous studies. A summary of results is presented in Fig. 7.

For brain tumors, resective surgery is a primary therapeutic tool. In general, hard tumors are difficult to remove and most often require manual dissection, whereas soft tumors can be removed by suction; therefore, prior knowledge of tumor stiffness plays an important role during preoperative planning, determining surgical approach and resection strategy for optimum posttherapeutic outcomes.[48–50] To date, only MR imaging has been capable of qualitatively characterizing brain tumor stiffness[51] (Fig. 8), since US-based techniques cannot penetrate the bony skull[52]. Stiffness measurements of solid intracranial tumors were first performed in 2007 using MRE (Fig. 9) and showed large variability in viscoelasticity.[37] Studies of meningiomas reported that MRE stiffness correlated with surgical evaluations of tumor consistency, but there were challenges for small and heterogeneous tumors.[53,54] One study used MRE-based slip interface imaging (SII) based on octahedral shear strain (OSS) maps, to predict the degree of meningioma-brain adhesions correlating with surgical findings.[55] A recent review of MRE application in brain tumors compared 19 original research studies that were conducted on groups of 4 to 34 patients, including 184 patients with metastases.[35,56,57] This study noted that the group mean tumor stiffness of meningiomas and pituitary adenomas correlated with intraoperative findings, but the pooled data analysis showed significant overlap between shear modulus values across brain tumor types. These overlaps limit the applicability of MRE for diagnostic purposes and highlight the need for further rigorous studies.

A reproducibility study of MRE in patients with pseudotumors was performed before and after lumbar puncture, compared with healthy volunteers.[18] The results showed good reproducibility of brain stiffness estimation in all subjects and significant stiffness differences between patients and healthy volunteers. However, there was no significant correlation between opening and closing CSF pressures and brain stiffness despite interval CSF drainage. These findings are similar to other studies pre/post-lumbar puncture in MS,[44] emphasizing that CSF pressure is one of many factors influencing brain stiffness, and that the brain may take time to adapt biomechanically.

POTENTIAL APPLICATIONS IN THE PEDIATRIC BRAIN

The mechanical properties of an organ are based on tissue composition and structural arrangement; therefore, MRE is a potential biomarker for changes in the brain during fetal, neonatal, childhood, and adolescent development. So far, there have been no formal MRE studies in the human fetal and neonatal population, and only one postnatal study in rats.[58] In recent years, there have been only a handful of MRE brain studies published in children and adolescents.[10–12,59]

Brain MRE of rats has been performed between 9 and 42 days (6 weeks) after birth, which represents the neonatal to juvenile age range.[58] Mechanical properties of brain tissue were measured using MRE at each developmental stage, as shown in Fig. 10A. There was a rapid increase in brain size between weeks 1 and 2, followed by slower growth thereafter relative to body size. Spatial variability in shear modulus was noted between different brain regions in each animal, with considerable variability among animals for the same brain regions. The shear modulus in the cortical gray matter increased during the first 2 weeks and remained stable for the next 4 weeks, followed by a significant decrease during the sixth week. Shear modulus of deep gray matter gradually increased from week 1 to 4 and was significantly lower in week 6. These results are summarized in Fig. 10B, C. The rate of stiffness change was higher during the period equivalent to infancy and early childhood in humans, than in the period equivalent to adolescence in humans.

Over the last several decades, through a large number of research studies and technological advancements, understanding of brain structural

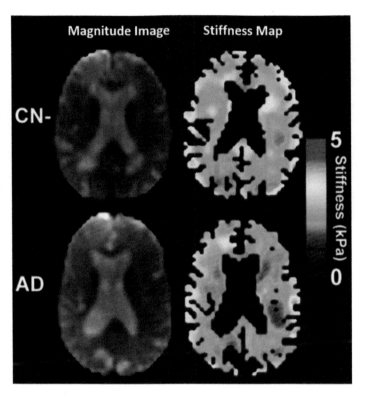

Fig. 6. Brain MRE with SE-EPI pulse sequence (axial plane, repetition time/echo time (TR/TE) 5 1500/61.3 milliseconds). Top row shows a cognitively normal control (CN), and bottom row shows a male patient with AD. EPI magnitude images for each patient are in the left column and stiffness maps in the right column. (Reproduced From M. C. Murphy et al., "Decreased brain stiffness in Alzheimer's disease determined by magnetic resonance elastography," J. Magn. Reson. Imaging, vol. 34, no. 3, pp. 494–498, 2011, https://doi.org/10.1002/jmri.22707.)

and functional developmental changes has vastly improved.[59–61] Studies that examine brain structural changes in cortical and subcortical regions have reported significant heterogeneity in developmental timing of each brain region.[60,62,63] A multifrequency MRE study to characterize the brain tissue stiffness in children compared with adults was performed by Yeung and colleagues.[12] Stiffness values did not correlate with age in gray matter and white matter regions, and there were no significant differences in global brain stiffness between adolescent and adult brains. However, the caudate and putamen of the adolescent brain were significantly stiffer

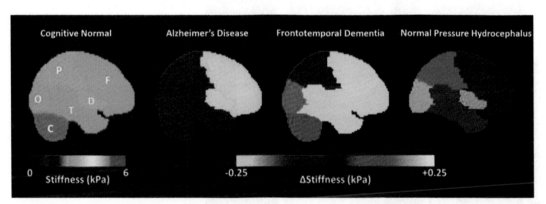

Fig. 7. Stiffness changes caused by different forms of dementia, based on sagittal views of a lobar brain atlas including frontal lobe (F), parietal lobe (P), temporal lobe (T), occipital lobe (O), deep gray and white matter (D), and cerebellum (C). The panels show cognitively normal subjects and various dementia subtypes. (Data from M. ElSheikh et al., "MR elastography demonstrates unique regional brain stiffness patterns in dementias," Am. J. Roentgenol., vol. 209, no. 2, pp. 403–408, 2017, doi:10.2214/AJR.16.17455.)

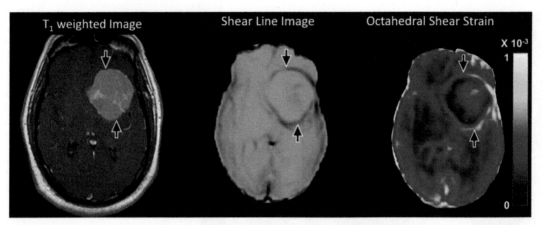

Fig. 8. Meningioma with a complete slip interface at imaging and no adhesions at surgery. (A) T1- weighted image with contrast shows a large left medial sphenoid wing meningioma. The tumor-brain interface is clearly defined by the (B) shear line image and (C) octahedral shear strain (OSS) maps, with arrows indicating the presence of a slip interface with no adhesion. Surgical findings showed that the dissection plane was nearly completely extrapial, with no tumor-brain adhesions encountered. (Reproduced from Z. Yin et al., "Slip interface imaging based on MR-elastography preoperatively predicts meningioma–brain adhesion," J. Magn. Reson. Imaging, vol. 46, no. 4, pp. 1007–1016, 2017, https://doi.org/10.1002/jmri.25623.)

than in adults, whereas other regions were softer. In pediatric subjects, the stiffness of white matter and gray matter was very similar, in contrast to earlier studies that found white matter to be stiffer than gray matter[22] (**Fig. 11**).

Another MRE study of healthy children used multifrequency stimulation to identify age and sex discrepancies in brain mechanical properties[11] (**Fig. 12**). This study concluded that there were no significant differences in whole-brain stiffness over the age range. There was a significant increase in microstructural parameters of white matter with age, thought to caused by age-related alignment and geometrical organization of white

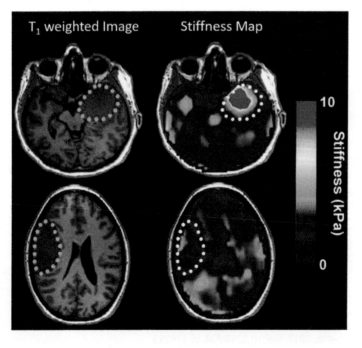

Fig. 9. MRE of firm (top) and soft (bottom) meningiomas (dotted outline). On the left are T1-weighted anatomic images and their respective stiffness maps. (Reproduced From M. C. Murphy et al., "Preoperative assessment of meningioma stiffness by magnetic resonance elastography," J. Neurosurg., vol.118, no. 3, p. 643, 2013, https://doi.org/10.3171/2012.9.JNS12519.Preoperative.)

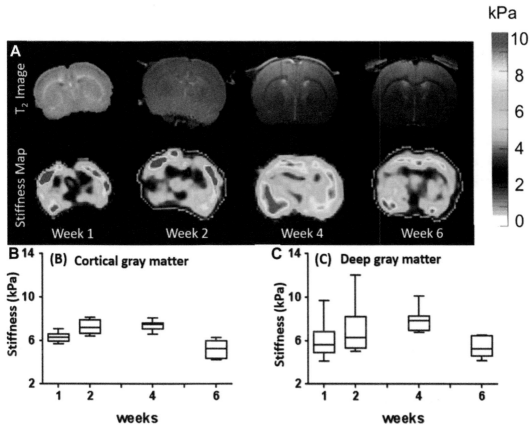

Fig. 10. (A) Development of rat brain with T2-weighted coronal MR at the level of foramina of Monro in the upper row (images acquired week 1 to 6), and MRE stiffness maps in the middle row. Complex shear modulus for (B) cortical gray matter and (C) deep gray matter shown in plots B and C in the bottom row. Longitudinal changes assessed using a generalized linear model with pairwise comparisons of means between weeks. (Images are reproduced from A. C. Pong et al., "Longitudinal measurements of postnatal rat brain mechanical properties in-vivo," J. Biomech., vol. 49, no. 9, pp.1751–1756, 2016, https://doi.org/10.1016/j.jbiomech.2016.04.005.)

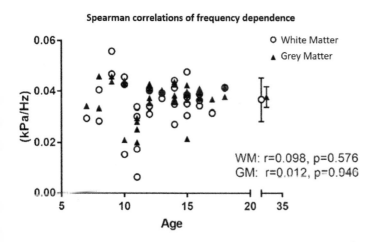

Fig. 11. Scatter plots of pediatric patients (7–18 years old) showing age versus frequency dependence stiffness for white matter (WM) and gray matter (GM). Spearman correlations show no significant age dependence. Adult data is plotted as the mean. (Adapted from J.Yeung et al., "Paediatric brain tissue properties measured with magnetic resonance elastography" Biomechanics and Modeling in Mechanobiology (2019) 18:1497–1505. https://doi.org/10.1007/s10237-019-01157-x)

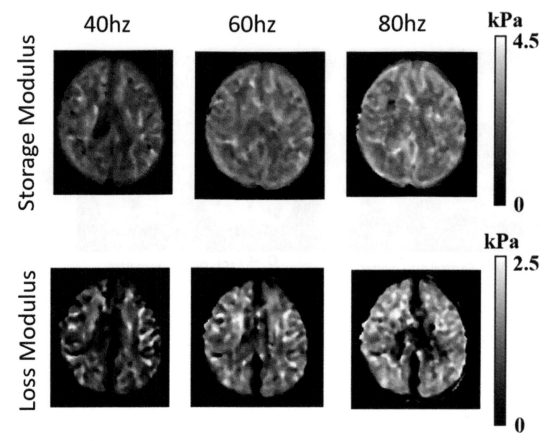

Fig. 12. Healthy children with estimated storage modulus and loss modulus at vibrating frequencies of 40 Hz, 60 Hz, and 80 Hz. (Adapted from E.Ozkaya et al., "Viscoelasticity of children and adolescent brains through MR elastography," Journal of the Mechanical Behavior of Biomedical Materials 115 (2021) 104229, https://doi.org/10.1016/j.jmbbm.2020.104229).

matter. This study also found that the female children and adolescent brains were significantly stiffer than their male counterparts, in line with earlier studies.[10,12]

A brain MRE study on children with cerebral palsy was recently published[10] and reported a direct relationship between brain stiffness and dynamic balance reactions. This study identified 12 distinct regions, 10 of which are known to be important for balance and locomotion.[64,65] Higher brain stiffness was noted in locomotive control regions, as shown in **Fig. 13**, which was an indication of higher balance recovery. Another MRE study in children with CP also reported that the stiffness of cerebral gray matter is significantly lower than in typically developing (TD) children, while the damping ratio of gray matter is significantly higher in CP.[66]

Researchers are expanding the scope of MRE into other territories, for example the relationship between brain structure and function. One study showed that the hippocampal damping ratio is a significant predictor of relational memory and behavioral performance.[67]

CURRENT LIMITATIONS AND FUTURE DIRECTIONS

As an emerging diagnostic technique, initial pediatric brain MRE studies promise to provide additional information about tissue characteristics. In the adult population, MRE studies have shown good test-retest repeatability in measuring stiffness, with typical errors of 1% for the whole brain, 2% for cerebral lobes, and 3% to 7% for deep gray matter.[35] However, MRE is still investigational, particularly in diagnosing small tumors with limited image resolution, as well as cystic tumors which cannot propagate shear waves.[37,57] Other challenges for MRE include metallic hardware, such as cerebral aneurysm clips and cochlear implants. Because MRE is performed with additional

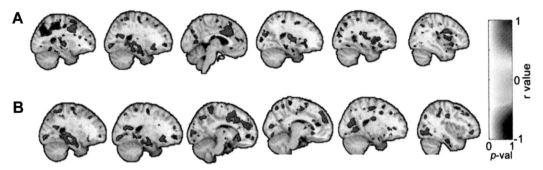

Fig. 13. Cerebral palsy with voxel-wise correlation coefficient maps showing clusters of regions in which brain stiffness significantly correlated with (A) anterior and (B) single-step threshold balance reaction tasks. (Images adapted from G.McIlvain et al., "Brain Stiffness Relates to Dynamic Balance Reactions in Children With Cerebral Palsy" Journal of Child Neurology 2020, Vol. 35(7) 463-471. doi:10.1177/0883073820909274)

hardware, large patients may have issues fitting into the MR bore and head coil. A major challenge in pediatric brain MRE is the image acquisition time of 4 to 10 minutes, which may be too long for young children without sedation. Because MRE is a motion-sensitive technique, patient motion during image acquisition introduces phase errors and image artifacts, resulting in miscalculation of stiffness maps. Although small motions can be addressed with motion navigator and correction techniques,[68,69] large motions lead to significant errors. Furthermore, in order to resolve small tumors, higher-frequency vibrations are needed but can lead to attenuation of waves in deep brain structures. Using lower-frequency vibrations generates longer wavelengths, which may violate infinite medium assumptions when inverting the wave data to produce robust stiffness estimates. An appropriate frequency should be selected to balance these competing considerations. Finally, the standard mechanical drivers used for adult patients should not be used in young children because (1) standard drivers may not provide optimal coupling between the patient body surface and the driver, leading to ineffective power delivery; and (2) comparatively high power can potentially cause mechanical or thermal injury. Therefore, it is essential to use a separate passive driver with reduced power (up to 50% of what is used for adult patients).

CLINICS CARE POINTS

- Viscoelastic properties of the brain provide insight into many disease states such as multiple sclerosis, neurogenerative disease, brain tumors, and cerebral palsy.

- MRE-derived brain tumor stiffness and adhesions to surrounding tissue are useful information for surgical planning.

- Brain stiffness measurements during pediatric development may aid in the diagnosis of neurodevelopmental disorders.

DISCLOSURE

The authors have nothing to disclose.

REFERENCES

1. Moran PR. A flow velocity zeugmatographic interlace for NMR imaging in humans. Magn Reson Imaging 1982;1:197–203.
2. Lenroot RK, Giedd JN. Brain development in children and adolescents: insights from anatomical magnetic resonance imaging. Neurosci Biobehav Rev 2006;30(6):718–29.
3. Hedner J, Lundell KH, Breese GR. Development variations in CSF monoamine metabolites during childhood. Biol Neonate 1986;49(4):190–7.
4. Klingberg T, Vaidya CJ, Gabrieli JDE, et al. Myelination and organization of the frontal white matter in children: a diffusion tensor MRI study. Neuroreport 1999;10(13):2817–21.
5. Jernigan TL, Baaré WFC, Stiles J, et al. Chapter 5 - Postnatal brain development: Structural imaging of dynamic neurodevelopmental processes. In: Braddick O, Atkinson J, Innocenti GM, editors. Progress in Brain Research. Volume 189. Elsevier; 2011. p. 77–92. https://doi.org/10.1016/B978-0-444-53884-0.00019-1.
6. Schmithorst VJ, Yuan W. White matter development during adolescence as shown by diffusion MRI. Brain Cogn 2010;72(1):16–25.

7. Toledo E, Lebel A, Becerra L, et al. The young brain and concussion: imaging as a biomarker for diagnosis and prognosis. Neurosci Biobehav Rev 2012; 36(6):1510–31.

8. Himmelmann K, Horber V, De La Cruz J, et al. MRI classification system (MRICS) for children with cerebral palsy: development, reliability, and recommendations. Dev Med Child Neurol 2017;59(1): 57–64.

9. Robinson MN, Peake LJ, Ditchfield MR, et al. Magnetic resonance imaging findings in a population-based cohort of children with cerebral palsy. Dev Med Child Neurol 2009;51(1):39–45.

10. McIlvain G, Tracy JB, Chaze CA, et al. Brain stiffness relates to dynamic balance reactions in children with cerebral palsy. J Child Neurol 2020; 35(7):463–71.

11. Ozkaya E, Fabris G, Macruz F, et al. Viscoelasticity of children and adolescent brains through MR elastography. J Mech Behav Biomed Mater 2021;115: 104229.

12. Yeung J, Jugé L, Hatt A, et al. Paediatric brain tissue properties measured with magnetic resonance elastography. Biomech Model Mechanobiol 2019;18(5): 1497–505.

13. Parker KJ, Doyley MM, Rubens DJ. Corrigendum: imaging the elastic properties of tissue: the 20 year perspective. Phys Med Biol 2012;57(16): 5359–60.

14. Lewa CJ, de Certaines JD. MR imaging of viscoelastic properties. J Magn Reson Imaging 1995; 5(2):242–4.

15. Lewa CJ, De Certaines JD. Viscoelastic property detection by elastic displacement NMR measurements. J Magn Reson Imaging 1996;6(4):652–6.

16. Sabet AA, Christoforou E, Zatlin B, et al. Deformation of the human brain induced by mild angular head acceleration. J Biomech 2008;41(2):307–15.

17. Muthupillai R, Lomas DJ, Rossman PJ, et al. Magnetic resonance elastography by direct visualization of propagating acoustic strain waves. Science 1995; 269(5232):1854–7.

18. Kolipaka A, Wassenaara PA, Cha S, et al. Magnetic resonance elastography to estimate brain stiffness: measurement reproducibility and its estimate in pseudotumor cerebri patients. Clin Imaging 2018; 51:114–22.

19. Kenyhercz WE, Raterman B, Illapani VS, et al. Quantification of aortic stiffness using magnetic resonance elastography: measurement reproducibility, pulse wave velocity comparison, changes over cardiac cycle, and relationship with age. Magn Reson Med 2016;75(5):1920–6.

20. Gandhi D, Kalra P, Raterman B, et al. Magnetic resonance elastography-derived stiffness of the kidneys and its correlation with water perfusion. NMR Biomed 2020;33(4):1–12.

21. Fakhouri F, Dong H, Kolipaka A. Magnetic resonance elastography of the lungs: a repeatability and reproducibility study. NMR Biomed 2019;32(7): 1–10.

22. Hiscox LV, Johnson CI, Barnhill E, et al. Magnetic resonance elastography (MRE) of the human brain: technique, findings and clinical applications. Phys Med Biol 2016;61(24):R401–37.

23. Yin M, Chen J, Glaser KJ, et al. Abdominal magnetic resonance elastography. Top Magn Reson Imaging 2009;20(2):79–87.

24. Graff KF. Wave motion in elastic solids. New York: Dover; 1991.

25. Burlew M. A new ultrasound tissue-equivalent material. Radiology 1980;134(2):517–20.

26. Manduca A, Oliphant TE, Dresner MA, et al. Magnetic resonance elastography: non-invasive mapping of tissue elasticity. Med Image Anal 2001; 5(4):237–54.

27. Romano A, Scheel M, Hirsch S, et al. In vivo waveguide elastography of white matter tracts in the human brain. Magn Reson Med 2012;68(5):1410–22.

28. Romano A, Guo J, Prokscha T, et al. In vivo waveguide elastography: effects of neurodegeneration in patients with amyotrophic lateral sclerosis. Magn Reson Med 2014;72(6):1755–61.

29. Kalra P, Raterman B, Mo X, et al. Magnetic resonance elastography of brain: comparison between anisotropic and isotropic stiffness and its correlation to age. Magn Reson Med 2019;82(2):671–9.

30. Kaur H, Hindman NM, Al-Refaie WB, et al. ACR appropriateness criteria® suspected liver metastases. J Am Coll Radiol 2017;14(5):S314–25.

31. Kim DK, Choi JY, suk Park M, et al. Clinical feasibility of mr elastography in patients with biliary obstruction. Am J Roentgenol 2018;210(6):1273–8.

32. Kruse SA, Dresner MA, Rossman PJ, et al. "Palpation of the brain" using magnetic resonance elastography. International Society for Magnetic Resonance in Medicine. Philadelphia, May 22–28, 1999. p. 258.

33. McCracken PJ, Manduca A, Felmlee J, et al. Mechanical transient-based magnetic resonance elastography. Magn Reson Med 2005;53(3):628–39.

34. Green M, Sinkus R, Cheng S, et al. 3D MR-elastography of the brain at 3 Tesla. ISMRM 13th Scientific Meeting & Exhibition. Miami Beach, May 7-13, 2005. p. 427.

35. Murphy MC, Huston J, Ehman RL. MR elastography of the brain and its application in neurological diseases. Neuroimage 2019;187:176–83.

36. Kruse SA, Rose GH, Glaser KJ, et al. Magnetic resonance elastography of the brain. Neuroimage 2008; 39(1):231–7.

37. Xu L, Lin Y, Han JC, et al. Magnetic resonance elastography of brain tumors: preliminary results. Acta Radiol 2007;48(3):327–30.

38. Nagashima T, Shirakuni T, Rapoport SI. A two-dimensional, finite element analysis of vasogenic brain edema. Neurol Med Chir (Tokyo) 1990;30(1):1–9.

39. Kruse SA, Ehman RL. 2D approximation of 3D wave propagation in MR elastography of the brain. Proceedings of the 11th ISMRM Scientific Meeting and Exhibition. Toronto, 2003. p. 1084.

40. Arani A, Murphy MC, Glaser KJ, et al. Measuring the effects of aging and sex on regional brain stiffness with MR elastography in healthy older adults. Neuroimage 2015;111:59–64.

41. Sack I, Beierbach B, Wuerfel J, et al. The impact of aging and gender on brain viscoelasticity. Neuroimage 2009;46(3):652–7.

42. Sack I, Streitberger KJ, Krefting D, et al. The influence of physiological aging and atrophy on brain viscoelastic properties in humans. PLoS One 2011;6(9):e23451.

43. Wuerfel J, Paul F, Beierbach B, et al. MR-elastography reveals degradation of tissue integrity in multiple sclerosis. Neuroimage 2010;49(3):2520–5.

44. Streitberger KJ, Sack I, Krefting D, et al. Brain viscoelasticity alteration in chronic-progressive multiple sclerosis. PLoS One 2012;7(1):1–7.

45. Perry DC, Datta S, Sturm VE, et al. Reward deficits in behavioural variant frontotemporal dementia include insensitivity to negative stimuli. Brain 2017;140(12):3346–56.

46. Murphy MC, Huston J 3rd, Jack CR Jr, et al. Decreased brain stiffness in Alzheimer's disease determined by magnetic resonance elastography. J Magn Reson Imaging 2011;34(3):494–8. https://doi.org/10.1002/jmri.22707.

47. ElSheikh M, Arani A, Perry A, et al. MR elastography demonstrates unique regional brain stiffness patterns in dementias. Am J Roentgenol 2017;209(2):403–8.

48. Itamura K, Chang KE, Lucas J, et al. Prospective clinical validation of a meningioma consistency grading scheme: association with surgical outcomes and extent of tumor resection. J Neurosurg 2019;131(5):1356–60.

49. Zada G, Du R, Laws ER. "Defining the 'edge of the envelope': patient selection in treating complex sellar-based neoplasms via transsphenoidal versus open craniotomy: clinical article. J Neurosurg 2011;114(2):286–300.

50. Zada G, Yashar P, Robison A, et al. A proposed grading system for standardizing tumor consistency of intracranial meningiomas. Neurosurg Focus 2013;35(6):1–6.

51. Meyer F, Hoover J, Morris J. Use of preoperative magnetic resonance imaging T1 and T2 sequences to determine intraoperative meningioma consistency. Surg Neurol Int 2011;2(1):142.

52. Chauvet M, Imbault D, Capelle M, et al. In vivo measurement of brain tumor elasticity using intraoperative shear wave elastography. Ultraschall Med 2016;37:584–90.

53. Hughes JD, Fattahi N, Van Gompel J, et al. Higher-resolution magnetic resonance elastography in meningiomas to determine intratumoral consistency. Neurosurgery 2015;77(4):653–9.

54. Murphy MC, et al. Preoperative assessment of meningioma stiffness by magnetic resonance elastography. J Neurosurg 2013;118(3):643.

55. Yin Z, Hughes JD, Trzasko JD, et al. "Slip interface imaging based on MR-elastography preoperatively predicts meningioma–brain adhesion. J Magn Reson Imaging 2017;46(4):1007–16.

56. Bunevicius A, Schregel K, Sinkus R, et al. REVIEW: MR elastography of brain tumors. Neuroimage Clin 2020;25:102109.

57. Di Ieva A, Grizzi F, Rognone E, et al. Magnetic resonance elastography: a general overview of its current and future applications in brain imaging. Neurosurg Rev 2010;33(2):137–45.

58. Pong AC, Jugé L, Cheng S, et al. Longitudinal measurements of postnatal rat brain mechanical properties in-vivo. J Biomech 2016;49(9):1751–6.

59. Johnson CL, Telzer EH. Magnetic resonance elastography for examining developmental changes in the mechanical properties of the brain. Dev Cogn Neurosci 2018;33:176–81.

60. Mills KL, Goddings AL, Herting MM, et al. Structural brain development between childhood and adulthood: convergence across four longitudinal samples. Neuroimage 2016;141:273–81.

61. Lebel C, Beaulieu C. Longitudinal development of human brain wiring continues from childhood into adulthood. J Neurosci 2011;31(30):10937–47.

62. Lebel C, Gee M, Camicioli R, et al. Diffusion tensor imaging of white matter tract evolution over the lifespan. Neuroimage 2012;60(1):340–52.

63. Raznahan A, Shaw PW, Lerch JP, et al. Longitudinal four-dimensional mapping of subcortical anatomy in human development. Proc Natl Acad Sci U S A 2014;111(4):1592–7.

64. Wittenberg E, Thompson J, Nam CS, et al. Neuroimaging of human balance control: a systematic review. Front Hum Neurosci 2017;11:1–25.

65. la Fougère C, Zwergal A, Rominger A, et al. Real versus imagined locomotion: a [18F]-FDG PET-fMRI comparison. Neuroimage 2010;50(4):1589–98.

66. Chaze CA, McIlvain G, Smith DR, et al. Altered brain tissue viscoelasticity in pediatric cerebral palsy measured by magnetic resonance elastography. Neuroimage Clin 2019;22:101750. https://doi.org/10.1016/j.nicl.2019.101750.

67. Schwarb H, Johnson CL, McGarry MDJ, et al. Medial temporal lobe viscoelasticity and relational memory performance. Neuroimage 2016;132: 534–41.

68. Fehlner A, Hirsch S, Weygandt M, et al. Increasing the spatial resolution and sensitivity of magnetic resonance elastography by correcting for subject motion and susceptibility-induced image distortions. J Magn Reson Imaging 2017;46(1):134–41.

69. Murphy MC, Huston III J, Glaser KJ, et al. Phase correction for interslice discontinuities in multislice EPI MR elastography. ISMRM 20th Annual Meeting & Exhibition. Melbourne, Australia, 2012. p. 3426.

Amide Proton Transfer–Weighted MR Imaging of Pediatric Central Nervous System Diseases

Hong Zhang, MD, PhD[a], Jinyuan Zhou, PhD[b], Yun Peng, MD, PhD[a],*

KEYWORDS

- APT-weighted imaging • CEST imaging • Pediatric brain development
- Hypoxic-ischemic encephalopathy • Intracranial infection • Brain tumors

KEY POINTS

- Amide proton transfer (APT)-weighted imaging is a molecular MR imaging technique that generates image contrast based on endogenous cellular proteins and peptides, using standard clinical MR imaging scanners.
- APT-weighted MR imaging is of value in assessing pediatric brain myelination and neonatal hypoxic-ischemic encephalopathy.
- APT-weighted MR imaging demonstrates excellent agreement with gadolinium-enhanced T$_1$-weighted MR imaging for the detection of intracranial infectious lesions and distinction of high- from low-grade intracranial tumors, as well as neoplasia from infection.

INTRODUCTION

Magnetic resonance (MR) imaging is the workhorse for imaging pediatric central nervous system (CNS) diseases. Widely used MR imaging sequences include T2-weighted (T2W), T1-weighted (T1W), fluid-attenuated inversion recovery, diffusion-weighted imaging (DWI), and gadolinium-enhanced T1-weighted imaging (Gd-T1W), in which the observed MR imaging signal comes from hydrogen atoms in "free" water in tissue. Amide proton transfer-weighted (APTw) imaging[1–3] is a chemical exchange saturation transfer (CEST)-based molecular MR imaging technique[4–7] that is sensitive to endogenous mobile proteins and peptides in tissue, such as those dissolved in the cytoplasm.[8] Early data have demonstrated that APTw imaging adds important value to standard MR imaging sequences in the clinical setting.[3] APTw imaging can be used to detect malignant brain tumors based on increased cell density (thus, increased protein concentration)[9–12] and acute cerebral ischemia because of tissue acidosis or decreased pH (thus, decreased exchange rate).[13–15] In particular, APTw imaging is based on endogenous contrast agents, so no exogenous contrast agent injection is required. This is beneficial to reduce contrast agent load and eliminate the need for intravenous injection, particular benefits for pediatric patients. In this article, the authors briefly introduce the technical background of APTw imaging and review its clinical applications to pediatric CNS diseases.

[a] Department of Radiology, Beijing Children's Hospital, Capital Medical University, National Center for Children's Health, 56 Nan Li Shi Road, Xi Cheng District, Beijing, 100045, China; [b] Division of MR Research, Department of Radiology, Johns Hopkins University School of Medicine, 600 N. Wolfe Street, Park 336, Baltimore, MD 21287, USA
* Corresponding author.
E-mail address: ppengyun@yahoo.com

Magn Reson Imaging Clin N Am 29 (2021) 631–641
https://doi.org/10.1016/j.mric.2021.06.012
1064-9689/21/© 2021 Elsevier Inc. All rights reserved.

AMIDE PROTON TRANSFER-WEIGHTED MR IMAGING PRINCIPLES AND TECHNIQUES

APTw imaging can be achieved by a saturation transfer experiment with a relatively low radiofrequency (RF) irradiation power (**Fig. 1**). Technically, the APT effect is measured as a reduction in bulk water intensity because of the chemical exchange of water protons with magnetically labeled backbone amide protons of endogenous mobile proteins. Thus, specific protein information is obtained indirectly through the bulk water signal usually used in imaging. Such labeling is accomplished using selective RF irradiation at the MR frequency of the backbone amide protons, ~3.5 ppm downfield of the water resonance,[16] causing saturation (or signal destruction) that is transferred to water protons.

When performing such experiments in tissue, direct water saturation and conventional magnetization transfer contrast (MTC, a well-known and large MR imaging contrast[17,18]) will interfere with the measurements. In theory, the sum of all saturation effects is generally called the magnetization transfer ratio, $MTR = 1 - S_{sat}/S_0$, where S_{sat} and S_0 are the signal intensities with and without selective irradiation. The APTw signal is usually measured through the MTR asymmetry analysis at 3.5 ppm[1-3]:

$$MTR_{asym}(3.5\,ppm) = MTR(+3.5\,ppm) - MTR(-3.5\,ppm) = \frac{S_{sat}(-3.5\,ppm) - S_{sat}(+3.5\,ppm)}{S_0} = APTR$$

$$+ MTR'_{asym}(3.5\,ppm)$$

where APTR is the proton transfer ratio for the amide protons associated with mobile cellular proteins and peptides in tissue, and $MTR'_{asym}(3.5\,ppm)$ is any remaining asymmetry, including the inherent MTR_{asym} of the solid-phase magnetization transfer effect[19] and nuclear Overhauser enhancement (NOE) effect of the upfield nonexchangeable protons (such as aliphatic protons) of cellular macromolecules and metabolites.[20,21] The presence of $MTR'_{asym}(3.5\,ppm)$ greatly complicates APT quantification in vivo. APT images defined by $MTR_{asym}(3.5\,ppm)$ are often called APT-weighted images.[22]

The importance of APTw imaging is that endogenous cellular protein information can be obtained sensitively through standard clinical MR imaging scanners. The APTw imaging sequence can be incorporated into any standard clinical MR imaging examination protocol for the brain. The early 2-dimensional, single-slice acquisition protocol can provide high-quality B_0 magnetic field inhomogeneity-corrected APTw images with a scan time of approximately 3 minutes.[23,24] Recently, 3-dimensional (3D) APTw technology[25-27] has been developed to improve the coverage of lesions, providing more information and a better signal-to-noise ratio. The scanning time of a 3D APTw sequence that covers a large part of the brain is approximately 3 to 8 minutes. The APTw imaging sequence is now available commercially as a product sequence through 1 vendor,[28] and the other vendors have "works-in-progress" packages. Currently, the commonly used RF power for APTw imaging at 3 T is about 2 μT, with a total RF saturation time of about 0.8 to 2 seconds (possibly with interpulse delays).[3]

There are several challenging issues for clinical APTw imaging[3]: (i) The APT effect is affected by several factors, including amide proton concentration, tissue pH, water proton concentration, and the T_1 relaxation of water.[29] However, according to previous articles,[30] the contributions of tissue water content and T_1 to the APTw signal are mostly compensated in many diseases.[30] Notably, some recent studies[31,32] have clearly indicated that the APT effect in tissue is roughly not affected by water T_1 at the saturation power of 2 μT. (ii) The APTw signal quantified based on the MTR asymmetry analysis is contaminated by the upfield NOE signals (including the conventional MTC asymmetry).[19] Thus, the APTw signal intensity (% of the bulk water signal intensity) is often negative (difficult to understand). Moreover, B_0 inhomogeneity remains a critical issue in MTR asymmetry-based APTw imaging, which may cause artifacts in APTw images. (iii) The APT effect is small. New APTw imaging techniques are needed to increase image spatial resolution, contrast, and signal-to-noise ratio that would be more suitable for imaging small lesions. (iv) APTw MR imaging signals could be generated by various sources of mobile proteins and peptides in living tissues. When reviewing APTw images, referring to conventional structural MR images to identify APT_w hyperintensity artifacts, such as cysts, liquefactive necrosis, hemorrhages, and vessels, is necessary for accurate interpretation.

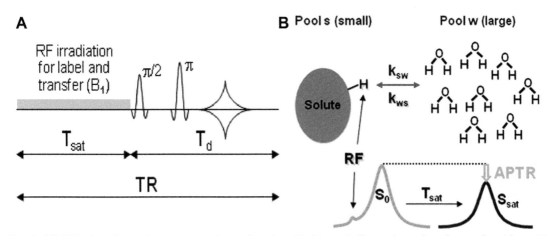

Fig. 1. (*A*) APTw imaging pulse sequence. Saturation time (T_{sat}) is typically on the order of seconds, with an RF saturation power (B_1) of 2 μT. (*B*) APTw signal enhancement principle. The small pool (s) reflects dilute exchangeable amide protons (~3.5 ppm downfield of the water resonance), and the large pool (w) reflects bulk water protons. The RF irradiation selectively saturates exchangeable protons in the small pool, which subsequently exchanges with unsaturated protons of the larger water pool (rate k_{sw}). Once on the solute, these protons become saturated, and the process repeats itself. The bulk water signal decreases significantly due to progressive saturation transfer, enabling detection of low solute concentrations. APTR, Amide Proton Transfer Ratio; T_d, Relaxation Delay; TR, Time of Repetition. ([*B*] Reproduced with permission from Zhou et al. Progr NMR Spectr 2006;48:109-136.)

CLINICAL APPLICATIONS TO PEDIATRIC CENTRAL NERVOUS SYSTEM DISEASES
Brain Development

Brain development is a complicated and lifelong process, with each developmental period associated with a different degree of brain maturity. Biochemical and physiologic maturity patterns may show different trends of APTw signal changes over time. The main manifestations of pediatric brain development are neuroglial cell proliferation and myelination. Neuroglial cell proliferation both precedes and contributes to myelination. The use of APTw imaging technology for the assessment of pediatric brain development has been reported in a few studies.[33–35] Zhang and colleagues[33] performed APTw imaging in 82 children between the ages of 2 and 190 months. The results showed that APT signals in the corpus callosum, frontal and occipital lobes, and centrum semiovale followed an exponentially decreasing curve with age, with the most significant changes occurring within the first year of life (**Fig. 2**). Decreasing protein mobility (from mobile proteins to semisolid proteins, such as the shift of the myelin basic protein from the oligodendroglial cytoplasm to the myelin sheath) may explain the decreasing APTw signal intensity observed during brain myelination. In a recent report in 51 pediatric patients with developmental delay (DD), Tang and colleagues[34] reported that children with DD and delayed myelination on MR imaging showed higher APTw values than normal controls, especially in white matter.

This may be related to the decreased conversion of myelin basic protein to myelin sheaths in the oligodendroglial cytoplasm. Therefore, APTw imaging can be used as a potential imaging method with which to evaluate brain development and myelination at the molecular level.

In another study, Zheng and colleagues[35] performed APTw imaging in 38 neonates (gestational age 27–41 weeks) to evaluate the development of the neonatal brain with gestational age. The results showed that APTw values in the frontal white matter, basal ganglia, and occipital white matter were significantly different, and that the APTw signal positively correlated linearly with gestational age. This may be related to increasing protein content during the process of neuroglial cell proliferation.

Neonatal Hypoxic-Ischemic Encephalopathy

Neonatal hypoxic-ischemic encephalopathy (HIE) results from a cascade of pathophysiological processes caused by global cerebral ischemia-hypoxia-reperfusion injury. The metabolic changes in brain tissue often appear earlier than morphologic changes, such that metabolic imaging may be helpful for early diagnosis. Zheng and colleagues[36] performed an APTw imaging study on a model of hypoxic-ischemic brain injury in neonatal piglets. The results showed that the APTw values immediately decreased after hypoxic-ischemic insult because of metabolic acidosis, then increased gradually, and ultimately exceeded those of the control group at 48 to

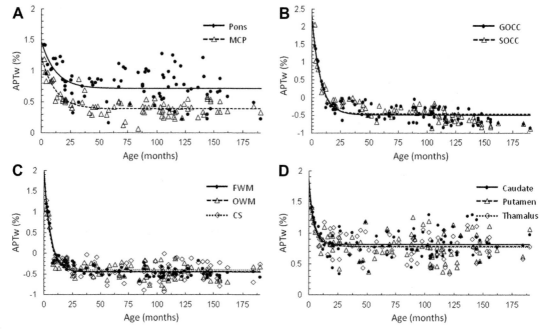

Fig. 2. Experimental and fitted age-related changes in APTw values within different brain regions in neurodevelopmentally normal children. (*A*) Pons ($R^2 = 0.235$) and middle cerebellar peduncle (MCP; $R^2 = 0.641$). (*B*) Genu (GOCC; $R^2 = 0.786$) and splenium of corpus callosum (SOCC; $R^2 = 0.734$). (*C*) Frontal white matter (FWM; $R^2 = 0.874$); occipital white matter (OWM; $R^2 = 0.735$); and centrum semiovale (CS; $R^2 = 0.685$). (*D*) Caudate ($R^2 = 0.222$); putamen ($R^2 = 0.188$); and thalamus ($R^2 = 0.221$). (Reproduced with permission from Zhang et al. Eur Radiol 2016;26:3368-3376.)

72 hours. In another study in 30 mild HIE neonates within 2 to 7 days after birth, Chen and colleagues[37] reported that the APTw values of mild HIE neonates in several regions were higher than that of the control group. This may be because most mild HIE neonates have experienced hypoxia and ischemia before APTw imaging, with subsequent recovery of aerobic metabolism. The pH value temporarily decreases and then increases, causing rebound alkalosis. Therefore, APTw imaging can be used to evaluate neonatal brain injury at the internal environmental and molecular levels.

Brain Infection

Intracranial infection in children continues to be a worldwide health problem, particularly in poor and developing countries. Gd-T1W imaging has been widely regarded as the most sensitive imaging study for the detection of intracranial infection.[38–40] However, the use of gadolinium-based contrast agents has contraindications. Furthermore, gadolinium deposition in the brain and other organs is a potential concern.[41,42] A molecular endogenous contrast imaging technique would be preferred, especially in children. In a recent study in 28 pediatric patients with 84 infectious lesions (24 brain abscesses, 28 viral encephalitis, and 32 meningitis),[43] it was reported that APTw

images demonstrated excellent agreement with Gd-T1W images, and the detection of infectious lesions was not significantly different from Gd-T1W images. APTw MR imaging enables the detection of infectious lesions at a level similar to that of Gd-T1W and represents a contrast-free means for evaluation of intracranial infection. Two examples of APTw, MTR, and conventional MR images of intracranial infection in children are shown in **Figs. 3** and **4**.

Brain Tumors

Brain tumors are among the most common solid tumors and a leading cause of death is a potential concern in the pediatric population.[44] Unlike brain tumors in adults, brain tumors in children predominate in the posterior fossa, with distinct molecular subtypes and pathologic features. Accurate preoperative diagnosis can contribute to appropriate therapeutic strategies and possibly better survival; however, this remains challenging because of diverse histologic presentations and biologic behaviors.

Currently, the most often used application of APTw imaging is for adult brain tumors. APTw MR has shown promising diagnostic value in distinguishing between tumor core and peritumoral edema,[23] glioma grading,[45–47] and evaluation of

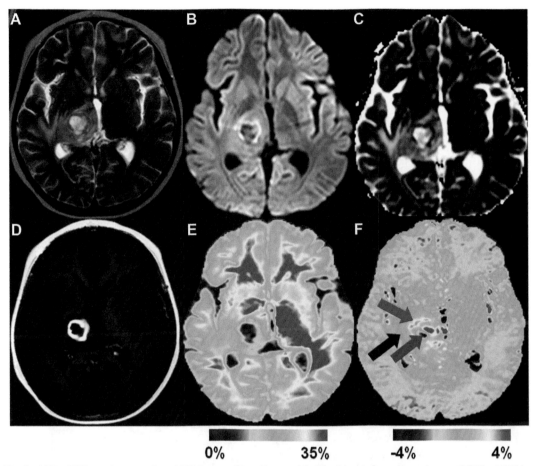

0%   35%   -4%   4%

Fig. 3. APTw, MTR, and conventional MR images for a 7-year-old girl with a tuberculous abscess. (*A*) The T2W image shows an irregular lesion with surrounding edema in the right thalamus. (*B*) DWI and (*C*) ADC map show restricted diffusion along the periphery and some contents of the lesion. (*D*) Gd-T1W image demonstrates an enhancing rim and nonenhancing necrotic center. (*E*) MTR signals are low in the gadolinium-enhancing rim and surrounding edema. (*F*) APTw image shows that the enhancing rim (*red arrow*) is hyperintense, whereas the necrotic region (*pink arrow*) and surrounding edema (*black arrow*) have equally low APTw signals. (Reproduced with permission from Zhang et al. Biomed Res Int 2020;2020: P6418343.)

glioma treatment effects.[48–51] Jiang and colleagues[52] have also demonstrated that APTw MR can differentiate primary CNS lymphoma from high-grade gliomas. APTw can also distinguish grade II gliomas of IDH-wild-type and IDH-mutant type, which is helpful when determining patient prognosis.[53] Notably, APTw MR–guided stereotactic biopsy can identify high-grade regions with high-cell density and cell proliferation in heterogeneous gliomas, which is helpful in improving the accuracy of tumor tissue sampling by neurosurgical neuronavigation.[9,12]

A major draw of APTw imaging in pediatric brain tumors is the avoidance intravenous gadolinium contrast. The authors have used a 3D APTw imaging sequence to evaluate the diagnostic performance of APTw imaging compared with DWI in children with brain tumors. Thirty-five children with brain tumors (19 boys and 16 girls; age range, 3–172 months) were included in the study. Two examples are shown in **Figs. 5** and **6**. The mean APTw values of high-grade brain tumors were higher than that of low-grade brain tumors, and the difference was statistically significant. Mean APTw was positively correlated with the Ki-67 expression level. The authors found that, although the maximum and minimum APTw values of high-grade brain tumors were slightly higher than those of low-grade brain tumors, the difference was not statistically significant. Receiver operating characteristic curve analysis showed that the diagnostic accuracy of mean APTw for the identification of high-grade brain tumors was low, which may be due to the special pathologic features of brain tumors in children. The apparent diffusion coefficient

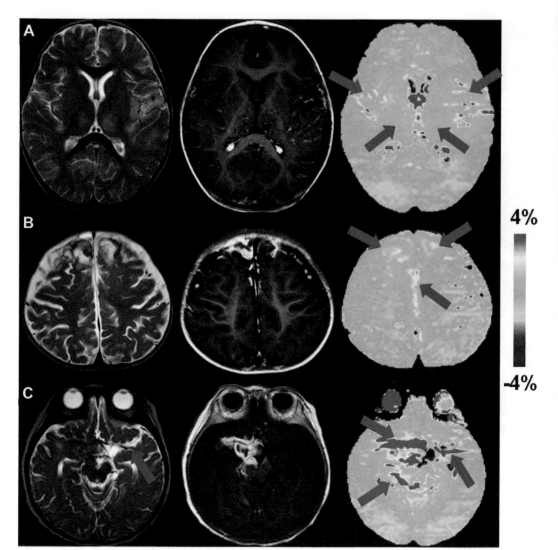

Fig. 4. APTw and conventional MR images for 3 patients with meningitis. (*A*) T2W, Gd-T1W, and APTw images (*left to right*) for a 17-month-old girl with viral meningoencephalitis. The gadolinium-enhancing thalamic lesions (*pink arrows*) and leptomeninges (*red arrows*) show slight hyperintensity on the APTw image. (*B*) T2W, Gd-T1W, and APTw images for a 9-month-old girl with pyogenic meningitis. Consistent with Gd-T1W, the APTw image shows hyperintensity over the frontal convexities (*red arrows*) and adjacent cerebral falx (*pink arrow*). (*C*) T2W, Gd-T1W, and APTw images for a 7-month-old boy with tuberculous meningitis. The enhancing leptomeninges show hyperintensity on the APTw image (*red arrows*), along with the left sylvian vallecula and temporal lobe (*pink arrow*) associated with the left middle cerebral artery. (Reproduced with permission from Zhang et al. Biomed Res Int 2020;2020:P6418343.)

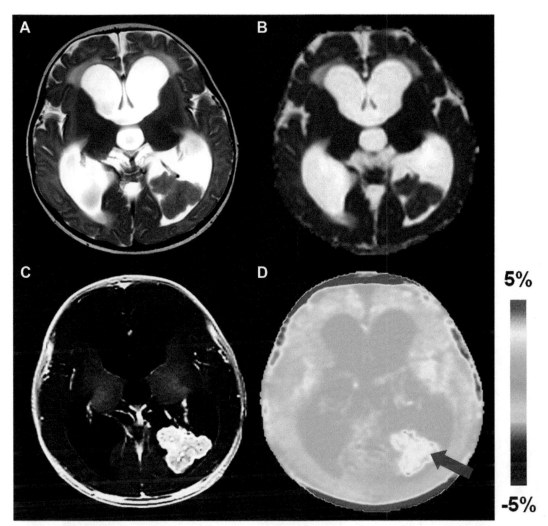

Fig. 5. APTw and conventional MR images for a 3-month-old boy with choroid plexus papilloma (World Health Organization [WHO] grade I). (*A*) T2W image shows an irregular tumor (*pink arrow*) in the left lateral ventricle. (*B*) ADC map with mean tumor value of 1.23×10^{-3} mm^2/s. (*C*) Gd-T1W image reveals obvious postcontrast enhancement. (*D*) APTw image shows a slightly elevated signal. The mean APTw value of the mass was 2.49%. All data were acquired on a Philips Ingenia 3.0 T CX MR imaging system.

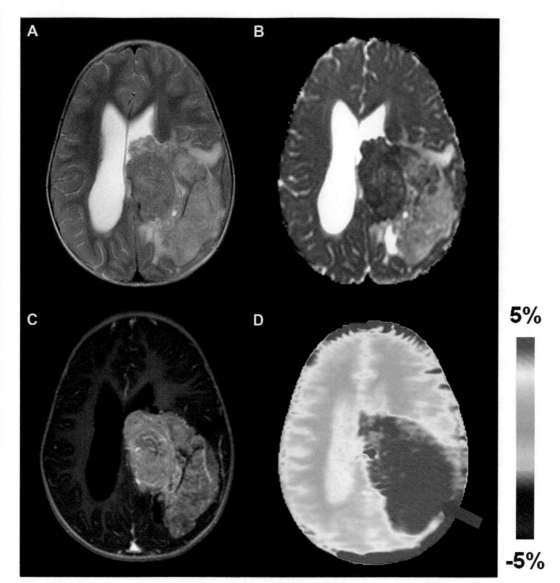

Fig. 6. APTw and conventional MR images for a 24-month-old girl with choroid plexus carcinoma (WHO grade III). (A) T2W image shows a large irregular mass (*pink arrow*) in the left lateral ventricle. (B) ADC map shows mean tumor value of 0.91×10^{-3} mm²/s. (C) Gd-T1W image reveals marked postcontrast enhancement. (D) APTw image shows a markedly high signal. The mean APTw value of the mass was 4.2%. All data were acquired on a Philips Ingenia 3.0 T CX MR imaging system.

(ADC) value had a higher diagnostic accuracy. The most common low-grade brain tumors in children are pilocytic astrocytoma, pilomyxoid astrocytoma, and diffuse astrocytoma. These low-grade tumors usually have microcysts, mucoid degeneration, or microvascular hyperplasia,[54] which can cause an increase in APTw signal and reduce the diagnostic accuracy for tumor grading. However, at present there are few articles in the literature, and the value of APTw

imaging in pediatric brain tumors requires further study.

Finally, the authors have explored the potential of APTw imaging in differentiating infectious and neoplastic lesions in children. The results showed that the APTw values of infectious lesions were significantly lower than that of neoplastic lesions. The best cutoff value for APTw in the discrimination of neoplastic and infective masses was 2.30%, with respective sensitivity and specificity of 88.6% and 70.8%, and an area under the curve of 0.857.

SUMMARY

APTw imaging is a relatively new protein-based molecular MR imaging technique. The technique has the potential for noninvasive protein content imaging and pH imaging. APTw MR imaging, which does not require intravenous contrast, has great potential as an alternative to gadolinium-enhanced MRI in the pediatric population. Brain tumors in children show a large histopathologic spectrum, such that grading and differential diagnosis of brain tumors with APTw requires further study. In the future, APTw imaging may be applied to more pediatric CNS diseases, such as infection, stroke, demyelinating disorders, traumatic brain injury, and metabolic encephalopathies.

DISCLOSURE

An imaging device used in the study described in this article is manufactured by Philips. Under a license agreement between Philips and the Johns Hopkins University, Dr J. Zhou and the University are entitled to fees and royalties from Philips. Dr J. Zhou is also a paid scientific speaker for Philips. This arrangement has been reviewed and approved by the Johns Hopkins University in accordance with its conflict of interest policies.

REFERENCES

1. Zhou J, Payen J, Wilson DA, et al. Using the amide proton signals of intracellular proteins and peptides to detect pH effects in MRI. Nat Med 2003;9: 1085–90.
2. Zhou J, Lal B, Wilson DA, et al. Amide proton transfer (APT) contrast for imaging of brain tumors. Magn Reson Med 2003;50:1120–6.
3. Zhou J, Heo H-Y, Knutsson L, et al. APT-weighted MRI: techniques, current neuro applications, and challenging issues. J Magn Reson Imaging 2019. https://doi.org/10.1002/jmri.26645.
4. Ward KM, Aletras AH, Balaban RS. A new class of contrast agents for MRI based on proton chemical exchange dependent saturation transfer (CEST). J Magn Reson 2000;143:79–87.
5. Zhou J, van Zijl PC. Chemical exchange saturation transfer imaging and spectroscopy. Progr NMR Spectr 2006;48:109–36.
6. Sherry AD, Woods M. Chemical exchange saturation transfer contrast agents for magnetic resonance imaging. Annu Rev Biomed Eng 2008;10:391–411.
7. Jones KM, Pollard AC, Pagel MD. Clinical applications of chemical exchange saturation transfer

8. Yan K, Fu Z, Yang C, et al. Assessing amide proton transfer (APT) MRI contrast origins in 9L gliosarcoma in the rat brain using proteomic analysis. Mol Imaging Biol 2015;17:479–87.
9. Jiang S, Eberhart CG, Zhang Y, et al. Amide proton transfer-weighted MR image-guided stereotactic biopsy in patients with newly diagnosed gliomas. Eur J Cancer 2017;83:9–18.
10. Choi YS, Ahn SS, Lee SK, et al. Amide proton transfer imaging to discriminate between low- and high-grade gliomas: added value to apparent diffusion coefficient and relative cerebral blood volume. Eur Radiol 2017;27:3181–9.
11. Togao O, Hiwatashi A, Yamashita K, et al. Grading diffuse gliomas without intense contrast enhancement by amide proton transfer MR imaging: comparisons with diffusion- and perfusion-weighted imaging. Eur Radiol 2017;27:578–88.
12. Jiang S, Eberhart CG, Lim M, et al. Identifying recurrent malignant glioma after treatment using amide proton transfer-weighted MR imaging: a validation study with image-guided stereotactic biopsy. Clin Cancer Res 2019;25:552–61.
13. Sun PZ, Zhou J, Sun W, et al. Detection of the ischemic penumbra using pH-weighted MRI. J Cereb Blood Flow Metab 2007;27:1129–36.
14. Harston GW, Tee YK, Blockley N, et al. Identifying the ischaemic penumbra using pH-weighted magnetic resonance imaging. Brain 2015;138:36–42.
15. Heo HY, Zhang Y, Burton TM, et al. Improving the detection sensitivity of pH-weighted amide proton transfer MRI in acute stroke patients using extrapolated semisolid magnetization transfer reference signals. Magn Reson Med 2017;78:871–80.
16. Mori S, Eleff SM, Pilatus U, et al. Proton NMR spectroscopy of solvent-saturable resonance: a new approach to study pH effects in situ. Magn Reson Med 1998;40:36–42.
17. Wolff SD, Balaban RS. Magnetization transfer contrast (MTC) and tissue water proton relaxation in vivo. Magn Reson Med 1989;10:135–44.
18. Henkelman RM, Stanisz GJ, Graham SJ. Magnetization transfer in MRI: a review. NMR Biomed 2001;14: 57–64.
19. Hua J, Jones CK, Blakeley J, et al. Quantitative description of the asymmetry in magnetization transfer effects around the water resonance in the human brain. Magn Reson Med 2007;58:786–93.
20. Ling W, Regatte RR, Navon G, et al. Assessment of glycosaminoglycan concentration in vivo by chemical exchange-dependent saturation transfer (gagCEST). Proc Natl Acad Sci U S A 2008;105(7): 2266–70.
21. Zhou J, Hong X, Zhao X, et al. APT-weighted and NOE-weighted image contrasts in glioma with

different RF saturation powers based on magnetization transfer ratio asymmetry analyses. Magn Reson Med 2013;70(2):320–7.

22. Zhou J, Blakeley JO, Hua J, et al. Practical data acquisition method for human brain tumor amide proton transfer (APT) imaging. Magn Reson Med 2008;60:842–9.

23. Wen Z, Hu S, Huang F, et al. MR imaging of high-grade brain tumors using endogenous protein and peptide-based contrast. NeuroImage 2010;51: 616–22.

24. Li C, Peng S, Wang R, et al. Chemical exchange saturation transfer MR imaging of Parkinson's disease at 3 Tesla. Eur Radiol 2014;24(10):2631–9.

25. Zhu H, Jones CK, van Zijl PCM, et al. Fast 3D chemical exchange saturation transfer (CEST) imaging of the human brain. Magn Reson Med 2010;64:638–44.

26. Heo HY, Xu X, Jiang S, et al. Prospective acceleration of parallel RF transmission-based 3D chemical exchange saturation transfer imaging with compressed sensing. Magn Reson Med 2019;82:1812–21.

27. Zhang Y, Heo HY, Jiang S, et al. Fast 3D chemical exchange saturation transfer imaging with variably-accelerated sensitivity encoding (vSENSE). Magn Reson Med 2019;82:2046–61.

28. U.S. Food and Drug Administration. Available at: https://www.accessdata.fda.gov/cdrh_docs/pdf17/K172920.pdf.

29. Zhou J, Wilson DA, Sun PZ, et al. Quantitative description of proton exchange processes between water and endogenous and exogenous agents for WEX, CEST, and APT experiments. Magn Reson Med 2004;51(5):945–52.

30. Lee DH, Heo HY, Zhang K, et al. Quantitative assessment of the effects of water proton concentration and water T1 changes on amide proton transfer (APT) and nuclear Overhauser enhancement (NOE) MRI: the origin of the APT imaging signal in brain tumor. Magn Reson Med 2017;77(2):855–63.

31. Heo HY, Lee DH, Zhang Y, et al. Insight into the quantitative metrics of chemical exchange saturation transfer (CEST) imaging. Magn Reson Med 2017;77(5):1853–65.

32. Zu Z. Towards the complex dependence of MTRasym on T1w in amide proton transfer (APT) imaging. NMR Biomed 2018;31(7):e3934.

33. Zhang H, Kang H, Zhao X, et al. Amide proton transfer (APT) MR imaging and magnetization transfer (MT) MR imaging of pediatric brain development. Eur Radiol 2016;26(10):3368–76.

34. Tang X, Zhang H, Zhou J, et al. Brain development in children with developmental delay using amide proton transfer-weighted imaging and magnetization transfer imaging. Pediatr Investig 2020;4(4):250–6.

35. Zheng Y, Wang X, Zhao X. Magnetization transfer and amide proton transfer MRI of neonatal brain development. Biomed Res Int 2016;2016:3052723.

36. Zheng Y, Wang XM. Measurement of lactate content and amide proton transfer values in the basal ganglia of a neonatal piglet hypoxic-ischemic brain injury model using MRI. AJNR Am J Neuroradiol 2017;38(4):827–34.

37. Chen S, Liu X, Mei Y, et al. Early identification of neonatal mild hypoxic-ischemic encephalopathy by amide proton transfer magnetic resonance imaging: a pilot study. Eur J Radiol 2019;119:108620.

38. Hedlund GL, Boyer RS. Neuroimaging of postnatal pediatric central nervous system infections. Semin Pediatr Neurol 1999;6(4):299–317.

39. Karagulle-Kendi AT, Truwit C. Neuroimaging of central nervous system infections. Handb Clin Neurol 2010;96:239–55.

40. Swinburne NC, Bansal AG, Aggarwal A, et al. Neuroimaging in central nervous system infections. Curr Neurol Neurosci Rep 2017;17(6):49.

41. Hu HH, Pokorney A, Towbin RB, et al. Increased signal intensities in the dentate nucleus and globus pallidus on unenhanced T1-weighted images: evidence in children undergoing multiple gadolinium MRI exams. Pediatr Radiol 2016;46(11):1590–8.

42. Roberts DR, Holden KR. Progressive increase of T1 signal intensity in the dentate nucleus and globus pallidus on unenhanced T1-weighted MR images in the pediatric brain exposed to multiple doses of gadolinium contrast. Brain Dev 2016;38(3):331–6.

43. Zhang H, Tang X, Lv Y, et al. Amide proton transfer-weighted (APTw) imaging of intracranial infection in children: initial experience and comparison with gadolinium-enhanced T1-weighted imaging. Biomed Res Int 2020;2020:6418343.

44. Panigrahy A, Bluml S. Neuroimaging of pediatric brain tumors: from basic to advanced magnetic resonance imaging (MRI). J Child Neurol 2009; 24(11):1343–65.

45. Zhou J, Zhu H, Lim M, et al. Three-dimensional amide proton transfer MR imaging of gliomas: initial experience and comparison with gadolinium enhancement. J Magn Reson Imaging 2013;38: 1119–28.

46. Togao O, Yoshiura T, Keupp J, et al. Amide proton transfer imaging of adult diffuse gliomas: correlation with histopathological grades. Neuro Oncol 2014; 16(3):441–8.

47. Sakata A, Okada T, Yamamoto A, et al. Grading glial tumors with amide proton transfer MR imaging: different analytical approaches. J Neurooncol 2015;122(2):339–48.

48. Zhou J, Tryggestad E, Wen Z, et al. Differentiation between glioma and radiation necrosis using molecular magnetic resonance imaging of endogenous proteins and peptides. Nat Med 2011;17:130–4.

49. Hong X, Liu L, Wang M, et al. Quantitative multiparametric MRI assessment of glioma response to

radiotherapy in a rat model. Neuro Oncol 2014; 16(6):856–67.

50. Ma B, Blakeley JO, Hong X, et al. Applying amide proton transfer-weighted MRI to distinguish pseudo-progression from true progression in malignant gliomas. J Magn Reson Imaging 2016;44(2):456–62.

51. Park JE, Kim HS, Park SY, et al. Identification of early response to anti-angiogenic therapy in recurrent glioblastoma: amide proton transfer-weighted and perfusion-weighted MRI compared with diffusion-weighted MRI. Radiology 2020;295(2):397–406.

52. Jiang S, Yu H, Wang X, et al. Molecular MRI differentiation between primary central nervous system lymphomas and high-grade gliomas using endogenous protein-based amide proton transfer MR imaging at 3 Tesla. Eur Radiol 2016;26(1):64–71.

53. Jiang S, Zou T, Eberhart CG, et al. Predicting IDH mutation status in grade II gliomas using amide proton transfer-weighted (APTw) MRI. Magn Reson Med 2017;78:1100–9.

54. Rodriguez FJ, Lim KS, Bowers D, et al. Pathological and molecular advances in pediatric low-grade astrocytoma. Annu Rev Pathol 2013;8:361–79.

Ultra-High-Field Imaging of the Pediatric Brain and Spinal Cord

Dinesh Kumar Deelchand, PhD[a], Mai-Lan Ho, MD[b], Igor Nestrasil, MD, PhD[c],*

KEYWORDS

- 7T • High field • Brain • Spinal cord • Pediatric • MR spectroscopy • Ultra-high-field

KEY POINTS

- Ultra-high field imaging provides superior signal-to-noise ratio, spatial resolution, and tissue contrast.
- Disadvantages include greater safety concerns, longer scanning times, and increased distortion and field inhomogeneity.
- Brain and spinal cord microstructure and function are revealed in greater detail, enabling superior lesion detection, delineation, and characterization.
- Greater accuracy in diagnostics, surgical planning, and treatment monitoring can impact clinical practice.

Neuroimaging at ultra-high-field (UHF) ($\geq$7 Tesla) provides superior signal-to-noise and contrast-to-noise ratios, as well as increased spatial resolution and tissue contrast. Trade-offs include greater safety concerns (higher specific absorption rate [SAR]), potentially longer scanning times, and increased distortion and field inhomogeneity. In this article, we discuss the technical considerations, challenges, and risks of ultra-high-field scanning in children, followed by practical clinical examples and a discussion of future potential in pediatric research.

TECHNICAL CONSIDERATIONS

Since the invention of MRI,[1] there have been a wealth of technical advancements including stronger magnetic (B_0) field strength, high performance and efficient gradient coils, better radiofrequency (RF) coils for transmission and reception, and faster acquisition and reconstruction techniques.[2] MR imaging techniques that have greatly benefited from these improvements include structural MR imaging, functional MR imaging[3] and diffusion MR imaging.[3] Functional MR imaging provides an indirect measure of brain activity by monitoring change in blood oxygen level–dependent response during specific tasks/stimuli or at rest. Diffusion MR imaging can be used to assess brain microstructure and white matter architecture. These techniques have been a major topic of research in the last decade, for example in the Human Connectome Project.

Proton (^{1}H) MR spectroscopy measures the biochemistry of several metabolites present in specific cell types, such as neuronal or glial, within the *in vivo* brain.[4,5] *N*-acetyl-aspartate, total creatine (creatine plus phosphocreatine), total choline (phosphorylcholine plus glycerophosphorylcholine), glutamate (Glu), and *myo*-inositol are the most commonly measured neurochemicals in the brain owing to their high concentrations or peak intensities.[6] Metabolites such as glutamine, γ-aminobutyric acid (GABA), lactate, and ascorbate are also present in the brain, but, owing to their

[a] Department of Radiology, Center for Magnetic Resonance Research, University of Minnesota, 2021 6th Street Southeast, Minneapolis, MN 55455, USA; [b] Department of Radiology, Nationwide Children's Hospital, 700 Children's Drive, Columbus, OH 43205, USA; [c] Masonic Institute for the Developing Brain, Division of Clinical Behavioral Neuroscience, Department of Pediatrics, University of Minnesota, 2025 East River Parkway, Minneapolis, MN 55414, USA
* Corresponding author.
E-mail address: nestr007@umn.edu

Magn Reson Imaging Clin N Am 29 (2021) 643–653
https://doi.org/10.1016/j.mric.2021.06.013
1064-9689/21/© 2021 Elsevier Inc. All rights reserved.

complex spectral pattern from J-coupling and low concentrations, cannot be reliably measured at low B_0 fields.[7] MR spectroscopy data can be measured using either single-voxel spectroscopy (SVS)[8] or multivoxel MR spectroscopic imaging.[9] SVS is the most commonly used technique, but is limited to a single volume of interest. In comparison, multivoxel data are acquired simultaneously from several volumes of interest covering a single or multiple slices. In general, SVS spectra have greater spectral quality owing to localization accuracy (better spatial response function), optimized B_0 inhomogeneity compensation, and efficient water suppression in the specific volume of interest.[10]

One of the most crucial components of an MR imaging scanner is the main B_0 field that dictates the signal-to-noise ratio (SNR) of the MR images. Based on this principle, MR researchers have been steadily moving toward UHF imaging. Studies have reported that the increase in SNR can scale supralinearly with B_0.[11–13] In the clinical settings, 1.5T and 3T scanners are routine, while in the research settings, UHF scanners (eg, 7, 8, and 9.4T) have been commonly used since the early 2000s. In 2017, the first 7T MR imaging scanner (Magnetom Terra, Siemens Healthineers, Erlangen, Germany) obtained 510(k) clearance from the US Food and Drug Administration for limited clinical use to scan the head and upper/lower extremities. Currently, all major MRI vendors offer a 7 Tesla MRI platform. The highest field human MR imaging scanners measure 10.5T,[14] located at the Center for Magnetic Resonance Center (University of Minnesota, Minneapolis, MN) (installed in 2014); and two 11.7T scanners (installed in 2019), located at the National Institutes of Health (Bethesda, MD) and NeuroSpin (CEA Paris-Saclay, France).

The gain in SNR with increasing B_0 produces higher spatial resolution, leading to improved tissue contrast in MR imaging. With multiple receive coils, the total scan time can be further reduced using simultaneous multislice[15] and parallel imaging techniques such as SENSE[16] and GRAPPA.[17] In MR spectroscopy studies, there is improved precision when quantifying neurochemicals, as reflected by the Cramer-Rao Lower bounds.[18] This improvement is related to an increase in chemical shift dispersion, resulting in less overlap between resonances. For example, C4 proton resonances of Glu and glutamine can be resolved at 7T and beyond in the brain.[19] In addition, J-coupled spectral patterns are simplified owing to an increase in spectral linewidth (mostly from microscopic susceptibility effects) with the magnetic field. For example, the C4 proton resonance of Glu will look like a singlet at 11.7T instead of multiplets at 3T.[18]

The major challenges when moving to UHF MR imaging/MR spectroscopy include increased SAR and inhomogeneous RF transmit (B_1^+) field. Because SAR increases roughly quadratically with B_0, all MR imaging scanners are required to operate within the RF safety limits imposed by the US Food and Drug Administration guidelines for participant safety during an MR imaging scan. Methods to decrease SAR include the use of longer repetition time, decreasing flip angles, or use of parallel imaging techniques. The B_1^+ inhomogeneity at UHF can be compensated when using multiple transmit RF coils with B_1^+ shimming techniques,[20] but this technique requires a system with multiple transmit channels. In clinical settings, this option is generally not feasible owing to additional scan time and patient SAR safety concerns. For a single transmit channel, the use of dielectric pads can partially mitigate the B_1^+ issue at UHF.[21]

Another challenge when going to UHF is that the transverse (T_2) relaxation times of water and metabolites become shorter. For instance, the apparent T_2 times of water tissue in the occipital lobe are reported to be 60 ms at 7T compared with 83 ms at 4T.[22] Interestingly, the T_2 relaxation times of metabolites with singlet peaks follow an exponential behavior with B_0 fields.[23] These findings suggest that short echo-time MR imaging/MR spectroscopy sequences are necessary to maintain the benefits of using UHF.

Several MR imaging pulse sequences are provided by MR vendors on UHF scanners, including 2-dimensional/3-dimensional ultrafast gradient echo and 2-dimensional/3-dimensional turbo spin-echo for T_1-weighted and T_2-weighted structural images. Many acquisition parameters, such as echo-time, repetition time, field of view, and number of slices, can be modified by end-users.

In MR spectroscopy studies, owing to the increase in chemical shift dispersion with B_0, higher bandwidth RF pulses are required to decrease chemical shift displacement errors.[8] Suitable pulse sequences at UHF include semi-LASER[24] and semi-adiabatic SPECIAL,[25] which utilize large bandwidth adiabatic refocusing pulses. In addition, gradient-modulated RF pulses such as FOCI[26] or GOIA[27] adiabatic pulses can be used to decrease the required B_1^+ fields,[28] thereby also decreasing the SAR.

Several considerations need to be taken into account when imaging children at UHF. One of the primary safety concerns is RF heating. Neonates and infants are most sensitive to these effects because they generally have a higher core body temperature, in addition to underdeveloped thermoregulation mechanisms. Furthermore, children have a greater body surface area to body weight ratio compared with adults, which results in more surface area exposure to the RF field and thus increased heating. All these effects may contribute to inaccurate prediction of SAR limits by conventional MR platforms. A final safety risk involves indwelling metallic devices that may malfunction in the magnetic field and cause distortion and artifacts in the MR images.

It is often difficult for children to remain still during lengthy MR imaging exams, which can induce anxiety and/or claustrophobia. Motion in MR imaging results in ghosting or blurring, thereby degrading image quality. In MR spectroscopy, motion results in inaccurate volume-of-interest localization and degrades the spectral quality. During diagnostic MR scans, sedation or general anesthesia may be required, leading to higher patient costs and risks of adverse events.[29,30] Strategies for minimizing sedation include child life specialists to prepare children for MRI, having a parent present in the examination room, and the use of video goggles to watch movies while in the scanner.[30,31] Prospective motion correction techniques can utilize external devices, for example, optical camera[32] and field probes[33] or internal image-based navigators based on spiral[34] or volumetric echo-planar imaging.[35]

Safety Precautions

Appropriate safety screening is a *conditio sine qua non* for all individuals before entering the MR scanner. Safety information is available for the majority of metallic devices and implants at 1.5 and 3T field strengths, but only selected models have undergone standardized testing at 7T and may thus require additional local testing and physicist expertise.[36]

Exposure to high or ultra-high magnetic fields also produces transient physiologic changes. These bioeffects are more pronounced at UHF and most commonly include nausea, vertigo, headache, tingling, numbness, visual disturbances such as magnetophosphenes (light spots in front of one's eyes), pain around tooth fillings, and electrogustatory effects (metallic taste).[37] Based on our experience, 7T tolerability is comparable to that at 3T in children greater than 8 years of age.

Practical Aspects of Pediatric Neuroimaging at Ultra-High-Field

At UHF, higher SNR, contrast-to-noise ratio, and spatial resolution of anatomic imaging, as well as enhanced sensitivity and spectral resolution of spectroscopy, has several exciting potential applications in the pediatric brain and spinal cord.

MR SPECTROSCOPY

[1]H MR spectroscopy with short TE at 7T field strength can quantify at least 18 established neurometabolites.[5] Reliable measures of lower-concentration metabolites (eg, gamma-aminobutyric acid (GABA) 1–2 mmol/L, glutathione [GSH] 2–3 mmol/L in human brain)[38] create opportunities to diagnose diseases with greater sensitivity, longitudinally track disease status, predict patient prognosis, and monitor therapeutic response.

Disruption of neurotransmitter balances occurs in many neurologic or psychiatric conditions including mood disorders, autism spectrum disorder, addiction, epilepsy, sleep, and movement disorders. For example, inhibitory GABA has been detected in the striatum at lower concentrations in individuals with autism spectrum disorder, in depressed (not remitted) patients with major depressive disorder,[39,40] and attention deficit hyperactivity disorder at 7T.[41,42] Excitatory Glu is increased in children with Tourette syndrome,[43] and can be either increased or decreased in autism spectrum disorder.[40]

Quantification of neurotransmitters is clinically relevant in the diagnosis and treatment monitoring of epilepsy. Therapeutic effects have been shown in patients with focal epilepsy responsive to the antiepileptic drug levetiracetam.[44] The patients showed a gradual increase of GABA concentration corresponding to drug dose titration. Similar findings have been detected for other antiepileptic drugs, such as topiramate or gabapentin.[45]

Measurement of neurotransmitter concentrations may also serve for therapeutic response monitoring in noninvasive brain stimulation. Repetitive transcranial direct current or magnetic brain stimulations can modulate cortical activity in a broad spectrum of conditions including mood disorders, motion disorders, and obesity.[46,47] In feasibility studies of healthy volunteers, brain stimulation was followed by changes in GABA and Glu concentrations assessed by ^{1}H MR spectroscopy,[46,47] representing potential biomarkers for efficacy monitoring.

MR spectroscopy can yield detailed biochemical information regarding brain metabolism in neurologic conditions. This knowledge can be used for clinical diagnosis and management, for example tumor grading directing image-guided surgery or radiation.[48] The SVS approach is ideal for small to medium-sized lesions, but multivoxel spectroscopy covering larger areas can better assess heterogeneous or diffuse tumors. Hypoxia and ischemia in tumor, stroke, and metabolic conditions result in increased lactate concentrations that can be assessed by MR spectroscopy in UHF[5] serving as a marker of anaerobic glycolysis.

Another low concentration neurometabolite detected on MR spectroscopy at UHF is GSH. GSH is an indicator of oxidative status and intrinsic cell protection to products of oxidative stress, such as reactive oxygen species. Oxidative stress plays a pivotal role in apoptosis and neurodegeneration, implicated in many neurologic disorders (Fig. 1). The quantification of GSH is challenging at conventional field strengths owing to overlap with resonances of other more concentrated compounds,[5,49,50] but can be reliably detected at UHF. In a study of an antioxidant agent, N-acetylcysteine (NAC), GSH concentrations measured by ^{1}H MR spectroscopy on 7T were boosted by orally administered NAC. This study served as a proof of concept, showing the effects of NAC on GSH concentration in brain and the ability to monitor treatment response by MR spectroscopy.[51]

Beyond ^{1}H MR spectroscopy, other nuclei can be targeted to explore energy metabolism using ^{13}C, [17]O, and ^{31}P, or electrolytes and cell viability using [23]Na, [35]Cl, and [39]K.[52–54] The clinical benefits of X-nuclei MR imaging and spectroscopy are still emerging.

HIGH SPATIAL AND CONTRAST RESOLUTION

Increased lesion conspicuity and detection owing to fine structural detail can be achieved by UHF (Fig. 2). For epilepsy, 7T can better reveal lesions in 1.5T or 3T MR imaging-negative cases. About 30% of patients with drug-resistant focal epilepsy have negative findings when scanned at lower magnetic field strength. Utilization of standardized protocols as recommended by the 7T Epilepsy Task Force provides optimal presurgical assessment with UHF for epileptogenic focus detection and characterization (Figs. 3 and 4). Mesoscopic-level functional cortical mapping of the eloquent cortex helps to minimize postoperative morbidity.[55,56]

Surgical planning before deep brain stimulation benefits from enhanced substructure anatomic detail possible at UHF, which can identify the subthalamic nucleus,[57] pars interna of globus pallidus,[58] thalamic nuclei,[59] and other targets to treat pediatric and adult movement disorders.[60]

In neuro-oncology, UHF has a number of diagnostic and surgical planning applications (Fig. 4). These include pituitary imaging for more sensitive detection of microadenomas, brain metastases, leptomeningeal infiltration, neoplasia involving the orbits or posterior fossa, and follow-up evaluation of postoperative changes versus tumor. Susceptibility-weighted imaging or T2* contrast also permit visualization of tumor hemorrhage and microvascularity[61] (Fig. 5).

Susceptibility-weighted imaging and quantitative susceptibility mapping measure the intrinsic magnetic susceptibility of tissue. The magnitude signal loss and phase information help characterize iron- or calcium-rich tissues, detect blood products, and visualize macro- and micro-vasculature.[62,63] Traumatic brain injury, arteriovenous malformations (Fig. 6), vascular dementia, multiple sclerosis, and tumors can all be better characterized with susceptibility-weighted imaging. Central vein visualization in multiple sclerosis is useful for lesion characterization (Fig. 7).[61,62]

MR ANGIOGRAPHY

Digital subtraction angiography is the gold standard for neurovascular assessment, but is far more invasive than MR angiography or CT angiography.[39] At UHF, higher SNR and longer T1 relaxation times leading to augmented vessel-background tissue signal differences result in improved MR angiography image quality.[61] Small perforating vessels can be detected on the submillimeter scale. Potential evaluation of vessel lumina and walls may further elucidate disease pathophysiology in a number of conditions.[64]

STRUCTURAL AND FUNCTIONAL CONNECTIVITY

Presurgical planning can benefit from the increased sensitivity and resolution of advanced techniques for structural (diffusion-weighted imaging and tractography) and functional (fMRI) connectivity. Clinical fMRI at 7T shows higher functional sensitivity than 3T when mapping eloquent areas.[65] Neuronal networks may be specifically altered in various neuropsychiatric disorders, potentially useful for diagnostics and treatment monitoring. Tractography-assisted surgical neuronavigation enhances characterization of brain subregional anatomy and identification of white matter tracts for precise resection or electrode placement.[58,59,66,67]

CHEMICAL EXCHANGE SATURATION TRANSFER

In chemical exchange saturation transfer (CEST), tissues containing exchangeable solute ^{1}H protons are selectively saturated using an RF pulse. Repeated transfer (chemical exchange) of RF excitation occurs from saturated solute protons to

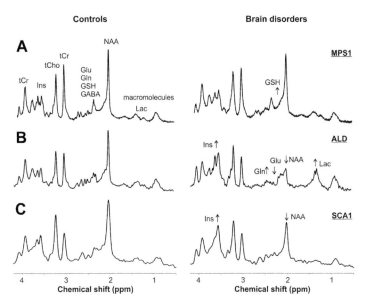

Fig. 1. Representative in vivo proton MR spectra acquired for different brain disorders. (*A*) Left, healthy control (11-year-old girl); right, patient with mucopolysaccharidosis type I (mild form, Scheie syndrome) (MPS1: 12-year-old girl). Data were acquired from the right hippocampus (4.3 mL) at 7T using semi-LASER sequence (TE/TR = 26/5000 ms, 96 transients). Dielectric padding was used for the acquisition. A higher GSH concentration in MPS versus control (1.365 vs 0.997 mmol/L; CRLB <7%) may indicate a protective response against the oxidative stress previously reported in lysosomal diseases. (*B*) Left, asymptomatic patient with adrenoleukodystrophy (ALD; 6-year-old); right, patient with cerebral ALD (9-year-old). Data were acquired from the occipital white matter at 4T using STEAM (TE/TR = 5/4500 ms). Changes in *N*-acetylaspartate (NAA), myo-inositol, glutamate (Glu), glutamine (Gln), and lactate (Lac) were observed in the lesion in ALD patient compared with a normal WM region in asymptomatic patient. (*C*) Left, a healthy control (47-year-old man); right, patient with spinocerebellar ataxia type 1 (SCA1; 47-year-old man). Data were acquired from the pontine (4 mL) at 3T using semi-LASER (TE/TR = 28/5000 ms, 64 transients). Changes in NAA and *myo*-inositol levels are clearly visible between the control and the patient.

protons in the surrounding bulk water, reaching an eventual equilibrium that can be detected as bulk water signal attenuation.[68,69] UHF benefits in CEST imaging include increased chemical shift dispersion resulting in better separation of metabolites with similar MR properties (spectral overlap), for example Glu and amide. Another factor is longer T1 relaxation time of water, allowing a longer accumulation of saturated protons in the water pool with more detectable CEST effect.[52,69]

Amide (NH) or amine (NH$_2$) proton transfers are associated with intracellular pH. Altered pH can be seen in conditions such as cerebrovascular stroke, tumors, neurodegeneration, or multiple sclerosis. Creatine, lactate, glutamate, glutamine, glycogene, urea, and exogenous agents (eg, D-glucose or iopamidol) are other molecules or compounds that are under development for potential clinical translation.[70]

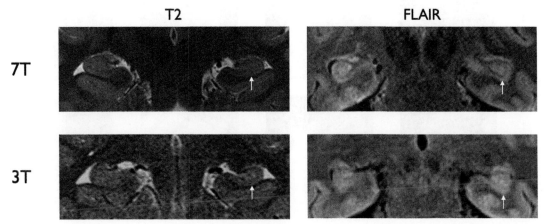

Fig. 2. Mesial temporal sclerosis at 3T and 7T field strengths. Coronal T2-weighted and fluid-attenuated inversion recovery (FLAIR) images of left mesial temporal sclerosis (*arrows*). At 7T, increased spatial and contrast resolution better demonstrates the subtle hippocampal volume loss and disruption of internal architecture.

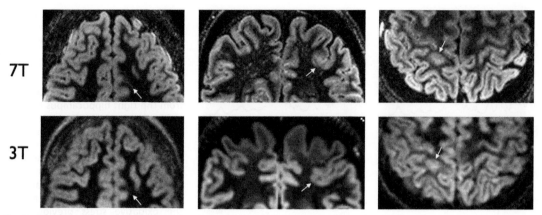

Fig. 3. Multiple examples of cortical dysplasia at 3T and 7T field strengths using fluid-attenuated inversion recovery (FLAIR). At 7T, improved spatial and contrast resolution better demonstrates dysgyria, gray-white blurring, and transmantle signal abnormality (*arrows*).

SPINAL CORD IMAGING

MR imaging and spectroscopy of the spinal cord, which measures 1.0 to 1.5 cm in diameter, can benefit from UHF. Clinical application remains challenging owing to RF B_1 field inhomogeneities, physiologic noise effects, suboptimal RF coils, and B_0 field shimming.[71] As advanced imaging of the spinal cord at 3T has increased,[72–75] exploratory imaging of the spinal cord at UHF continues to progress. Recently, imaging of the spinal cord in 7T has been used for manual lesion quantification in multiple sclerosis. Lesions were most commonly identified near the central canal and subpial CSF interface.[76] 7T feasibility studies have also investigated anatomic T1 mapping with MP2RAGE sequence and ^{1}H MR spectroscopy with semi-LASER sequence.[77,78]

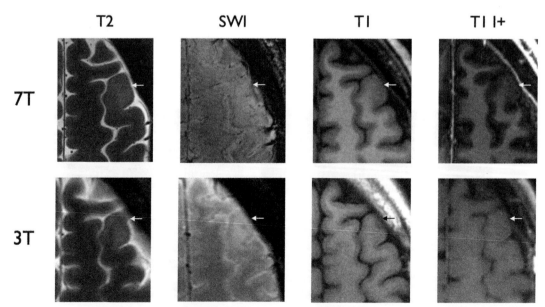

Fig. 4. Low-grade glioma at 3T and 7T field strengths. Axial T2-weighted, susceptibility weighted imaging (SWI), T1-weighted, and postcontrast T1-weighted images of a left frontal peripheral glioma (*arrows*). At 7T, there is improved spatial and contrast resolution with demonstration of cortical and venous mesoarchitecture.

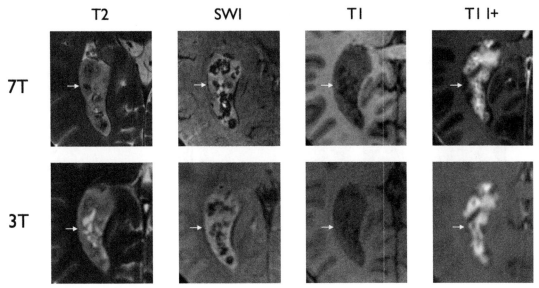

Fig. 5. Choroid plexus papilloma at 3T and 7T field strengths. Axial T2-weighted, susceptibility-weighted imaging (SWI), T1-weighted, and postcontrast T1-weighted images of choroid plexus papilloma in the right lateral ventricle (*arrows*). At 7T, multinodular enhancement, intratumoral hemorrhage, and tumor microstructure are better demonstrated.

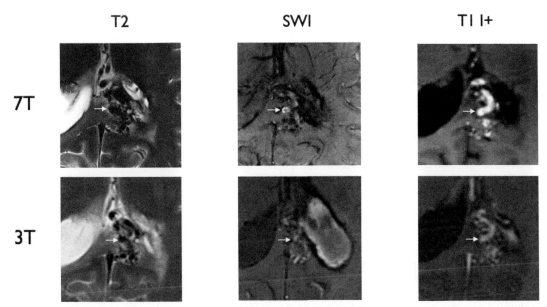

Fig. 6. Arteriovenous malformation at 3T and 7T field strengths. Axial T2-weighted, susceptibility-weighted imaging (SWI), and postcontrast T1-weighted images of a left splenial arteriovenous malformation (*arrows*). At 7T, there is improved delineation of lesion angioarchitecture.

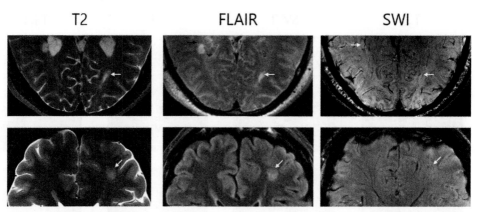

Fig. 7. Multiple sclerosis at 7T field strength. Axial T2-weighted, fluid-attenuated inversion recovery (FLAIR), and susceptibility-weighted imaging (SWI) show demyelinating lesions with central vein sign *(arrows)*.

SUMMARY

UHF imaging is gaining momentum in both clinical and research settings as an application-specific and problem-solving tool. Improved characterization of anatomic microstructure and function offers improved disease understanding, diagnosis, and follow-up. Ongoing development of novel imaging contrasts and translation of cutting-edge sequences will aid more accurate, sensitive, and precise diagnosis, interventional planning, and follow-up for a variety of pathologic conditions.

CLINICS CARE POINTS

- Ultra-high-field advantages for structural MR imaging include improved spatial and contrast resolution, MR angiography, and susceptibility-weighted imaging.

- UHF offers benefits for advanced sequences such as structural and functional connectivity, MR spectroscopy, and chemical exchange saturation transfer.

- In children, the diagnostic benefits of UHF must be balanced against safety considerations, longer scan times, and greater image artifacts.

SOURCES OF FUNDING

I. Nestrasil was supported by the Million Dollar Bike Ride from the University of Pennsylvania, PA, USA (MDBR-17–123-MPS; 303052MPS1-16–003–02); Sanofi Genzyme, Cambridge, MA, USA (GZ-2014-11270), and National MPS Society (project #00067088).

ACKNOWLEDGMENTS

The authors thank Prof. Gülin Öz (CMRR, University of Minnesota) for providing the ALD proton MR spectra in **Fig. 1**.

DISCLOSURE

D.K. Deelchand has nothing to disclose. M.L. Ho is principal investigator on the Radiological Society of North America Research Scholar Grant, Society for Pediatric Radiology Pilot Award, and American Society of Head and Neck Radiology William N. Hanafee Award, for work unrelated to this article. I. Nestrasil is consultant for ICON and Quantims; received research support from National MPS Society, Sanofi Genzyme, Biomarin, and Shire/Takeda.

REFERENCES

1. Mayor S. Nobel prize in medicine awarded to MRI pioneers. BMJ 2003;327:827.
2. Hamilton J, Franson D, Seiberlich N. Recent advances in parallel imaging for MRI. Prog Nucl Magn Reson Spectrosc 2017;101:71–95.
3. Norris CD, Quick SE, Parker JG, et al. Diffusion MR imaging in the head and neck: principles and applications. Neuroimaging Clin N Am 2020; 30:261–82.
4. De Graaf, Robin A. In vivo NMR spectroscopy: principles and techniques – 2nd edition. Chichester, West Sussex: John Wiley & Sons Ltd; 2007.
5. Oz G, Alger JR, Barker PB, et al. Clinical proton MR spectroscopy in central nervous system disorders. Radiology 2014;270(3):658–79.
6. Tkáč I, Oz G, Adriany G, et al. In vivo 1H NMR spectroscopy of the human brain at high magnetic fields: metabolite quantification at 4T vs. 7T. Magn Reson Med 2009;62:868–79.

7. Deelchand DK, Adanyeguh IM, Emir UE, et al. Two-site reproducibility of cerebellar and brainstem neurochemical profiles with short-echo, single-voxel MRS at 3T. Magn Reson Med 2015;73:1718–25.

8. Öz G, Deelchand DK, Wijnen JP, et al. Working group on advanced single voxel HM. Advanced single voxel 1H magnetic resonance spectroscopy techniques in humans: experts' consensus recommendations. NMR Biomed 2020;34:e4236.

9. Maudsley AA, Andronesi OC, Barker PB, et al. Advanced magnetic spectroscopic neuroimaging: Experts' consensus recommendations. NMR Biomed 2021;34:e4309.

10. Deelchand DK, Kantarci K, Öz G. Improved localization, spectral quality, and repeatability with advanced MRS methodology in the clinical setting. Magn Reson Med 2018;79:1241–50.

11. Pohmann R, Speck O, Scheffler K. Signal-to-noise ratio and MR tissue parameters in human brain imaging at 3, 7, and 9.4 tesla using current receive coil arrays. Magn Reson Med 2016 Feb;75(2):801–9.

12. Guérin B, Villena JF, Polimeridis AG, et al. The ultimate signal-to-noise ratio in realistic body models. Magn Reson Med 2017;78:1969–80.

13. Wiggins GC, Potthast A, Triantafyllou C, et al. Eight-channel phased array coil and detunable TEM volume coil for 7 T brain imaging. Magn Reson Med 2005;54:235–40.

14. Sadeghi-Tarakameh A, DelaBarre L, Lagore RL, et al. In vivo human head MRI at 10.5T: a radiofrequency safety study and preliminary imaging results. Magn Reson Med 2020;84:484–96.

15. Barth M, Breuer F, Koopmans PJ, et al. Simultaneous multislice (SMS) imaging techniques. Magn Reson Med 2016;75:63–81.

16. Pruessmann KP, Weiger M, Scheidegger MB, et al. SENSE: sensitivity encoding for fast MRI. Magn Reson Med 1999;42:952–62.

17. Griswold MA, Jakob PM, Heidemann RM, et al. Generalized autocalibrating partially parallel acquisitions (GRAPPA). Magn Reson Med 2002;47:1202–10.

18. Deelchand DK, Iltis I, Henry P-G. Improved quantification precision of human brain short echo-time 1H magnetic resonance spectroscopy at high magnetic field: a simulation study. Magn Reson Med 2014;72:20–5.

19. Tkáč I, Andersen P, Adriany G, et al. In vivo 1H NMR spectroscopy of the human brain at 7 T. Magn Reson Med 2001;46:451–6.

20. Padormo F, Beqiri A, Hajnal JV, et al. Parallel transmission for ultrahigh-field imaging. NMR Biomed 2016;29:1145–61.

21. van Gemert J, Brink W, Webb A, et al. High-permittivity pad design tool for 7T neuroimaging and 3T body imaging. Magn Reson Med 2019;81:3370–8.

22. Michaeli S, Garwood M, Zhu XH, et al. Proton T2 relaxation study of water, N-acetylaspartate, and creatine in human brain using Hahn and Carr-Purcell spin echoes at 4T and 7T. Magn Reson Med 2002;47:629–33.

23. Deelchand DK, Moortele P-FVd, Adriany G, et al. In vivo 1H NMR spectroscopy of the human brain at 9.4 T: initial results. J Magn Reson 2010;206:74–80.

24. Öz G, Tkac I. Short-echo, single-shot, full-intensity proton magnetic resonance spectroscopy for neurochemical profiling at 4 T: validation in the cerebellum and brainstem. Magn Reson Med 2011;65:901–10.

25. Xin L, Tkáč I. A practical guide to in vivo proton magnetic resonance spectroscopy at high magnetic fields. Anal Biochem 2017;529:30–9.

26. Ordidge RJ, Wylezinska M, Hugg JW, et al. Frequency offset corrected inversion (FOCI) pulses for use in localized spectroscopy. Magn Reson Med 1996;36:562–6.

27. Tannus A, Garwood M. Adiabatic pulses. NMR Biomed 1997;10:423–34.

28. Deelchand DK, Berrington A, Noeske R, et al. Across-vendor standardization of semi-LASER for single-voxel MRS at 3T. NMR Biomed 2019;34:e4218.

29. Andre JB, Bresnahan BW, Mossa-Basha M, et al. Toward quantifying the prevalence, severity, and cost associated with patient motion during clinical MR examinations. J Am Coll Radiol 2015;12:689–95.

30. Greene DJ, Koller JM, Hampton JM, et al. Behavioral interventions for reducing head motion during MRI scans in children. Neuroimage 2018;171:234–45.

31. Öz G, Tkáč I, Charnas LR, et al. Assessment of adrenoleukodystrophy lesions by high field MRS in non-sedated pediatric patients. Neurology 2005;64:434–41.

32. Zaitsev M, Dold C, Sakas G, et al. Magnetic resonance imaging of freely moving objects: prospective real-time motion correction using an external optical motion tracking system. Neuroimage 2006;31:1038–50.

33. Aranovitch A, Haeberlin M, Gross S, et al. Motion detection with NMR markers using real-time field tracking in the laboratory frame. Magn Reson Med 2020;84:89–102.

34. White N, Roddey C, Shankaranarayanan A, et al. PROMO: real-time prospective motion correction in MRI using image-based tracking. Magn Reson Med 2010;63:91–105.

35. Tisdall MD, Hess AT, Reuter M, et al. Volumetric navigators for prospective motion correction and selective reacquisition in neuroanatomical MRI. Magn Reson Med 2012;68:389–99.

36. Shellock FG. 2021. Available at: http://mrisafety.com/. Accessed February 23, 2021.

37. Hoff MN, McKinney At, Shellock FG, et al. Safety considerations of 7-T MRI in clinical practice. Radiology 2019;292(3):509–18.

38. Prinsen H, de Graaf RA, Mason GF, et al. Reproducibility measurement of glutathione, GABA, and glutamate: towards in vivo neurochemical profiling of multiple sclerosis with MR spectroscopy at 7T. J Magn Reson Imaging 2017;45(1):187–98.

39. Schur RR, Draisma LW, Wijnen JP, et al. Brain GABA levels across psychiatric disorders: a systematic literature review and meta-analysis of (1) H-MRS studies. Hum Brain Mapp 2016;37(9):3337–52.

40. Rojas DC, Becker KM, Wilson LB. Magnetic resonance spectroscopy studies of glutamate and GABA in autism: implications for excitation-inhibition imbalance theory. Curr Dev Disord Rep 2015;2(1):46–57.

41. Puts NA, Ryan M, Oeltzschner G, et al. Reduced striatal GABA in unmedicated children with ADHD at 7T. Psychiatry Res Neuroimaging 2020;301:111082.

42. Hai T, Swansburg R, Kahl CK, et al. Magnetic resonance spectroscopy of gamma-aminobutyric acid and glutamate concentrations in children with attention-deficit/hyperactivity disorder. JAMA Netw Open 2020;3(10):e2020973.

43. Mahone EM, Puts NA, Edden RAE, et al. GABA and glutamate in children with Tourette syndrome: a (1)H MR spectroscopy study at 7T. Psychiatry Res Neuroimaging 2018;273:46–53.

44. Doelken MT, Hammen T, Bogner W, et al. Alterations of intracerebral gamma-aminobutyric acid (GABA) levels by titration with levetiracetam in patients with focal epilepsies. Epilepsia 2010;51(8):1477–82.

45. Levy LM, Degnan AJ. GABA-based evaluation of neurologic conditions: MR spectroscopy. AJNR Am J Neuroradiol 2013;34(2):259–65.

46. Grohn H, Gillick BT, Tkac I, et al. Influence of repetitive transcranial magnetic stimulation on human neurochemistry and functional connectivity: a pilot MRI/MRS study at 7 T. Front Neurosci 2019;13:1260.

47. Heimrath K, Brechmann A, Blobel-Luer R, et al. Transcranial direct current stimulation (tDCS) over the auditory cortex modulates GABA and glutamate: a 7 T MR-spectroscopy study. Sci Rep 2020;10(1):20111.

48. Li Y, Park I, Nelson SJ. Imaging tumor metabolism using in vivo magnetic resonance spectroscopy. Cancer J 2015;21(2):123–8.

49. Srinivasan R, Ratiney H, Hammond-Rosenbluth KE, et al. MR spectroscopic imaging of glutathione in the white and gray matter at 7 T with an application to multiple sclerosis. Magn Reson Imaging 2010;28(2):163–70.

50. Terpstra M, Henry PG, Gruetter R. Measurement of reduced glutathione (GSH) in human brain using LCModel analysis of difference-edited spectra. Magn Reson Med 2003;50(1):19–23.

51. Holmay MJ, Terpstra M, Coles LD, et al. N-Acetylcysteine boosts brain and blood glutathione in Gaucher and Parkinson diseases. Clin Neuropharmacol 2013;36(4):103–6.

52. Budinger TF, Bird MD. MRI and MRS of the human brain at magnetic fields of 14T to 20T: technical feasibility, safety, and neuroscience horizons. Neuroimage 2018;168:509–31.

53. Kraff O, Quick HH. 7T: physics, safety, and potential clinical applications. J Magn Reson Imaging 2017;46(6):1573–89.

54. Niesporek SC, Nagel AM, Platt T. Multinuclear MRI at ultrahigh fields. Top Magn Reson Imaging 2019;28(3):173–88.

55. Opheim G, van der Kolk A, Bloch KM, et al. 7T epilepsy task force consensus recommendations on the use of 7T MRI in clinical practice. Neurology 2021;96(7):327–41.

56. Kreidenhuber R, De Tiege X, Rampp S. Presurgical functional cortical mapping using electromagnetic source imaging. Front Neurol 2019;10:628.

57. Duchin Y, Shamir RR, Patriat R, et al. Patient-specific anatomical model for deep brain stimulation based on 7 Tesla MRI. PLoS One 2018;13(8):e0201469.

58. Patriat R, Cooper SE, Duchin Y, et al. Individualized tractography-based parcellation of the globus pallidus pars interna using 7T MRI in movement disorder patients prior to DBS surgery. Neuroimage 2018;178:198–209.

59. Xiao Y, Zitella LM, Duchin Y, et al. Multimodal 7T imaging of thalamic nuclei for preclinical deep brain stimulation applications. Front Neurosci 2016;10:264.

60. Elkaim LM, Alotaibi NM, Sigal A, et al. Deep brain stimulation for pediatric dystonia: a meta-analysis with individual participant data. Dev Med Child Neurol 2019;61(1):49–56.

61. Rutland JW, Delman BN, Gill CM, et al. Emerging use of ultra-high-field 7T MRI in the study of intracranial vascularity: state of the field and future directions. AJNR Am J Neuroradiol 2020;41(1):2–9.

62. Reichenbach JR, Schweser F, Serres B, et al. Quantitative susceptibility mapping: concepts and applications. Clin Neuroradiol 2015;25(Suppl 2):225–30.

63. Ladd ME, Bachert P, Meyerspeer M, et al. Pros and cons of ultra-high-field MRI/MRS for human application. Prog Nucl Magn Reson Spectrosc 2018;109:1–50.

64. De Cocker LJ, Lindenholz A, Zwanenburg JJ, et al. Clinical vascular imaging in the brain at 7T. Neuroimage 2018;168:452–8.

65. Beisteiner R, Robinson S, Wurnig M, et al. Clinical fMRI: evidence for a 7T benefit over 3T. Neuroimage 2011;57(3):1015–21.

66. Liebrand LC, van Wingen GA, Vos FM, et al. Spatial versus angular resolution for tractography-assisted planning of deep brain stimulation. Neuroimage Clin 2020;25:102116.

67. Shapey J, Vos SB, Vercauteren T, et al. Clinical applications for diffusion MRI and tractography of cranial nerves within the posterior fossa: a systematic review. Front Neurosci 2019;13:23.

68. van Zijl PC, Yadav NN. Chemical exchange saturation transfer (CEST): what is in a name and what isn't? Magn Reson Med 2011;65(4):927–48.

69. Wu B, Warnock G, Zaiss M, et al. An overview of CEST MRI for non-MR physicists. EJNMMI Phys 2016;3(1):19.

70. Jones KM, Pollard AC, Pagel MD. Clinical applications of chemical exchange saturation transfer (CEST) MRI. J Magn Reson Imaging 2018;47(1):11–27.

71. Barry RL, Vannesjo SJ, By S, et al. Spinal cord MRI at 7T. Neuroimage 2018;168:437–51.

72. Nestrasil I, Labounek R, Nguyen C, et al. Intraspinal space restriction at the occipito-cervical junction alters cervical spinal cord diffusion MRI metrics in mucopolysacharidoses patients. Mol Genet Metab 2020;129(2):S115.

73. Pisharady PK, Eberly LE, Cheong I, et al. Tract-specific analysis improves sensitivity of spinal cord diffusion MRI to cross-sectional and longitudinal changes in amyotrophic lateral sclerosis. Commun Biol 2020;3(1):370.

74. van de Stadt SIW, van Ballegoij WJC, Labounek R, et al. Spinal cord atrophy as a measure of severity of myelopathy in adrenoleukodystrophy. J Inherit Metab Dis 2020;43(4):852–60.

75. Labounek R, Valosek J, Horak T, et al. HARDI-ZOOMit protocol improves specificity to microstructural changes in presymptomatic myelopathy. Sci Rep 2020;10(1):17529.

76. Ouellette R, Treaba CA, Granberg T, et al. 7 T imaging reveals a gradient in spinal cord lesion distribution in multiple sclerosis. Brain 2020;143(10):2973–87.

77. Massire A, Rasoanandrianina H, Guye M, et al. Anterior fissure, central canal, posterior septum and more: new insights into the cervical spinal cord gray and white matter regional organization using T1 mapping at 7T. Neuroimage 2020;205:116275.

78. Henning A, Koning W, Fuchs A, et al. (1) H MRS in the human spinal cord at 7 T using a dielectric waveguide transmitter, RF shimming and a high density receive array. NMR Biomed 2016;29(9):1231–9.

3D Modeling and Advanced Visualization of the Pediatric Brain, Neck, and Spine

Sanjay P. Prabhu, MBBS, DCH, FRCR, DABR

KEYWORDS

- 3D printing • Virtual reality • Advanced visualization • Augmented reality • Pediatric neuroimaging
- Cinematic rendering • Simulation • Volume rendering technique

KEY POINTS

- Acquisition of a high-quality volumetric imaging data set is the most crucial step in creating an accurate 3D model for advanced visualization or printing.
- Advanced visualization tools include "on-screen" technologies like volumetric rendering and cinematic rendering, "beyond the screen" technologies like AR and VR, and the creation of physical 3D printed models.
- Image acquisition, segmentation, mesh creation, and printing are the steps required to create a clinically useful 3D printed model.
- Advanced visualization tools help surgical planning and simulation, trainee and patient/family education, and patient preparation for surgical or image-guided intervention.
- Although there is emerging literature documenting the added value of advanced visualization tools in managing pediatric neurologic disease, there is further need for cost-benefit analysis of these applications and their impact on patient outcomes.
- Technological advancements will help enhance newer applications' functionality and make them more accessible to physicians and patients, potentially translating to tangible therapeutic impact.

INTRODUCTION

Advances in cross-sectional imaging techniques have enabled rapid imaging of the pediatric brain, head and neck, and spine with excellent spatial and contrast resolution. Improvements in scanner hardware and newer pulse sequences, motion correction techniques, and image reconstructions augmented by artificial intelligence have allowed rapid scanning in young children, often avoiding sedation and general anesthesia.[1,2] As imaging acquisition becomes faster and imaging data sets increase exponentially in size, radiologists face the challenges of reviewing thousands of images generated from these studies, delivering informative reports summarizing essential findings, and helping clinicians formulate effective treatment plans.

We have seen the steady evolution and increasing use of "on-screen" visualization techniques like volume rendering technique (VRT) over the past 3 decades.[3] Newer image rendering alternatives like cinematic rendering can display high-density and high-contrast tissues with ultra-realistic detail.[4,5] These techniques can help radiologists synthesize and convey the information in a cogent format to the clinician.[6] In turn, clinicians use these reconstructions to plan appropriate treatment, discuss findings with multidisciplinary

Neuroradiology Division, Department of Radiology, Boston Children's Hospital, Harvard Medical School, SIM-Peds3D Print, 300 Longwood Avenue, Boston, MA 02115, USA
E-mail address: sanjay.prabhu@childrens.harvard.edu

Magn Reson Imaging Clin N Am 29 (2021) 655–666
https://doi.org/10.1016/j.mric.2021.06.014
1064-9689/21/© 2021 Elsevier Inc. All rights reserved.

teams, and convey findings to patients and their caregivers.

The ready availability of advanced visualization platforms on PACS (picture archiving and communication systems) workstations or even standard laptops through server-based or cloud-based solutions has enabled greater adoption of these techniques. Also, radiologists and clinicians can access these highly informative visualizations on mobile platforms in the clinic, operating room, or multidisciplinary meetings.[7]

More recently, physical 3-dimensional (3D)-printed models, created using data from imaging studies, have emerged as an extension of the more common volume-rendered reconstructions traditionally displayed on 2-dimensional (2D) screens.[8] These models provide tangible information about the depth of various anatomic structures and their spatial relation to one another.

Developments in enhanced viewing technologies that provide depth perception through binocular vision are also available, including virtual reality (VR) and augmented reality (AR).[9,10] Many institutions have access to these technologies and are exploring new ways to deploy them in the clinical and radiology departments.

This review starts with a brief overview of how to tailor imaging techniques for optimal 3D reconstructions, followed by a brief review of standard and newer "on-screen" techniques, including volume rendering and cinematic rendering. We then discuss the process of creating 3D printed models for surgical simulation and education. Finally, we highlight current uses and potential future use cases for VR and AR applications in a pediatric neuroimaging setting.

TECHNICAL BACKGROUND
Optimizing Imaging Protocols for 3D Modeling and Advanced Visualization

The first and arguably most crucial step in creating an accurate 3D model for viewing on any advanced visualization platform is acquiring a high-quality volumetric imaging data set highlighting the anatomic structures of interest and differentiating them from surrounding structures. If a structure is not imaged optimally or not included in the field of view, it is impossible to accurately segment and visualize it in the 3D model. The radiologist can play a critical role by optimizing imaging studies, thereby enabling accurate delineation of the anatomic structures. The need to avoid repeat imaging is vital in the pediatric population to minimize the risk of radiation exposure in computed tomography (CT) or avoid

sedation for repeat magnetic resonance imaging (MRI) studies.

For CT, volumetric images acquired with a slice thickness of 1 to 2 mm or lower are ideal for creating 3D models. Other parameters like smaller voxel sizes, lower slice thickness, and sharp kernel settings appropriate for capturing sufficient image detail may necessitate more manual segmentation and postprocessing due to image noise.[11] Conversely, larger voxel size and soft reconstruction kernels facilitate faster and more automated segmentation, enabling the creation of smoother 3D models, but may limit anatomic detail. In addition, a lower tube potential (kV) can increase the degree of enhancement of iodinated contrast media for vascular studies.

Most advanced visualization software and 3D printing applications are tailored for images generated from CT. However, in pediatric-focused practices, many vascular, soft tissue, and osseous anatomic models for surgical planning are created using MRI data. Ideally, 3D printed models from MRI also benefit from volumetric isotropic imaging data sets without significant gaps between slices.[11] Accurate segmentation to delineate osseous, soft tissue, or vascular structures remains a time-consuming process on MRI, even when using the most advanced software tools. More recently, the black bone sequences using zero echo-time and T1-weighted volumetric interpolated breath-hold examination sequences have helped with better visualization of cortical bone and can potentially lower segmentation time.[12,13]

When imaging is optimized, it is possible to merge data from different sequences and modalities into the same model, either for visualization on a screen or to create a 3D printed model (**Fig. 1**).

Advanced Data Visualization

3D models generated from imaging studies can be visualized using standard "on-screen" technologies, physical 3D printed models, and "beyond the screen" technologies like AR and VR. We discuss each of these technologies in detail. However, at the outset, we emphasize that these visualizations serve as adjuncts to 2D reconstructions and should not be considered as a stand-alone tool, at least in the diagnostic arena.

Standard "On-Screen" Advanced Visualization

VRT is the most widely used 3D display technique in clinical practice. VRT relies on ray tracing and local light source principles—for every pixel on the screen, a single virtual ray of light is cast through the volume and intersects a series of

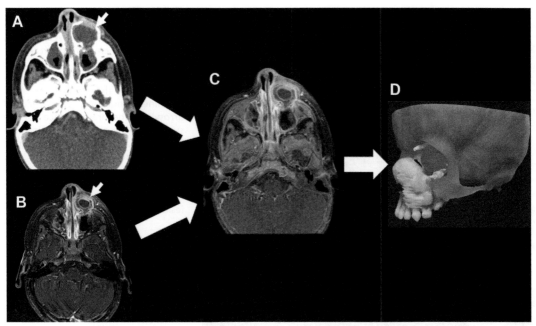

Fig. 1. Combining multiple modalities to create 3D printed models: (*A*) contrast-enhanced maxillofacial CT and (*B*) postcontrast fat-saturated T1-weighted MRI obtained in a 2-year-old boy with recurrent maxillary myxoma (*arrow*). (*C*) Fused image produced by overlaying and coregistering the CT with the MRI was used to help segment the mass. (*D*) 3D printed model created using the segmented data helped the surgeon clarify relationships to the surrounding structures and plan surgical resection.

voxels along its path. This technique allows visualization of larger volumes on a single image, with simultaneous evaluation of distant structures and their spatial relationships. The main limitation of the VRT technique is its failure to consider complex light paths, such as scattering and light extinction, which results in more artificial-appearing images.[5,14]

Cinematic rendering is a recently introduced 3D reconstruction technique that produces photorealistic images from cross-sectional imaging data. In contrast to VRT, algorithms used in cinematic rendering rely on path-tracing methods and a complex global lighting model that simulates a natural lighting environment in which different paths of light travel from all possible directions. Various cinematic effects like soft shadows, depth of field, refraction, and absorption can be achieved using this technique.[5]

Potential applications of cinematic rendering technique in pediatric neuroimaging include a more realistic depiction of skull fractures and deformities (**Fig. 2**); optimal visualization of vascular lesions (**Fig. 3**) and tumors in the brain, head, and neck; and display of spine deformities. There are no systematic studies documenting advantages of cinematic rendering over VRT or 3D printed models in pediatric neuroimaging.

3D PRINTING
What is 3D Printing?

Physical 3D printed models, created using data from imaging studies, have emerged as an extension of the more common volume-rendered reconstructions displayed on 2D screens. 3D printed models provide tangible information about the depth of various anatomic structures and their spatial relationships to one another. With the depth inherent in a physical model, our brains engage in true binocular vision, and the sensory input of touch (haptic feedback) complements this. This experience enables a more robust understanding of anatomic spatial relationships than is afforded by 2D projections.

How is a 3D Printed Model Created?

The process of creating a patient-specific 3D printed model is summarized in **Fig. 4**.

Optimal image acquisition is the most important first step in creating a 3D printed model. This step is followed by image segmentation. Segmentation refers to the process of isolating structures of interest from the rest of the imaged anatomy to create patient-specific, highly accurate computer models of organs and tissue. There are several commercial and open-source image segmentation

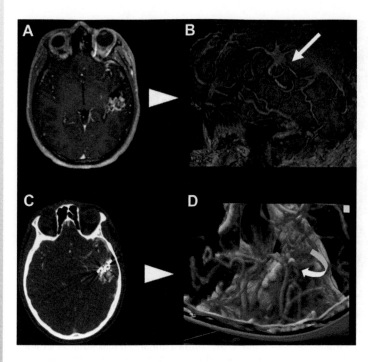

Fig. 2. VRT and cinematic rendering: (A) postcontrast volumetric T1-weighted image in a 13-year-old boy with a partially embolized left temporal lobe arteriovenous malformation was used to create (B) surface reconstructions of the brain that show prominent engorged vessels (straight arrow) on the brain surface for the surgeon to be aware of while planning the approach. (C) CT angiogram images were used to create highly targeted (D) cinematic rendered reconstructions of the lesion (curved arrow) to help the surgeon examine the lesion in detail.

tools used to create files suitable for 3D printing.[15] Most 3D printing facilities use specialized commercial or open-source software packages designed for use with a 3D printer, each with its own advantages and disadvantages. No single segmentation technique is suitable for all images and applications, and almost all the tools have a learning curve. The key points to bear in mind when choosing a software tool for image segmentation are ease of use, ability to segment the most commonly printed structures in one's practice, availability of training to deal with segmentation challenges, and cost. For most models involving nonosseous structures, multiple components,

and/or MRI-based models, at least some manual segmentation is required to print anatomic structures of interest as separate objects. Patient-specific segmented images designated for 3D printing should be reviewed carefully, ideally by the radiologist or surgeon familiar with the anatomy and the planned use of the model.[16] Errors in 3D printed models most often result from inaccuracies in segmentation. Even when an expert checks segmentation, there is inherent variation in the degree of accuracy of the printed models due to overestimation or underestimation of small nonuniform structures (eg, soft tissue structures), irrespective of the segmentation tool used.[17] The

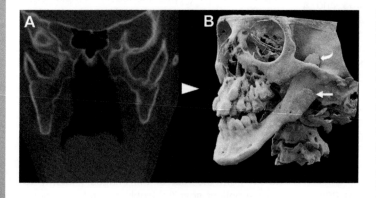

Fig. 3. Cinematic rendering: (A) maxillofacial CT in a 12-year-old girl presenting with bilateral temporomandibular ankyloses following failure of multiple procedures for micrognathia associated with the Robin sequence. (B) Cinematic rendering provides exquisite detail of the condylar fusion to the skull base (shown only on the left on this oblique image), particularly at the lateral portions adjacent to the zygomatic arches (straight arrow) and the long coronoid processes touching the skull base (curved arrow). Note the large osseous protuberances extending from the pterygoid plates attaching the mandibular rami (black arrows).

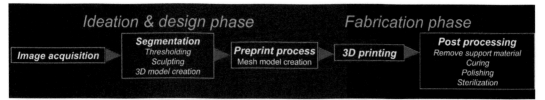

Fig. 4. Workflow to create a patient-specific 3D printed model.

best way to mitigate or minimize this is to use frequent quality checks on imaging scanners and have calibration tools that allow for quality checks on printed models at regular intervals.

The next step after segmentation is mesh creation, which generates a 3D computer-aided design model from the segmented anatomy. Mesh creation involves eliminating unwanted structures, removing artifacts, and fixing surface flaws. Other tweaks required include fixing holes to make the mesh watertight, removing discontinuous portions, and joining up elements artificially separated from the model during segmentation. Finally, structures segmented from another imaging study (eg, MRI) or hardware components may be added at this stage.

The refined mesh model is then sent to a printer in a variety of file formats. The most common file format used is the 3D Standard Tessellation Language (3DSTL) file format, which defines the surface geometry enclosing any 3D objects as a series of connected polygons.

The 3D printing process typically consists of depositing material layer by layer in a semiliquid, liquid, or powder form and solidifying using light energy (eg, ultraviolet light or laser), an electron beam, chemical binders, or heat and allowing the model to solidify at room temperature.[15] A detailed discussion of the types of printers for medical and radiology-specific applications is beyond the scope of this review and is discussed extensively by other investigators.[18,19]

APPLICATIONS OF 3D PRINTED MODELS IN PEDIATRIC NEUROIMAGING

We discuss the clinical applications of 3D printed models in pediatric neuroimaging under the following 3 sections.

Brain and Vessels

Bespoke patient-specific 3D printed models of the brain created using CT and MRI are used to plan complex pediatric neurosurgical procedures and facilitating trainee and patient/parent education.

Some examples from the authors' institutional archives include:

1. 3D printed models to plan brain tumor resections by showing the relationship of the tumor to surrounding vascular structures and white matter tracts.
2. 3D printed display of subdural electrodes registered to a brain model printed using a volumetric T1-weighted data set in a patient undergoing presurgical evaluation for intractable epilepsy (**Fig. 5**).
3. Surgical simulation of hemispherectomy in patients with unihemispheric disorders like Sturge-Weber syndrome or arterial infarction (**Fig. 6**).
4. Ultrarealistic endoscopic third ventriculostomy neurosurgical simulators created using a combination of 3D printing and casting processes to aid neurosurgical trainees indicated that these models could help distinguish between expert and novice skills to blinded observers.[20]
5. Use of high-fidelity 3D printed models of pediatric cerebrovascular conditions for planning neurointerventional procedures (**Fig. 7**). In a small study, our group showed that 3D printed models could help resect arteriovenous malformations without complications and resulted in a 30-min reduction in operative time (12%) in 2 cases compared with matched controls.[21]
6. A simulator created using a combination of 3D printing, sculpting, and molding for training radiology residents to perform neonatal brain ultrasonography showed improvements in technical knowledge and confidence and reduced anxiety in residents performing brain ultrasonography. In addition, objective measures of image quality improved.[22]

Head and Neck

Dental and maxillofacial surgeons were early adopters of 3D printing and have used these models to aid complex craniofacial reconstructions (**Fig. 8**) and fabricate customized autologous or synthetic grafts (**Fig. 9**). Pediatric-focused studies have been published demonstrating reduced intraoperative times, decreased procedural costs, and fewer complications when 3D printed models were used to plan complex pediatric craniofacial reconstructions.[23] Other examples

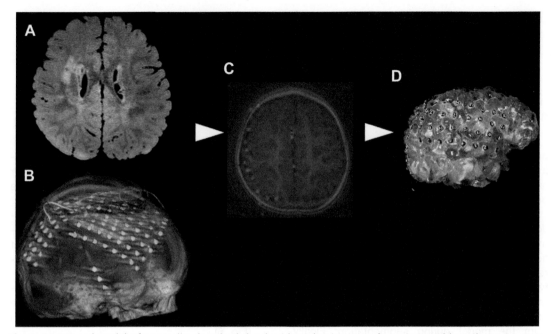

Fig. 5. 3D printed model of surgically placed subdural grids and strips to evaluate intractable epilepsy. Preoperative 3D fluid-attenuated inversion recovery sequence from (*A*) MRI and (*B*) CT obtained after placement of subdural electrodes was used to create (*C*) coregistered overlay image and (*D*) 3D printed model in a 9-month-old infant with tuberous sclerosis.

of the utility of 3D printed models in pediatric head and neck surgical procedures or training models include:

1. Creating 3D printed models of temporal bone anatomy for surgical simulation and trainee education, including planning of cochlear implantation in patients with a high risk for complications. Early results have been promising and have shown reduced operative time compared with cases of a similar degree of complexity.
2. Use of 3D printed models created from CT and MRI for planning resection of pediatric head and neck tumors. An example was shown earlier (see **Fig. 1**).
3. Use of 3D printed models of the unaffected ear of patients with unilateral microtia or to plan autologous ear reconstruction in patients with craniofacial microsomia.[24]
4. 3D printed models of the variant anatomy of pediatric paranasal sinuses, neck spaces, pharynx, and larynx for resident and trainee education.[25]
5. 3D printed model of complex fetal maxillofacial anatomy to determine the degree of upper airway obstruction using images from fetal MRI.[26]

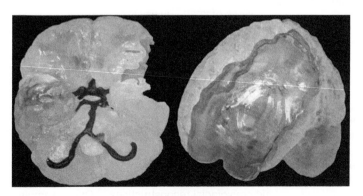

Fig. 6. 3D printed model of the brain in a 11-month-old infant with left middle cerebral artery infarction: model was used for planning functional hemispherectomy and parent counseling.

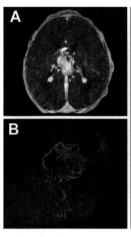

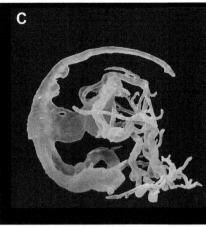

Fig. 7. 3D printed model in a newborn male infant with a vein of Galen malformation: (*A*) contrast-enhanced volumetric T1 and (*B*) magnetic resonance angiogram were used to create a model showing the various components of the malformation. (*C*) The printed model was used by the neuro-interventional radiologist to plan embolization. Of note, the model was printed at a 2-fold magnification to help optimally visualize the architecture of the malformation.

Spine

3D printed models can play an essential role in the correction of complex pediatric spine deformities and planning resection or biopsy of vertebral lesions. Example applications of 3D printing in the pediatric spine include:

1. Creation of patient-specific models for presurgical planning of correction of complex scoliosis (**Fig. 10**); in a study of 3D printed models in congenital spinal deformity secondary to myelomeningocele, Karlin and colleagues[27]

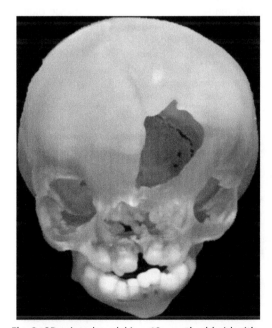

Fig. 8. 3D printed model in a 19-month-old girl with a Tessier facial cleft involving the nose and hypertelorism: the model was used to plan the osteotomy pattern and the nature of movements of the bilateral orbital maxillary complexes.

reported appreciation of anomalous anatomy on the physical model not mentioned on official imaging reports. This study also showed how the surgeon was able to precontour the rods based on the 3D model resulting in reduced operative time.[27]

2. Creation of patient-specific jigs or guides to optimize instrumentation placement during correction of complex cervical spine deformities (**Fig. 11**) and, more recently, thoracic and lumbar spine deformities (**Fig. 12**): a prospective controlled study showed that patient-specific pedicle guides allowed for more accurate placement of pedicle screws and potential reduction of operative time and intraoperative complications in patients with severe congenital scoliosis.

3. Creation of instrumentation or implants to fit a patient-specific or goal-specific need: 3D printed implants have been used in some adult centers to create patient-specific vertebral bodies, but there are no pediatric-specific applications to date.

4. Alteration of "off-the-shelf" implants or screws to fit a specific patient's anatomy using data from imaging studies: this application can be invaluable in pediatrics wherein the number of patients in each category may not be sufficient for the industrial manufacturer to create multiple sizes for each age group.

5. Planning image-guided biopsy of osseous lesions in and around the spine.

ENHANCED VIEWING PLATFORMS: VIRTUAL REALITY AND AUGMENTED REALITY

VR and AR are both simulations in which virtual elements substitute or supplement native sensory input.[10]

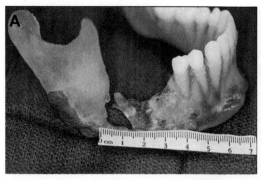
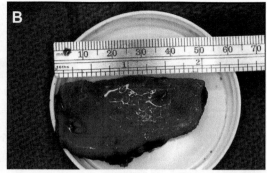

Fig. 9. 3D printed model for planning bone graft harvest: (*A*) 3D printed model in a 14-year-old boy with an osseous defect in the right hemimandible following prior ameloblastoma resection and instrumentation was used to plan (*B*) iliac crest graft harvest.

VR applications can be divided into nonimmersive, semi-immersive, or fully immersive VR. Nonimmersive VR refers to virtual surgical planning (VSP) on desktop computers.[28] Fully immersive VR applications immerse users in synthetic 3D environments via wearable screens, usually wearing a head-mounted display (HMD), and completely remove the real world from the user's field of view. The user interacts with the data through handheld devices or voice gestures and can maneuver around the virtual environment by moving his or her head or physically walking (tracked by external cameras). In semi-immersive VR, the outside world is only partially blocked from the user's field of view. A particular challenge of VR is the inability to head track accurately and the propensity to cause motion sickness. These challenges have been partially mitigated by newer iterations of VR technologies with faster frame rates and high-performance wireless HMDs.

AR differs from VR in that it superimposes virtual images onto the user's real-world environment, such that, the real world is not eliminated from the user's view and the user can interact with the virtual and real-world images simultaneously. User interaction with both virtual world in AR applications occurs through hand gestures, handheld controllers, or voice commands. In AR, the virtual image can be transparent like a hologram or appear solid. Early-stage AR technologies necessitated using HMDs and were marker based, requiring prior knowledge of a user's environment to overlay virtual 3D content into a scene and maintain it at a fixed target point (marker) in space. Newer markerless AR technologies merge digital data with input from dynamic real-world inputs registered to a physical space. These technologies allow an increased range of motion and a larger field of view. It is now possible to interact with a virtual image overlaid on the user's physical

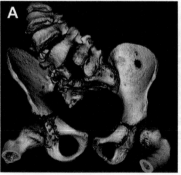
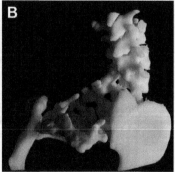
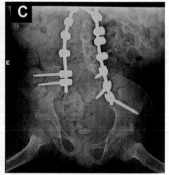

Fig. 10. 3D printed model in planning surgery for complex scoliosis: 10-year-old boy with complex congenital rotatory dextroscoliosis and myelomeningocele. Note the hypoplastic right S1 and S2 elements, incomplete fusion of the right L4-L5 posterior elements, L5 and S1 vertebra, left L5-S1 posterior elements, and absent lamina in the lumbosacral spine. Use of (*A*) volume rendering and (*B*) 3D model helped plan posterior spinal fusion and segmental instrumentation between T10 and the pelvis, pelvis fixation, L5 vertebrectomy, and L4 osteotomy. (*C*) Radiographs obtained in the sitting position demonstrate improved appearance of the spine after spinal fixation and instrumentation.

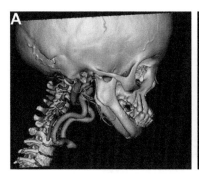 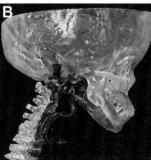

Fig. 11. 3D model for cervical spinal reconstructive surgery: (*A*) digital model for planning interactive on-screen visualization and (*B*) 3D printed model were created for planning occipitocervical fusion in a 28-year-old man with chondrodysplasia punctata. The model helped the surgeon avoid placing screws at C1 because the vertebral artery lay directly in the trajectory of the screws and shorten the size of the screws placed at C2, thereby avoiding damage to the vertebral artery because it became exposed medially over the C2 lamina.

environment using smartphones or tablets (**Fig. 13**). Current AR technology limitations include dependence on flat and textured surfaces, relative difficulty in converting imaging data into a form useable by AR compared with competing technologies like 3D printing, and slow adoption by clinicians. The quality of the AR experience is an essential requisite for successful deployment and acceptance. The use of AR systems in the operating room will potentially be encouraged by the availability of "surgery-specific" HMDs that would guarantee the accuracy required for surgical tasks, provide optimal ergonomics, and reduce the learning curve for interaction with the virtual objects.

CLINICAL APPLICATIONS OF VIRTUAL AND AUGMENTED REALITY AND POTENTIAL ADVANTAGES OVER 3D PRINTED MODELS

Despite the proven benefits of 3D printing, several limitations may preclude use in certain scenarios and hinder widespread adoption, including relatively long turnaround times, cost, and size constraints. Furthermore, there are technical constraints, including the requirement that the model mesh is watertight and the limitation posed by the printer and materials available at the point of care. Also, connectors or supports may need to be introduced between parts to ensure stability or maintain spatial relationships; this can affect

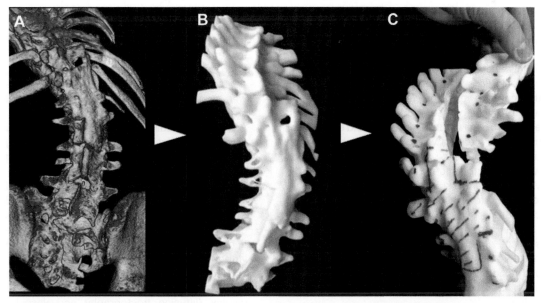

Fig. 12. 3D printed model for surgical simulation in complex scoliosis: (*A*) VRT created from a CT scan was complemented with (*B*) 3D printed model in a 14-year-old boy with complex scoliosis and myelomeningocele. (*C*) Markings made on the model by the surgeon and T9 through L1 posterior laminectomy and T11 vertebrectomy, simulating the first portion of the planned operation; this was eventually followed by bone grafting and fusion in the operating room.

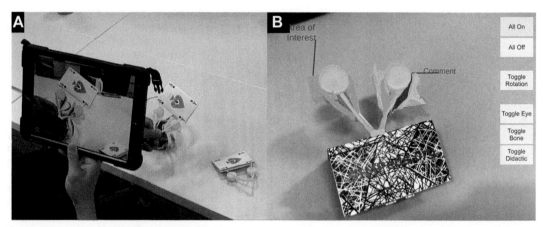

Fig. 13. Augmented reality for surgical planning and patient education: (*A*) AR display created using a tablet and off-the-shelf software to demonstrate the complexity of the anatomy in a 4-year-old girl with globe retraction due to retrobulbar fibrotic bands (accessory extraocular muscle/retractor bulbi). (*B*) Overlay of the colored extraocular muscles over the 3D printed model with the ability to actively annotate and change the structures seen using the on-screen display.

use in surgical simulation by altering anatomy, unless carefully tailored to consider the planned procedure.

VR and AR displays have some advantages over 3D printed models, including the ability to display complex models that would be challenging to print at actual scale due to large size, relative fragility, or cost. The constraints of material requirements do not limit viewing a segmented model in the VR or AR setting. Furthermore, layers of information can be overlaid in a single model and "peeled away" to reveal underlying layers, which one cannot always do with a physical model. An additional benefit is that a model can be enlarged and manipulated dynamically to allow interaction with the anatomic volume in ways that are not possible with physical printed models. For example, an enlarged virtual model of the globe and extraocular muscles in a patient with complex strabismus can be used to analyze the structural relationships within a small space. Finally, models in the AR/VR setting can be shared with colleagues in distant locations for instant feedback or real-time collaboration.

VR and AR applications have a potential role in surgical simulation, image-guided intervention, patient/family education, and medical student and resident education. Some of these applications as they relate to pediatric neuroimaging include:

1. VR and AR can help clarify complex spatial relationships between anatomic structures and pathologic lesions. For example, the use of an AR application has been described for brain tumor resection and cerebral aneurysm clipping in adult patients.[29,30]

2. On-screen VSP is used in some practices to aid surgical planning and decision making before pediatric craniofacial reconstructive surgery.[31]

3. Real-time AR reconstructions superimposed on patients for endovascular interventions and percutaneous procedures may help augment standard localization techniques.[10] Challenges to overcome in developing some of these applications include misregistration due to patient movement and respiratory and visceral motion. Improved AR image reconstruction is being developed to help mitigate these problems with more accurate lesion localization and real time tracking.

4. A novel VR reading room has been proposed using a commercially available HMD, allowing image interpretation in an optimal viewing environment.[32]

5. In addition to using AR models for surgical simulation in place of physical 3D printed models, surgeons can transpose 3D models of the segmented anatomy using AR on a patient to aid surgical navigation or to perform virtual-assisted surgeries, with colleagues giving feedback in real time. Specific examples in pediatric neuroimaging include using AR to display diffusion tractography and vascular data in relation to a tumor in eloquent areas of the brain.

6. Another role for AR and VR applications is in enabling patient education and obtaining

informed consent. For example, by overlaying the abnormal anatomy derived from imaging over a part of the body, the physician can show a child (and their parents) how the disorder might look in their body and potentially animate treatments to show how the proposed treatment protocols might work. Studies in adults have shown that patients primed with what to experience during the treatment and recovery process experienced decreased postprocedural pain and shorter length of stay and reported more positive affect.[33]

7. Multiple studies have demonstrated value in reducing the need for sedation for MRI. Immersive VR also benefits pediatric patients aged 4 to 6 years during intravenous line placement and other procedural interventions.[34] Some hospitals deliver VR-based education materials to the child at home before an MRI scan to acclimatize them with the scanner environment.[35]

8. VR and AR applications have a potential role in trainee education at all levels. Trainees can use VR environments to familiarize themselves with the procedure room, observe, and even actively participate in virtual procedures before performing the procedure on patients.[36,37] This approach can be especially helpful for complex or rare procedures that trainees encounter less frequently during their training.

SUMMARY

The judicious use of advanced visualization tools can enhance and add value to standard imaging techniques by providing a unique summary of the imaging data. These tools allow merging of information from different sequences or studies and provide the substrate for surgical planning, surgical simulation, trainee education, and personalized patient/family education. Radiologists can help harness the potential of these evolving technologies for patient care by optimizing image acquisitions and creating tailored advanced visualization artifacts (both virtual and physical) in conjunction with our clinical colleagues.

REFERENCES

1. Kozak BM, Jaimes C, Kirsch J, et al. MRI techniques to decrease imaging times in children. Radiographics 2020;40(2):485–502.
2. Gottumukkala RV, Kalra MK, Tabari A, et al. Advanced CT techniques for decreasing radiation dose, reducing sedation requirements, and optimizing image quality in children. Radiographics 2019;39(3):709–26.
3. Duran AH, Duran MN, Masood I, et al. The additional diagnostic value of the three-dimensional volume rendering imaging in routine radiology practice. Cureus 2019;11(9):e5579.
4. Rowe SP, Zinreich SJ, Fishman EK. 3D cinematic rendering of the calvarium, maxillofacial structures, and skull base: preliminary observations. Br J Radiol 2018;91(1086):20170826.
5. Eid M, De Cecco CN, Nance JW Jr, et al. Cinematic rendering in CT: a novel, lifelike 3d visualization technique. AJR Am J Roentgenol 2017;209(2):370–9.
6. Andriole KP, Wolfe JM, Khorasani R, et al. Optimizing analysis, visualization, and navigation of large image data sets: one 5000-section CT scan can ruin your whole day. Radiology 2011;259(2):346–62.
7. Wang KC, Filice RW, Philbin JF, et al. Five levels of PACS modularity: integrating 3D and other advanced visualization tools. J Digit Imaging 2011;24(6):1096–102.
8. Chepelev L, Wake N, Ryan J, et al. Radiological Society of North America (RSNA) 3D printing Special Interest Group (SIG): guidelines for medical 3D printing and appropriateness for clinical scenarios. 3d Print Med 2018;4(1):11.
9. Ficarra B. Virtual reality, augmented reality, and mixed reality. In: Carroll WM, editor. New York: Springer Publishing Company; 2020. p. 95–126.
10. Elsayed M, Kadom N, Ghobadi C, et al. Virtual and augmented reality: potential applications in radiology. Acta Radiol 2020;61(9):1258–65.
11. Leng S, McGee K, Morris J, et al. Anatomic modeling using 3D printing: quality assurance and optimization. 3D Printing Med 2017;3(1):6.
12. Delso G, Wiesinger F, Sacolick LI, et al. Clinical evaluation of zero-echo-time MR imaging for the segmentation of the skull. J Nucl Med 2015;56(3):417–22.
13. Lu A, Gorny KR, Ho ML. Zero TE MRI for craniofacial bone imaging. AJNR Am J Neuroradiol 2019;40(9):1562–6.
14. Zhang Q, Eagleson R, Peters TM. Volume visualization: a technical overview with a focus on medical applications. J Digit Imaging 2011;24(4):640–64.
15. Parthasarathy J, Krishnamurthy R, Ostendorf A, et al. 3D printing with MRI in pediatric applications. J Magn Reson Imaging 2020;51(6):1641–58.
16. Matsumoto JS, Morris JM, Foley TA, et al. Three-dimensional physical modeling: applications and experience at mayo clinic. Radiographics 2015;35(7):1989–2006.
17. George E, Liacouras P, Rybicki FJ, et al. Measuring and establishing the accuracy and reproducibility of 3D printed medical models. Radiographics 2017;37(5):1424–50.
18. Jamroz W, Szafraniec J, Kurek M, et al. 3D printing in pharmaceutical and medical applications - recent

achievements and challenges. Pharm Res 2018; 35(9):176.

19. Mitsouras D, Liacouras P, Imanzadeh A, et al. Medical 3D printing for the radiologist. Radiographics 2015;35(7):1965–88.

20. Weinstock P, Rehder R, Prabhu SP, et al. Creation of a novel simulator for minimally invasive neurosurgery: fusion of 3D printing and special effects. J Neurosurg Pediatr 2017;20(1):1–9.

21. Weinstock P, Prabhu SP, Flynn K, et al. Optimizing cerebrovascular surgical and endovascular procedures in children via personalized 3D printing. J Neurosurg Pediatr 2015;16(5):584–9.

22. Tsai A, Barnewolt CE, Prabhu SP, et al. Creation and validation of a simulator for neonatal brain ultrasonography: a pilot study. Acad Radiol 2017;24(1): 76–83.

23. Rogers-Vizena CR, Sporn SF, Daniels KM, et al. Cost-benefit analysis of three-dimensional craniofacial models for midfacial distraction: a pilot study. Cleft Palate Craniofac J 2017;54(5):612–7.

24. Mussi E, Furferi R, Volpe Y, et al. Ear Reconstruction Simulation: From Handcrafting to 3D Printing. Bioengineering (Basel) 2019;6(1).

25. Chen G, Jiang M, Coles-Black J, et al. Three-dimensional printing as a tool in otolaryngology training: a systematic review. J Laryngol Otol 2020;134(1): 14–9.

26. VanKoevering KK, Morrison RJ, Prabhu SP, et al. Antenatal three-dimensional printing of aberrant facial anatomy. Pediatrics 2015;136(5):e1382–5.

27. Karlin L, Weinstock P, Hedequist D, et al. The surgical treatment of spinal deformity in children with myelomeningocele: the role of personalized three-dimensional printed models. J Pediatr Orthop B 2017;26(4):375–82.

28. Douglas DB, Venets D, Wilke C, et al. Augmented reality and virtual reality: initial successes in diagnostic radiology. In: Mohamudally N, editor. State of the Art Virtual Reality and Augmented Reality Knowhow. IntechOpen; 2018. https://doi.org/10.5772/intechopen. 74317.

29. Alaraj A, Luciano CJ, Bailey DP, et al. Virtual reality cerebral aneurysm clipping simulation with real-time haptic feedback. Neurosurgery 2015;11(Suppl 2):52–8.

30. Gerard IJ, Kersten-Oertel M, Drouin S, et al. Combining intraoperative ultrasound brain shift correction and augmented reality visualizations: a pilot study of eight cases. J Med Imaging (Bellingham) 2018;5(2):021210.

31. Ganske IM, Schulz N, Livingston K, et al. Multimodal 3D simulation makes the impossible possible. Plast Reconstr Surg Glob Open 2018;6(4):e1751.

32. Sousa M, Mendes D, Paulo S, et al. VRRRRoom: virtual reality for radiologists in the reading room. In: Proceedings of the 2017 CHI Conference on Human Factors in Computing Systems. New York: Association for Computing Machinery; May 2017. p. 4057–62.

33. Kruzik N. Benefits of preoperative education for adult elective surgery patients. AORN J 2009; 90(3):381–7.

34. Schlechter AK, Whitaker W, Iyer S, et al. Virtual reality distraction during pediatric intravenous line placement in the emergency department: a prospective randomized comparison study. Am J Emerg Med 2021;44:296–9.

35. Ashmore J, Di Pietro J, Williams K, et al. A free virtual reality experience to prepare pediatric patients for magnetic resonance imaging: cross-sectional questionnaire study. JMIR Pediatr Parent 2019;2(1): e11684.

36. Perez-Escamirosa F, Medina-Alvarez D, Ruiz-Vereo EA, et al. Immersive virtual operating room simulation for surgical resident education during COVID-19. Surg Innov 2020;27(5):549–50.

37. Gallagher AG, Ritter EM, Champion H, et al. Virtual reality simulation for the operating room: proficiency-based training as a paradigm shift in surgical skills training. Ann Surg 2005;241(2): 364–72.

Statement of Ownership, Management, and Circulation
(All Periodicals Publications Except Requester Publications)

UNITED STATES POSTAL SERVICE

1. Publication Title	2. Publication Number	3. Filing Date
MAGNETIC RESONANCE IMAGING CLINICS OF NORTH AMERICA	011 – 909	9/18/2021

4. Issue Frequency	5. Number of Issues Published Annually	6. Annual Subscription Price
FEB, MAY, AUG, NOV	4	$404.00

7. Complete Mailing Address of Known Office of Publication (Not printer) (Street, city, county, state, and ZIP+4®)
ELSEVIER INC.
230 Park Avenue, Suite 800
New York, NY 10169

Contact Person: Malathi Samayan
Telephone (Include area code): 91-44-4299-4507

8. Complete Mailing Address of Headquarters or General Business Office of Publisher (Not printer)
ELSEVIER INC.
230 Park Avenue, Suite 800
New York, NY 10169

9. Full Names and Complete Mailing Addresses of Publisher, Editor, and Managing Editor (Do not leave blank)

Publisher (Name and complete mailing address)
DOLORES MELONI, ELSEVIER INC.
1600 JOHN F KENNEDY BLVD. SUITE 1800
PHILADELPHIA, PA 19103-2899

Editor (Name and complete mailing address)
JOHN VASSALLO, ELSEVIER INC.
1600 JOHN F KENNEDY BLVD. SUITE 1800
PHILADELPHIA, PA 19103-2899

Managing Editor (Name and complete mailing address)
PATRICK MANLEY, ELSEVIER INC.
1600 JOHN F KENNEDY BLVD. SUITE 1800
PHILADELPHIA, PA 19103-2899

10. Owner (Do not leave blank. If the publication is owned by a corporation, give the name and address of the corporation immediately followed by the names and addresses of all stockholders owning or holding 1 percent or more of the total amount of stock. If not owned by a corporation, give the names and addresses of the individual owners. If owned by a partnership or other unincorporated firm, give its name and address as well as those of each individual owner. If the publication is published by a nonprofit organization, give its name and address.)

Full Name	Complete Mailing Address
WHOLLY OWNED SUBSIDIARY OF REED/ELSEVIER, US HOLDINGS	1600 JOHN F KENNEDY BLVD. SUITE 1800 PHILADELPHIA, PA 19103-2899

11. Known Bondholders, Mortgagees, and Other Security Holders Owning or Holding 1 Percent or More of Total Amount of Bonds, Mortgages, or Other Securities. If none, check box ▶ ☐ None

Full Name	Complete Mailing Address
N/A	

12. Tax Status (For completion by nonprofit organizations authorized to mail at nonprofit rates) (Check one)
The purpose, function, and nonprofit status of this organization and the exempt status for federal income tax purposes:
☒ Has Not Changed During Preceding 12 Months
☐ Has Changed During Preceding 12 Months (Publisher must submit explanation of change with this statement)

PS Form 3526, July 2014 [Page 1 of 4 (see instructions page 4)] PSN: 7530-01-000-9931 PRIVACY NOTICE: See our privacy policy on www.usps.com

---

13. Publication Title	14. Issue Date for Circulation Data Below
MAGNETIC RESONANCE IMAGING CLINICS OF NORTH AMERICA	MAY 2021

15. Extent and Nature of Circulation		Average No. Copies Each Issue During Preceding 12 Months	No. Copies of Single Issue Published Nearest to Filing Date
a. Total Number of Copies (Net press run)		363	322
b. Paid Circulation (By Mail and Outside the Mail)	(1) Mailed Outside-County Paid Subscriptions Stated on PS Form 3541 (Include paid distribution above nominal rate, advertiser's proof copies, and exchange copies)	260	250
	(2) Mailed In-County Paid Subscriptions Stated on PS Form 3541 (Include paid distribution above nominal rate, advertiser's proof copies, and exchange copies)	0	0
	(3) Paid Distribution Outside the Mails Including Sales Through Dealers and Carriers, Street Vendors, Counter Sales, and Other Paid Distribution Outside USPS®	66	59
	(4) Paid Distribution by Other Classes of Mail Through the USPS (e.g. First-Class Mail®)	0	0
c. Total Paid Distribution (Sum of 15b (1), (2), (3), and (4)) ▶		346	309
d. Free or Nominal Rate Distribution (By Mail and Outside the Mail)	(1) Free or Nominal Rate Outside-County Copies included on PS Form 3541	17	13
	(2) Free or Nominal Rate In-County Copies Included on PS Form 3541	0	0
	(3) Free or Nominal Rate Copies Mailed at Other Classes Through the USPS (e.g. First-Class Mail)	0	0
	(4) Free or Nominal Rate Distribution Outside the Mail (Carriers or other means)	0	0
e. Total Free or Nominal Rate Distribution (Sum of 15d (1), (2), (3) and (4)) ▶		17	13
f. Total Distribution (Sum of 15c and 15e) ▶		363	322
g. Copies not Distributed (See instructions to Publishers #4 (page #3)) ▶		0	0
h. Total (Sum of 15f and g) ▶		363	322
i. Percent Paid (15c divided by 15f times 100) ▶		95.31%	95.96%

* If you are claiming electronic copies, go to line 16 on page 3. If you are not claiming electronic copies, skip to line 17 on page 3

PS Form 3526, July 2014 (Page 2 of 4)

16. Electronic Copy Circulation	Average No. Copies Each Issue During Preceding 12 Months	No. Copies of Single Issue Published Nearest to Filing Date
a. Paid Electronic Copies ▶		
b. Total Paid Print Copies (Line 15c) + Paid Electronic Copies (Line 16a) ▶		
c. Total Print Distribution (Line 15f) + Paid Electronic Copies (Line 16a) ▶		
d. Percent Paid (Both Print & Electronic Copies) (16b divided by 16c × 100) ▶		

☒ I certify that 50% of all my distributed copies (electronic and print) are paid above a nominal price.

17. Publication of Statement of Ownership
☒ If the publication is a general publication, publication of this statement is required. Will be printed in the NOVEMBER 2021 issue of this publication. ☐ Publication not required.

18. Signature and Title of Editor, Publisher, Business Manager, or Owner

Malathi Samayan – Distribution Controller
Malathi Samayan
Date: 9/18/2021

I certify that all information furnished on this form is true and complete. I understand that anyone who furnishes false or misleading information on this form or who omits material or information requested on the form may be subject to criminal sanctions (including fines and imprisonment) and/or civil sanctions (including civil penalties).

PS Form 3526, July 2014 (Page 3 of 4) PRIVACY NOTICE: See our privacy policy on www.usps.com

Moving?

Make sure your subscription moves with you!

To notify us of your new address, find your **Clinics Account Number** (located on your mailing label above your name), and contact customer service at:

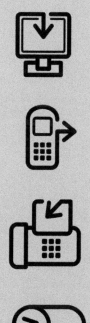

Email: journalscustomerservice-usa@elsevier.com

800-654-2452 (subscribers in the U.S. & Canada)
314-447-8871 (subscribers outside of the U.S. & Canada)

Fax number: 314-447-8029

Elsevier Health Sciences Division
Subscription Customer Service
3251 Riverport Lane
Maryland Heights, MO 63043

*To ensure uninterrupted delivery of your subscription, please notify us at least 4 weeks in advance of move.

ELSEVIER

Moving?

**Make sure your subscription
moves with you!**

Printed and bound by CPI Group (UK) Ltd, Croydon, CR0 4YY

08/05/2025

01864697-0010